Pediatri cket

Authors:
Daniel R. Neuspiel, MD, MPH, FAAP
Director, Ambulatory Pediatrics
Levine Children's Hospital
Adjunct Clinical Professor of Pediatrics
University of North Carolina School of Medicine
Medical Director, Myers Park Pediatrics
1350 S. Kings Dr., 2nd Floor
Charlotte, NC 28207

Editing: Dominik Stauber, MD, Shantanu Patil, MD, Bhagyashree Ghugari, MD, Jayateerth Korti, MD
Cover Illustration: Alexander Storck, Petra Rau, Rohit Kumar
Production: Alexander Storck, Dominik Schmook
Publisher: Börm Bruckmeier Publishing LLC, www.media4u.com

111 ½ Eucalyptus Drive
El Segundo, CA 90245
www.media4u.com | Ph: (310) 414 8300

IMPORTANT NOTICE – PLEASE READ!
This book is based on information from sources believed to be reliable, and every effort has been made to make the book as complete and accurate as possible and to describe generally accepted practices based on information available as of the printing date, but its accuracy and completeness cannot be guaranteed. Despite the best efforts of the author and publisher, the book may contain errors, and the reader should use the book only as a general guide and not as the ultimate source of information about the subject matter.
This book is not intended to reprint all of the information available to the author or publisher on the subject, but rather to simplify, complement, and supplement other available sources. The reader is encouraged to read all available material and to consult the package insert and other references to learn as much as possible about the subject.
This book is sold without warranties of any kind, expressed or implied, and the publisher and author disclaim any liability, loss, or damage caused by the content of this book.
IF YOU DO NOT WISH TO BE BOUND BY THE FOREGOING CAUTIONS AND CONDITIONS, YOU MAY RETURN THIS BOOK TO THE PUBLISHER FOR A FULL REFUND.

Printed in China through Colorcraft Ltd., Hong Kong
ISBN 978-1-59103-267-0

Preface

This Pediatrics pocket is divided into 16 chapters, guiding the readers in an easy-to-follow style, offering evidence-based guidance on management and treatment issues. Each of the chapters provides adequate coverage of most commonly seen pediatric disorders in day-to-day clinical practice.

Topics include: common acute symptoms, normal lab values, critical and emergency care, neonatology, genetic conditions, cardiovascular disorders, neurology and normal development, gastroenterology and nutrition, infectious diseases, respiratory disorders and SIDS, renal disorders, allergy/immunology, rheumatic disorders, hematology/oncology, endocrine disorders, psychosocial and behavioral problems, and injuries.

The pocket is arranged in a short, comprehensive, and tabular format. For easy and quick access, it includes illustrative diagrams, algorithms, and scales wherever required and several handy tables detailing commonly used pediatric medications as well as other information which does not need to be committed to memory. I hope that you will find the book helpful in providing comprehensive quality care for pediatric disorders.

The book is based on the latest recommendations from the American Academy of Pediatrics and aims to assist students, residents, pediatricians, family physicians, and midlevel providers of health care to children. This book is dedicated to the optimal health of all the world's children.

We welcome critical comments and constructive suggestions from the readers. Please contact us at info@media4u.com.

The authors and the publisher December, 2013

Daniel R. Neuspiel, MD, MPH, FAAP
Director, Ambulatory Pediatrics, Levine Children's Hospital, Charlotte, NC
Clinical Professor of Pediatrics, University of North Carolina School of Medicine

Contents

Contents

Contents

1 Common Acute Symptoms

1.1 Fever

(see reference [1])
→ Rectal temperature ≥38°C under 3 months, ≥39°C if 3-36 months

1.1.1 Management of fever according to age

Age	Investigations	Management
0-27 days of age or <3 months: With toxic appearance or baseline high risk	• CBC, UA, blood, urine cultures, CSF studies, and culture • Optional: Chest x-ray, HSV studies, stool culture	• Hospitalize • Parenteral antibiotics: – Ampicillin – Acyclovir if concern for HSV – Cefotaxime or Gentamycin
28-60 days of age: With baseline low risk	• CBC, UA, blood, urine cultures, CSF studies, and culture • Optional: Chest x-ray, HSV studies, stool culture	**If abnormal labs or x-ray:** • Hospitalize • Parenteral antibiotics: – Ceftriaxone – Ampicillin or vancomycin if concern for Listeria, gram-positive cocci, or Enterococcus **If normal labs:** • Follow-up in 24 h • Assure access to telephone and transportation • Consider ceftriaxone 50 mg/kg IV/IM
61-90 days of age	**Option 1** • Blood and urine culture, UA • Optional: CBC, CSF studies/culture, stool culture, rapid viral testing, chest x-ray	See 28-60 days of age with baseline low risk for management with abnormal or normal labs
	Option 2	See age 3-36 month for management

Age (cont.)	Investigations	Management
3-36 months: Healthy, no underlying conditions, nontoxic	**UA and urine culture in:** • All children ≤6 months • Girls <24 months if fever ≥2 days, age <12 months, no other source fever • Uncircumcised boys <12 months • Temp 38.3°C-38.9°C with ≥2 risk factors above	IF UA suggests UTI: • Antibiotic treatment →25 • See follow-up below
	Chest x-ray: • DO if hypoxia, tachypnea, respiratory distress, abnormal breath sounds • Consider if no other source, T ≥39°C and WBC >20,000/ mm^3 • Prolonged cough or fever	IF chest x-ray suggests pneumonia: • Antibiotic treatment →18 • See follow-up below
3-36 months: High-risk patient*	**Option 1** • Blood culture	• Consider ceftriaxone
	Option 2 • Blood culture • CBC with differential	If WBC >15,000: • Treat with ceftriaxone • See follow-up below
3-36 months: Low-risk patient	• At least 2 PCV and no high-risk criteria: No blood testing	• See follow-up below

***HIGH-RISK patient → ANY of the below:**

- Temp ≥ 40°C
- Prolonged gastroenteritis
- Contacts with meningococcal disease
- Petechiae
- <2 doses PCV
- Abnormal UA if <18 months

Follow-up
• Assess clinical stability before discharge • Ensure follow-up care availability • Follow-up in 24-48 h if symptoms persist • Immediate follow-up in case the condition worsens or positive blood cultures

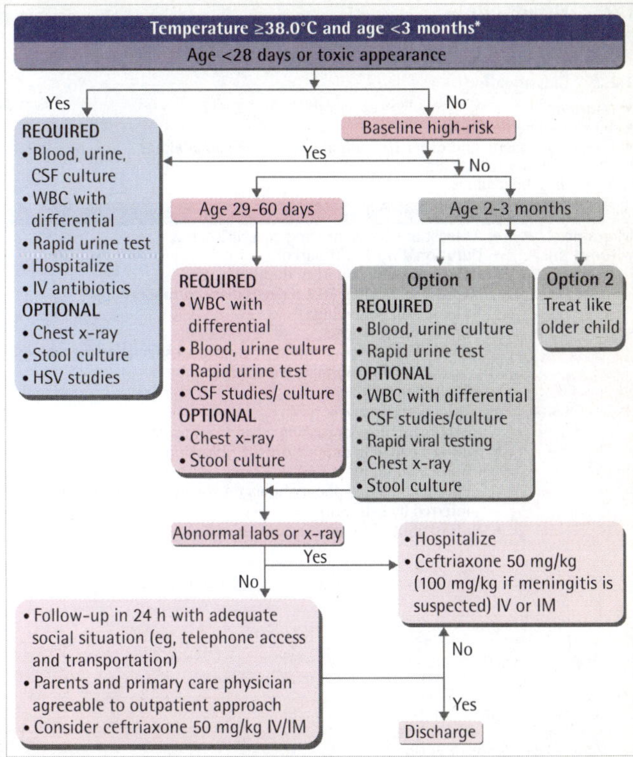

Temperature ≥38.0°C and age <3 months*
Age <28 days or toxic appearance
Yes
No
REQUIRED
• Blood, urine, CSF culture
• WBC with differential
• Rapid urine test
• Hospitalize
• IV antibiotics
OPTIONAL
• Chest x-ray
• Stool culture
• HSV studies
Baseline high-risk
Yes
No
Age 29-60 days
Age 2-3 months
REQUIRED
• WBC with differential
• Blood, urine culture
• Rapid urine test
• CSF studies/ culture
OPTIONAL
• Chest x-ray
• Stool culture
Option 1
REQUIRED
• Blood, urine culture
• Rapid urine test
OPTIONAL
• WBC with differential
• CSF studies/culture
• Rapid viral testing
• Chest x-ray
• Stool culture
Option 2
Treat like older child
Abnormal labs or x-ray
Yes
No
• Hospitalize
• Ceftriaxone 50 mg/kg (100 mg/kg if meningitis is suspected) IV or IM
• Follow-up in 24 h with adequate social situation (eg, telephone access and transportation)
• Parents and primary care physician agreeable to outpatient approach
• Consider ceftriaxone 50 mg/kg IV/IM
No
Yes
Discharge

1.2 Headache

(see reference [3])

1.2.1 Classification

- Migraine
- Tension-type headache
- Cluster headache and other trigeminal autonomic cephalalgias
- Other primary headaches
- Secondary headaches

Migraine	
Migraine without aura	• At least 5 attacks meeting criteria* below • Duration 4-72 h untreated: – Sleep considered part of duration – 1-72 h in children (1-2 h needs diary corroboration) • At least 2 of following: – Unilateral headache: 1. Bilateral most common in children, especially frontal 2. Exclusive occipital is worrisome – *Pulsating headache – *Moderate or severe pain – *Aggravation by or causing avoidance of routine physical activity • During headache at least one of following: – Nausea/vomiting – Photophobia and phonophobia (in young children may be inferred by behavior) • Not attributed to another disorder

Migraine	
Migraine with aura	• At least 2 attacks meeting criteria* • Aura with at least one of following, but no motor weakness: – Fully reversible visual symptoms (eg, flickering lights, spots or lines, numbness) – Fully reversible sensory symptoms (eg, pins and needles, numbness) – Fully reversible dysphasic speech disturbance • At least 2 of following: – Homonymous visual symptoms and/or unilateral sensory symptoms – At least one aura symptom develops gradually over ≥5 min and/or different aura symptoms occur in succession over ≥5 min – Each symptom lasts between 5-60 min • Headache begins during aura or follows aura within 60 min • Not attributed to another disorder
Childhood periodic syndromes	**ABC:** • **A**bdominal migraine • **B**enign paroxysmal vertigo of childhood • **C**yclical vomiting
Retinal migraine	• At least two attacks fulfilling criteria 2 & 3 • Full reversible monocular visual phenomena (eg, scintillation, scotomata or blindness) confirmed during an attack or later by the patient's drawing of a monocular field defect during an attack • Headache begins during the visual symptoms or follows them within 60 min (fulfilling criteria 2nd-4th for migraine without aura) • Normal ophthalmological examination between the attacks • Not attributed to another disorder
Probable migraine	• Without aura • With aura
Complications	• Chronic migraine • Status migrainosus • Seizures • Persistent aura without infarction • Migrainous infarction

*Criteria for migraine:
• Pulsating headache • Moderate or severe pain • Worse by or causing avoidance of routine physical activity

Tension Type Headache
• Infrequent episodic • Frequent episodic • Chronic • Probable

1.2.2 Evaluation of headache

Evaluation
• Detailed headache history: Length of time since onset, severity, quality, location, functional impact; review of systems; past medical, social, family history • Neurological examination • Consider neuroimaging if: – Abnormal neurologic examination (eg, focal findings, signs of increased intracranial pressure, significant alteration of consciousness), and/or coexistent seizures – Recent onset severe headache, change in type of headache, or associated features suggesting neurologic dysfunction

1.2.3 Treatment of headache

Treatment	
Acute	• NSAIDS (ibuprofen, naproxen) and acetaminophen • Triptans (sumatriptan, almotriptan, eletriptan, rizatriptan, zolmitriptan)
Prophylactic medication	• Antiepileptics (valproate sodium, topiramate, gabapentin, levetiracetam, zonisamide) • Antidepressants (amitriptyline) • Cyproheptadine • Antihypertensives (propranolol, timolol, verapamil)
Biobehavioral	• Efforts to improve treatment adherence • Lifestyle management: Identify triggers, nutrition, sleep, exercise • Psychological intervention, including relaxation

1.3 Meningitis

Age	Etiology	Treatment
0–28 days	Group B Streptococcus, Enterobacteriaceae (esp. E. coli), Listeria monocytogenes	Ampicillin and cefotaxime; or ampicillin and gentamycin
29–30 days	Group B Streptococcus, S. pneumoniae, H. influenzae, N. meningitidis, Enterobacteriaceae	Ampicillin and cefotaxime
Over 3 months	S. pneumoniae, H. influenzae, N. meningitidis	Cefotaxime or ceftriaxone. Add vancomycin for possible penicillin-resistant S. pneumoniae until susceptibility is known

1.4 Otitis Media

1.4.1 Acute otitis media (AOM) [4]

Acute otitis media	
Etiology	• S. pneumoniae • H. influenzae (nontypeable) • M. catarrhalis • Viruses
Diagnosis	• Confirm history of acute onset, identify signs of middle-ear effusion, and evaluate for presence of signs and symptoms of middle-ear inflammation • Perform pain assessment
Treatment	• If pain present, treat it • In uncomplicated, nonsevere AOM, observation without antibiotic treatment is an option if over 6 months with uncertain diagnosis or over 2 yrs in any child • If treating with antibiotic, amoxicillin at 80-90 mg/kg/day is recommended • If no response to management after 48-72 h, patient should be reassessed to confirm AOM and exclude other illness. If AOM is confirmed, patients initially untreated should start an antibiotic and those initially treated should change their antibiotic

Acute otitis media (cont.)	
Complication	• Chronic otitis media with hearing loss, labyrinthitis, cholesteatoma, mastoiditis • Meningitis, brain abscess, facial palsy, sinus thrombosis
Prevention	Clinicians should encourage the prevention of AOM through reducing modifiable risk factors: • Day care attendance • Breastfeeding less than 6 months • Supine bottle feeding or bottle propping • Pacifier use from 7-12 months • Passive tobacco smoke exposure • Lack of vaccination to influenza and pneumococcus

1.4.2 Otitis media with effusion (OME) [5]

Otitis media with effusion (OME)	
Diagnosis	• Primary diagnostic method for OME is pneumatic otoscopy • Tympanometry to confirm the diagnosis of OME • At each assessment of child, document the laterality, duration of effusion, presence, and severity of symptoms
Management	• Children with risk for speech, language, or learning problems must get more prompt evaluation of hearing, speech, language, and need for intervention Developmental risk factors include: – Permanent hearing loss independent of OME – Developmental delay – Suspected or diagnosed speech and language delay or disorder – Autism-spectrum disorder and other pervasive developmental disorders – Syndromes or craniofacial disorders that include cognitive, speech and language delays – Blindness or uncorrectable visual impairment – Cleft palate with or without associated syndrome • Low risk children may be managed with watchful waiting for 3 months from date of effusion onset or diagnosis • Antihistamines and decongestants are ineffective and not recommended • Antimicrobials and corticosteroids do not have long-term efficacy and are not recommended for routine management • Language testing should be conducted in children with hearing loss

Otitis media with effusion (OME)	
Management (cont.)	• Hearing test is recommended when OME persists for >3 months or any time that language delay, learning problems, or significant hearing loss is suspected • Low-risk children with persistent OME should be reexamined at 3- to 6- month intervals until the effusion is no longer present, significant hearing loss is identified, or structural abnormalities of the eardrum or middle ear are suspected • When referring to an otolaryngologist, audiologist, or speech-language pathologist, the clinician should document the effusion duration, specific reason for referral, and other relevant information • Tympanostomy tube insertion is the preferred initial surgical procedure • Repeat surgery consists of adenoidectomy plus myringotomy

1.5 Cough

Etiology & Management	
Common causes	• Infection • Sinusitis • Habit • Asthma/reactive airway disease • Croup/laryngotracheobronchitis • Bronchiolitis • Pneumonia • Allergic rhinitis • Inhaling a foreign body
High morbidity causes	• Asthma/reactive airway disease • Bacterial tracheitis • Bronchiolitis • Congestive heart failure • Croup/laryngotracheobronchitis • Foreign body • Laryngeal edema • Pertussis • Pneumonia • Toxic inhalation
Treatment	• Find and treat the cause • Viral infection usually subsides in a week or two • Refer to as an allergist in case of asthma/allergic rhinitis

1.6 Pneumonia

(see reference [6])

Clinical presentation		
Fever with chills, cough, rapid breathing, nasal congestion, poor appetite, chest & abdominal pain, in extreme cases cyanosis.		
Age	**Etiology**	**Treatment**
0–28 days	E. coli, GBS, S. aureus, L. monocytogenes, C. trachomatis	Ampicillin + gentamycin, or Ampicillin + cefotaxime
3weeks–4 months	C. trachomatis, S. pneumoniae, viruses	Erythromycin (PO), azithromycin (PO), cefotaxime (IV)
6 weeks–4 yrs	**Lobar:** S. pneumoniae	PO amoxicillin or clindamycin; IV ceftriaxone or cefotaxime
	Atypical: Bordetella pertussis or respiratory viruses	**Pertussis**: Erythromycin, azithromycin or clarithromycin **Influenza**: Zanamivir, oseltamivir, amantadine, rimantadine
≥4 yrs	**Lobar:** S. pneumoniae	PO amoxicillin or erythromycin; IV ceftriaxone or cefotaxime + macrolide; clarithromycin, azithromycin
	Atypical: Mycoplasma pneumoniae, Chlamydia pneumoniae, influenza	**Mycoplasma or Chlamydia**: Clarithromycin, azithromycin, doxycycline, erythromycin **Influenza**: Zanamivir or oseltamivir

1.7 Abdominal Pain

1.7.1 Acute abdominal pain

	Location	Referral	Quality	Associated Finding
Appendicitis	Periumbilical, migrating to right lower quadrant, then generalized with peritonitis	Back, or pelvis if retrocecal	Sharp, steady	Anorexia, nausea, vomiting, local tenderness, fever with peritonitis
Gastroenteritis (See →20)	Pain in particular area of belly	-	Cramping/ colicky	Diarrhea, vomiting, fever, signs of dehydration
Intussusception	Periumbilical, lower abdomen	-	Cramping, intermittent pain-free	Hematochezia, knees pulled-up
Intestinal obstruction	Periumbilical, lower abdomen	Back	Alternating cramping/ colic and pain-free	Distention, obstipation, emesis, increased bowel sounds, discomfort
Urolithiasis	Unilateral back	Back to groin	Sharp, intermittent, cramping	Hematuria, crystals in urine
UTI	Back	Bladder	-	Fever, chills, frequent urination
Pancreatitis	Epigastric, left upper quadrant	Back	Constant, sharp, boring	Nausea, emesis, tenderness

1.7.2 Chronic abdominal pain

Chronic abdominal pain		
Nonorganic	Functional abdominal pain	
Gastrointestinal tract	• Irritable bowel syndrome • IBD • Non-ulcer dyspepsia • Chronic constipation • Lactose intolerance • Peptic ulcer • Meckel's diverticulum	• Esophagitis • Recurrent intussusception • Hernia (internal, inguinal, or abdominal wall) • Chronic appendicitis or appendiceal mucocele • Parasitic infestation (esp. Giardia)

Chronic abdominal pain (cont.)		
Gallbladder and Pancreas	• Cholelithiasis, choledochal cyst • Recurrent pancreatitis	
Genitourinary tract	• UTI • Hydronephrosis • Urolithiasis	
Other	• Abdominal epilepsy • Gilbert syndrome • Familial Mediterranean fever	• Lead poisoning • Henoch-Schönlein purpura • Angioneurotic edema • Acute intermittent porphyria

1.8 Acute Gastroenteritis

1.8.1 Types and treatment

Types	Treatment
E. coli	• Antibiotics may increase risk of hemolytic-uremic syndrome in E. coli 0157: H7 • Hospitalize • Early fluid resuscitation
Salmonella	• Hospitalize • Rehydration • Antibiotics only for: – Infants <6 months – Bacteremia – Toxic appearance – Immunocompromised status • Cefotaxime, ceftriaxone, or azithromycin
Shigella	• TMP/SMX, ceftriaxone, PO cefixime, azithromycin
Yersinia	• Antibiotics only for: – Bacteremia – Extraintestinal infection – Immunocompromised status • TMP/SMX, aminoglycosides, cefotaxime, tetracycline (>8 yrs)
Campylobacter	• Azithromycin or erythromycin
Clostridium difficile	• Usually nosocomial • Metronidazole
Viruses	Prevent dehydration, ORS

1.8.2 Management of acute gastroenteritis with dehydration[7]

Indications for Medical Evaluation of Children with Acute Diarrhea
• Age <6 months or weight <8 kg • History of prematurity, chronic medical conditions, or concurrent illness • Fever ≥38°C if < 3 months or ≥39°C if 3-36 months • Visible blood in stool • High output, including frequent and substantial volumes of diarrhea • Persistent vomiting • Report of signs consistent with dehydration, eg, sunken eyes, decreased tears, dry mucous membranes, decreased urine output • Change in mental status • Suboptimal response to oral rehydration therapy (ORT) or inability of caregiver to administer ORT

Classification and Treatment of Dehydration*	
Types	**Treatment**
Minimal or no dehydration (<3% loss of body weight)	**No rehydration therapy necessary if:** • Alert mental status • Heart rate, breathing, eyes, tears, mouth moistness, skin turgor, capillary refill, extremity warmth, all normal • Urine output normal to decreased **Replace losses:** • <10 Kg: 60-120 mL ORS per diarrheal stool or vomiting episode • >10 Kg: 120-240 mL ORS per diarrheal stool or vomiting episode Continue breastfeeding, or resume age-appropriate normal diet after initial hydration, including adequate maintenance calories
Mild to moderate dehydration (3%-9% loss of body weight)	• Mental status: Normal, fatigued or restless, irritable • Heart rate normal to increased; pulses normal to decreased • Breathing normal to fast • Oral mucosa dry with slightly sunken, dry eyes • Skin recoil <2 sec; capillary refill >2 sec • Extremities feel cool • Decreased urine output • Rehydration with ORS: 50-100 mL/kg over 3-4 h **Replace losses**: – Same as minimal or no dehydration

Types (cont.)	Treatment
Severe dehydration (>9% loss of body weight)	• Mental status: apathetic, lethargic, unconscious • Tachycardia, to bradycardia when severe • Pulse: Weak, thready, or impalpable • Deep breathing • Deeply sunken eyes, no tears; parched oral mucosa • Skin recoil >2 sec; capillary refill >2 sec and minimal • Cold, mottled, cyanotic extremities • Urine output: minimal • Rehydration with normal saline or lactated Ringer's solution, 20 mL/kg IV boluses until perfusion and mental status improve, then 100 mL/kg ORS over 4 h or D5 1/2 normal saline IV at twice maintenance rates **Replace losses:** – Same as in minimal or no dehydration; if unable to drink, administer via NG tube or give D5 ¼ NS with 20 mEq/L of KCl IV

* Repeated weights most accurate

Principles of Appropriate Treatment for Diarrhea and Dehydration
• Continue breastfeeding in nursing infants • No unnecessary laboratory tests or medications should be administered • ORT should be used for rehydration except for initial treatment of severe dehydration, which should be performed rapidly within 3-4 h • Age-appropriate, unrestricted diet once dehydration is corrected • If formula-fed infant, diluting formula is not recommended, and special formula is usually not necessary • Additional ORT should be administered for ongoing losses

1.9 Chronic Diarrhea

(lasting ≥14 days) (see reference [8])

1.9.1 Etiology

Etiology of Chronic Diarrhea		
Anatomic abnormalities	• Hirschsprung's disease	• Short bowel syndrome
Infections	• Bacterial, viral, and protozoal • Small intestinal bacterial overgrowth	• Postenteritis syndrome • Tropical sprue • Whipple's disease
Abnormal digestion	• Cystic fibrosis • Shwachman-Diamond syndrome • Isolated pancreatic enzyme deficiency • Chronic pancreatitis • Johanson-Blizzard syndrome	• Pearson syndrome • Trypsinogen and enterokinase deficiency • Chronic cholestasis • Use of bile acid sequestrants • Primary bile acid malabsorption
Associated with exogenous substances	• Excess intake of: – Carbonated/ caffeinated drinks – Laxatives, antacids	• Diet foods with sorbitol, mannitol, or xylitol
Nutrient malabsorption	• Acrodermatitis enteropathica • Sucrase-isomaltase deficiency • Glucose-galactose malabsorption	• Fructose malabsorption • Short bowel • Cystic fibrosis • Lactase deficiency
Immune and inflammatory	• HIV • Autoimmune enteropathy • IgA or IgG deficiency • Food allergy • Inflammatory bowel disease	• IPEX syndrome • Primary and secondary immunodeficiencies • Celiac disease • Eosinophilic gastroenteritis
Structural defects	• Microvillus inclusion disease • Tufting enteropathy • Phenotypic diarrhea • Heparan-sulphate deficiency	• $\alpha_2\beta_1$ and $\alpha_6\beta_4$ integrin deficiency • Lymphangiectasia • Enteric anendocrinosis (neorogenin-3 mutation)
Defects of electrolyte and metabolite transport	• Congenital chloride/sodium diarrhea • Acrodermatitis enteropathica	• Selective folate deficiency • Abetalipoproteinemia

Etiology of Chronic Diarrhea (cont.)		
Motility disorders	• Hirschsprung disease • Thyrotoxicosis	• Chronic intestinal pseudo-obstruction
Neoplastic diseases	• Neuroendocrine hormone-secreting tumors • Zollinger-Ellison syndrome	• Mastocytosis • Pheochromocytoma • Lymphoma
Chronic nonspecific diarrhea	• Functional diarrhea • Toddler's diarrhea	• Irritable bowel syndrome

1.9.2 Evaluation

Evaluation of Children with Chronic Diarrhea	
Step 1	• Intestinal microbiology: – Stool cultures – Ova and parasites – Viral tests – H_2 breath test • Screen for celiac disease (transglutaminase 2 antibodies) • Noninvasive tests for intestinal and pancreatic function, sweat test, intestinal inflammation • Food allergy tests
Step 2	• Intestinal biopsy
Step 3	• Special investigations

1.10 Urinary Tract Infection (UTI)

(see reference [9])

1.10.1 Etiology

Etiology of UTI	
Bacteria	E. coli, Klebsiella, Proteus, Staphylococcus saprophyticus, Enterococcus
Viruses	Adenovirus and others

1.10.2 Evaluation

Evaluation of UTI	
• Obtain urine culture and urinalysis before administering antibiotic (in precontinent child, obtain culture through catheterization or suprapubic aspiration) • In nontoxic infants, assess likelihood of UTI prior to treatment:	
Boys	**Girls**
• **If circumcised**, 3 risk factors listed below needed for likelihood >1%, all 4 below needed for likelihood >2% • **If uncircumcised**, 2 risk factors listed below needed for likelihood > 1%, only 1 below needed for likelihood >2% – Nonblack race – Temp ≥39°C – Fever >24 h – No other source of infection	• 2 risk factors listed below needed for likelihood >1%; 3 risk factors listed below needed for likelihood >2% – White race – Age <12 months – Temp ≥39°C – Fever >2 days – No other source of infection
• If low likelihood of UTI, clinical follow-up monitoring without testing • If febrile infant is not in low-risk group, may either: – Obtain urine specimen for culture and urinalysis via catheterization or suprapubic aspiration, or – Obtain urinalysis, and if suggestive of UTI (positive leukocyte esterase, positive nitrite, or microscopic leukocytes or bacteria), then obtain urine for culture as above • To establish UTI diagnosis in infant, need both: – Urinalysis results suggestive of infection (see above), and – At least 50,000 colony-forming units per mL of uropathogen obtained via catheterization or suprapubic aspiration	

1.10.3 Treatment

Treatment of UTI
• Base initial choice of antibiotic on local antimicrobial sensitivity patterns • Adjust choice according to sensitivity testing of isolated organism • 7-14 days is optimal duration of treatment • Oral treatment options: – Cephalosporins: cephalexin, cefixime – Amoxicillin plus clavulanic acid – TMP/SMZ – Avoid nitrofurantoin in infants • Parenteral treatment options: – Cephalosporins: ceftriaxone, cefotaxime or ampicillin plus gentamycin

1.10.4 Follow-up

Follow-up of UTI
• Febrile infants with UTIs should have renal and bladder ultrasonography (RBUS) • Voiding cystourethrography should only be done if: – RBUS reveals hydronephrosis, scarring, or other findings suggestive of high-grade vesicoureteral reflux (VUR) or obstructive uropathy – Other atypical or complex clinical circumstances – A recurrence of febrile UTI occurs • Advise caregivers to seek medical attention within 48 h for future febrile illnesses to detect recurrent UTIs

1.11 Easy Bruising

Easy Bruising	
Brief discussion	• Easy bruising is usually associated with platelet disorders • Bruises are area of subcutaneous bleeding • A bruise is considered abnormal if it is out of proportion to offending trauma
Signs	• Petechiae • Purpura • Ecchymosis

Approach to the patient with easy bruising[10]

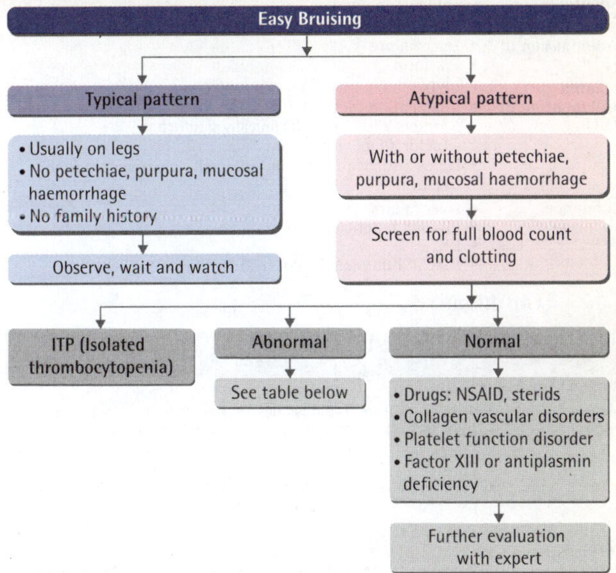

Reference: Reproduced from A Vora, M Makris, Personal practice: An approach to investigation of easy bruising, Arch Dis Child 2001;84:6 488-491, with permission from BMJ Publishing Group Ltd.

Abnormality of Clotting Screen[10]	
Abnormality	**Cause**
Isolated prolongation of PT	• Vitamin K deficiency (HDN, malabsorption) • Liver failure • Warfarin
Isolated prolongation of APTT	• vWD • Coagulation factor deficiencies: – Factors VIII, XI and XI: clinically significant – Factor XII: not significant • Lupus anticoagulant: Dilute Russell's viper venom time • Heparin
Combined abnormalities	• Liver failure • Vitamin K deficiency • DIC • Rare afibrinogenemia or dysfibrinogenemia

1.12 Exanthems

Etiology	Prodrome	Contagious Period	Rash	Incubation and Other Features
Rubeola (measles)				
Measles virus	**3–4 days** • High fever, • Cough • Coryza • Conjunctivitis	• 1-2 days before symptoms • 4 days after rash appears	• Red-brown morbilliform • Spreads from above downwards • Lasts 6-7 days	**8–12 days** • Koplik spots
Varicella				
Varicella virus	**1–2 days** • Fever • Rash • Anorexia • Headache	• 1-2 days before rash • 3-7 days after onset of rash, when all lesions crusted over	• Central • Vesicular	**10–21 days** • Secondary skin infections, • Pneumonia • Encephalitis

Etiology (cont.)	Prodrome	Contagious Period	Rash	Incubation and Other Features
Rubella (German measles)				
Rubella virus	**None, or 1–3 days** • Low-grade fever and malaise	Few days before to 7 days after onset rash	Pink, maculopapular	**14–21 days** • Tender postauricular and suboccipital lymph nodes
Erythema infectiosum (fifth disease)				
Parvo-virus B19	None	Not contagious after rash appears	Lacy maculopapular rash (trunk and extremities)	**4–28 days** • Slapped cheek appearance
Roseola infantum (exanthem subitum)				
Human herpes viruses 6 and 7	**3–4 days** • High fever and irritability	Unknown	Maculopapular rash (spares extremities)	**5–15 days** • Drop in fever with onset of rash
Hand-foot-mouth disease				
Entero-viruses (mainly coxsackievirus A16)	**None, or 3–4 days** • Mild fever	Fecal virus may last several weeks, respiratory to 1 week	Discrete red papules and vesicles (palms, soles, buttocks), with oropharyngeal ulcers	**3–6 days** • Mainly in summer and early fall
Rocky mountain spotted fever				
Rickettsia rickettsii	**2–4 days** • Headache • Anorexia • Myalgia • Restlessness • GI symptoms	No human-to-human transmission	Maculopapular rash, progressing to petechiae and purpura	**2–14 days** • Ticks are vectors • 5-20% have no rash

Etiology (cont.)	Prodrome	Contagious Period	Rash	Incubation and Other Features
Scarlet fever				
Group A β-hemolytic Streptococcus	**Within 1–4 days**	Up to 24 h after treatment started	Erythematous papules (trunk and proximal extremities); feels like fine sandpaper	Pastia lines: persistent red lines after light pressure
Kawasaki disease				
Unknown	**5 days** • Fever and irritability	No evidence	• Marked erythema (palms and sole) • Varying appearance	• Conjunctivitis • Tender lymphadenopathy • Strawberry tongue • Meatitis • Late desquamation • Coronary aneurysms

List of References

1 Ishimine P. The evolving approach to the young child who has fever and no obvious source. Emerg Med Clin N Am 2007; 25:1087-1115

2 Reprinted from Paul Ishimine, The Evolving Approach to the Young Child Who Has Fever and No Obvious Source, Emergency Medicine Clinics of North America, Vol. 25, Issue 4, Nov. 2007, Pages 1087-1115, with permission from Elsevier.

3 Hershey AD, Winner P, Kabbouche MA, Powers SW. Headaches. Curr Opin Pediatr 2007; 19:663-669

4 Subcommittee on Management of Acute Otitis Media, Steering Committee on Quality Improvement and Management, American Academy of Pediatrics. Diagnosis and management of acute otitis media. Pediatrics 2004;113: 1451-1465

5 Subcommittee on Otitis Media with Effusion, Steering Committee on Quality Improvement and Management, American Academy of Pediatrics. Otitis Media with Effusion. Pediatrics 2004; 113: 1412-1429

6 Antonyrajah B, Mukundan D. Fever without apparent source on clinical examination. Curr Opin Pediatr 2008; 20: 96-102

7 King CK, Glass R, Bresee JS, Duggan C. Managing acute gastroenteritis among children: Oral rehydration, maintenance, and nutritional therapy. MMWR, 2003: Vol. 52, No. RR-16, pp 3-18

8 Guarino A, Branski D. Chronic diarrhea, In Kliegman RM et al, eds. Nelson Textbook of Pediatrics, 19th ed. Philadelphia, Elsevier, 2011, pp 1339-1346

9 Subcommittee on Urinary Tract Infection, Steering Committee on Quality Improvement and Management, American Academy of Pediatrics. Urinary Tract Infection: Clinical Practice Guideline for the Diagnosis and Management of the Initial UTI in Febrile Infants and Children 2 to 24 Months. Pediatrics 2011; 128: 595-610

10 Reproduced from A Vora, M Makris, Personal practice: An approach to investigation of easy bruising, Arch Dis Child 2001;84:6 488-491, with permission from BMJ Publishing Group Ltd.

2 Normal Values

2.1 Vital Signs, Normal Parameters by Age

(see reference [11])

Age	Heart Rate	Respiratory Rate	Systolic Blood Pressure	Diastolic Blood Pressure
Premature newborn	120-170	40-75	55-75	35-45
0-3 months	100-150	35-55	65-85	45-55
3-6 months	90-120	30-45	70-90	50-65
6-12 months	80-120	25-40	80-100	55-65
1-3 yrs	70-110	20-30	90-105	55-70
3-6 yrs	65-110	20-25	95-110	60-75
6-12 yrs	60-95	14-22	100-120	60-75
>12 yrs	55-85	12-18	110-135	65-85

2.2 Hematology

(see reference [12])

2.2.1 Blood cell indices by age

Age	Hb (g/dL)*	HTC (%)*	MCV*	MCHC*	Retic	WBC** ($x10^3/\mu L$)	Platelets** ($10^3/\mu L$)
26-30 weeks premature	13.4 (11)	41.5 (34.9)	118.2 (106.7)	37.9 (30.6)	-	4.4 (2.7)	254 (180-327)
28 weeks premature	14.5	45	120	31	5-10	-	275
32 weeks premature	15.0	47	118	32	3-10	-	290
Term (cord)	16.5 (13.5)	51 (42)	108 (98)	33 (30)	3-7	18.1 (9-30)	290

Age (cont.)	Hb (g/dL)*	HTC (%)*	MCV*	MCHC*	Retic	WBC** (x10³/µL)	Platelets** (10³/µL)
1-3 days	18.5 (14.5)	56 (45)	108 (95)	33 (29)	1.8-4.6	18.9 (9.4-34)	192
2 weeks	16.6 (13.4)	53(41)	105 (88)	31.4 (28.1)	-	11.4 (5-20)	252
1 month	13.9 (10.7)	44 (33)	101 (91)	31.8 (28.1)	0.1-1.7	108 (4-19.5)	-
2 months	11.2 (9.4)	35 (28)	95 (84)	31.8 (28.3)	-	-	-
6 months	12.6 (11.1)	36 (31)	76 (68)	35 (32.7)	0.7-2.3	11.9 (6-17.5)	-
6 months-2 yrs	12.0 (10.5)	36 (33)	78 (70)	33 (30)	-	10.6 (6-17)	150-350
2-6 yrs	12.5 (11.5)	37 (34)	81 (75)	34 (31)	0.5-1	8.5 (5-15.5)	150-350
6-12 yrs	13.5 (11.50	40 (35)	86 (77)	34 (31)	0.5-1	8.1 (4.5-13.5)	150-350
12-18 yrs	-	-	-	34 (31)	0.5-1	7.8 (4.5-13.5)	150-350
Male	14.5 (13)	43 (36)	88 (78)	-	-	-	-
Female	14.0 (12)	41 (37)	90 (78)	-	-	-	-
Adult	-	-	90 (80)	34 (31)	-	7.4 (4.5-11)	150-350
Male	15.5 (13.5)	47 (41)	-	-	0.8-2.5	-	-
Female	14.0 (12)	41 (360)	-	-	0.8-4.1	-	-

*(- 2 SD); **(± 2 SD)

2.3 Chemistry

(see reference [13])

2.3.1 Alanine aminotransferase (ALT)

Age	U/L
0-7 days	6-40
8-30 days, male	10-40
8-30 days, female	8-32

Age (cont.)	U/L
1–12 months	12–45
1–19 yrs	5–45

2.3.2 Albumin

Age	g/dL
Premature, day 1	1.8–3
Full term, first week	2.5–3.4
8 days–1 yrs	1.9–4.9
1–3 yrs	3.4–4.2
4–19 yrs	3.5–5.6

2.3.3 Alkaline phosphatase

Age	Male (U/L)	Female (U/L)
1–9 yrs	145–420	145–420
10–11 yrs	140–560	140–560
12–13 yrs	200–495	105–420
14–15 yrs	130–525	70–130
16–19 yrs	65–260	50–130

2.3.4 Ammonia

Age group	µmol/L
Newborn	64–107
0–2 wk	56–92
Infant/child	21–50
Adult	11–32

2.3.5 Amylase

Age	U/L
0–3 months	0–30
3–6 months	0–50
6–12 months	0–80
>1 yr	30–100

2.3.6 Aspartate aminotransferase (AST)

Age	U/L
0-7 days (male)	30-100
0-7 days (female)	24-95
8-30 days	22-71
1-12 months	22-63
1-3 yrs	20-60
3-9 yrs	15-50
10-15 yrs	10-40
16-19 yrs, male	15-45
16-19 yrs, female	5-30

2.3.7 Bicarbonate

Type	mmol/L
Arterial	21-28
Venous	22-29

2.3.8 Bilirubin

Total Bilirubin	mg/dL (µmol/L)
Newborn	→77
1 month-adult	<1 (<17)

2.3.9 C-reactive protein

Age	Male (mg/dL)	Female (mg/dL)
0-90 days	0.08-1.58	0.09-1.58
3-12 months	0.08-1.12	0.05-0.79
1-3 yrs	0.08-1.12	0.08-1.12
4-10 yrs	0.06-0.79	0.5-1
11-14 yrs	0.08-0.76	0.06-0.81
15-18 yrs	0.04-0.79	0.06-0.79

2.3.10 Calcium

Calcium (ionized)	mg/dL (mmol/L)
Cord blood	5-6 (1.25-1.5)
Newborn, 3-24 h	4.3-5.1 (1.07-1.27)
Newborn, 24-48 h	4-4.7 (1-1.17)
Over 48 h	4.8-4.92 (1.12-1.23)
Calcium (total)	**mg/dL (mmol/L)**
Cord blood	9-11.5 (2.25-2.88)
Newborn, 3-24 h	9-10.6 (2.3-2.65)
Newborn, 24-48 h	7-12 (1.75-3)
4-7 days	9-10.9 (2.25-2.73)
Child	8.8-10.8 (2.2-2.7)
Adolescent-adult	8.4-10.2 (2.1-2.55)

2.3.11 Chloride

Age group	mmol/L
Newborn	97-110
Older	98-106

2.3.12 Creatine

Creatine kinase	U/L
5-8 h	214-1,175
24-33 h	130-1,200
72-100 h	87-725
Adult	5-130
Creatine clearance	**mL/min/1.73 m^2**
Newborn	40-65
1 month-40 yrs, male	97-137
1 month-40 yrs, female	88-128

2.3.13 Ferritin

Age	ng/mL (mcg/L)
0-4 weeks	25-200 (55-1300)
1-5 mo	50-200 (15-300)

Age (cont.)	ng/mL (mcg/L)
6 mo - 15 yrs	7-140
Adult male	18-300
Adult female	18-160

2.3.14 Folate

Folate (serum)	ng/mL (nmol/L)
Newborn	7-32 (15.9-72.4)
Older	1.8-9 (4.1-20.4)
Folate (whole blood)	**ng/mL (nmol/L)**
Normal value	150-450 (340-1,020)

2.3.15 Glucose

Serum glucose	mg/dL (mmol/L)
Cord blood	45-96 (2.5-5.3)
Premature	20-60 (1.1-3.3)
Neonate	30-60 (1.7-3.3)
1 day	40-60 (2.2-3.3)
1-30 days	50-90 (2.8-5)
Child	60-100 (3.3-5.5)
Adult	70-105 (3.9-5.8)
2 h post-prandial	<120 (<6.7)

2.3.16 Glucose tolerance test (GTT)

→ After 1.75 g/kg oral dose (max 75 g)

Time	Normal mg/dL (mmol/L)	Diabetic mg/dL (mmol/L)
Fasting	70-105 (3.9-5.8)	≥126 (≥7)
60 min	120-170 (6.7-9.4)	≥200 (≥11)
90 min	100-140 (5.6-7.8)	≥200 (≥11))
120 min	70-120 (3.9-6.7)	≥200 (≥11)

2.3.17 γ-Glutamyl transpeptidase (GGT)

γ-Glutamyl Transpeptidase	U/L
Cord blood	37-193
0-1 month	13-147
1-2 months	12-123
2-4 months	8-90
4 months-10 yrs	5-32
10-15 yrs	5-24

2.3.18 Immunoglobulin

Immunoglobulin A (IgA)	mg/dL
Cord blood	1.4-3.6
1-3 months	1.3-53
4-6 months	4.4-84
7 months-1 yr	11-106
2-5 yrs	14-159
6-10 yrs	33-236
Adult	70-312
Immunoglobulin E (IgE)	**IU/mL**
Male	0-230
Female	0-170
Immunoglobulin G (IgG)	**mg/dL**
Cord blood	636-1,606
1 month	251-906
2-4 months	176-601
5-12 months	172-1,069
1-5 yrs	345-1,236
6-10 yrs	608-1,572
Adult	639-1,349
Immunoglobulin M (IgM)	**mg/dL**
Cord blood	6.3-25
1-4 months	17-105
5-9 months	33-126

Immunoglobulin M (IgM) (cont.)	mg/dL
10 months–1 yr	41–173
2–8 yrs	43–207
9–10 yrs	52–242
Adult	56–352

2.3.19 Iron

Iron	μg/dL (μmol/L)
Normal value	22–184 (4–33)
Iron-binding capacity	**μg/dL (μmol/L)**
Infant	100–400 (17.9–71.6)
Older	250–400 (44.75–71.6)

2.3.20 L-lactate (whole blood)

Age	mg/dL (mmol/L)
1–12 months	10–21 (1.1–2.3)
1–7 yrs	7–14 (0.8–1.5)
7–15 yrs	5–8 (0.6–0.9)

2.3.21 Lactate dehydrogenase (LDH)

Age	U/L
<1 yr	170–580
1–9 yrs	150–500
10–19 yrs	120–330

2.3.22 LDH isoenzymes

LDH Isoenzymes (% total activity)	1–6 yrs	7–19 yrs
LD1	20–38	20–35
LD2	27–38	31–38
LD3	16–26	19–28
LD4	5–16	7–13
LD5	3–13	5–12

2.3.23 Lead

Lead (whole blood)	µg/dL (mmol/L)
Child	<10 (<0.48)

2.3.24 Lipase

Age	U/L
1–18 yrs	145-216

2.3.25 Magnesium

Age	mg/dL (mmol/L)
0–6 days	1.2-2.6 (0.48-1.05)
7 days–2 yrs	1.6-2.6 (0.65-1.05)
2–14 yrs	1.5-2.3 (0.6-0.95)

2.3.26 Osmolality

Age	mOsm/kg H_2O
All ages	275-295

2.3.27 Phosphorous (inorganic)

Age	mg/dL (mmol/L)
0–5 days	4.8-8.2 (1.55-2.65)
1–3 yrs	3.8-6.5 (1.25-2.10)
4–11 yrs	3.7-5.6 (1.2-1.8)
12–15 yrs	2.9-5.4 (0.95-1.75)
16–19 yrs	2.7-4.7 (0.9-1.5)

2.3.28 Potassium

Age	mmol/L
0–1 week	3.2-5.5
1 week–1 month	3.4-6
1–6 months	3.5-5.6
6 months–1 yr	3.5-6.1
>1 yr	3.3-4.6

2.3.29 Prealbumin

Age	mg/dL
0–5 days	6–21
1–5 yrs	14–30
6–9 yrs	15–30
10–13 yrs	20–36
14–19 yrs	22–45

2.3.30 Protein

Total protein	g/dL
Premature	4.3–7.6
Newborn	4.6–7.4
1–7 yrs	6.1–7.9
8–12 yrs	6.4–8.1
13–19 yrs	6.6–8.2

2.3.31 Pyruvate

Age	mmol/L
7–17 yrs	0.076 ± 0.026

2.3.32 Sodium

Age	mmol/L
Newborn	133–146
Infant	134–144
Child	134–143
Older	135–145

2.3.33 Thyroid-stimulating hormone (TSH)

Age	µIU/L
0–3 days	1–20
3–30 days	0.5–6.5
1–5 months	0.5–6
6 months–18 yrs	0.5–4.5

2.3.34 Thyrotropin-releasing hormone (TRH)

Age	pg/mL (pmol/L)
All ages	5-60 (14-165)

2.3.35 Thyroxine

Thyroxine-Binding Globulin (TBG)	mg/dL
Cord blood	1.4-9.4
1-4 weeks	1-9
1-12 months	2-7.6
1-5 yrs	2.9-5.4
5-10 yrs	2.5-5
10-15 yrs	2.1-4.6
Adult	1.5-3.4
Thyroxine (total)	**µg/dL (nmol/L)**
Newborn screen	6.2-22 (80-283)
0-3 days	8-20 (103-258)
3-30 days	5-15 (64-193)
31-365 days	6-14 (77-180)
1-5 yrs	4.5-11 (58-142)
6-18 yrs	4.5-10 (58-129)
Thyroxine (free)	**ng/dL (pmol/L)**
0-3 days	2-5 (25.7-64.3)
3-30 days	0.9-2.2 (11.6-28.3)
31 days-18 yrs	0.7-2 (9-25.7)

2.3.36 Triiodothyronine (T_3)

Triiodothyronine (T_3), (free)	pg/dL (pmol/L)
Cord blood	20-240 (0.3-3.7)
1-3 days	200-610 (3.1-9.4)
6 weeks	240-560 (3.7-8.6)
Adult	230-660 (3.5-10)
Triiodothyronine Resin Uptake (T_3RU)	
Newborn	26-36%
Older	26-35%

Triiodothyronine (T_3), (total)	ng/dL (nmol/L)
0-3 days	60-300 (0.9-4.7)
4-365 days	90-260 (1.4-4)
1-6 yrs	90-240 (1.4-3.7)
7-11 yrs	90-230 (1.4-3.6)
12-18 yrs	100-210 (1.5-3.3)

2.3.37 Urea nitrogen

Blood Urea Nitrogen (BUN)	mg/dL (mmol urea/L)
Cord blood	21-40 (7.5-14.3)
Premature (1 week)	3-25 (1.1-9)
Newborn	3-12 (1.1-4.3)
Infant or child	5-18 (1.8-6.4)
Older	7-18 (2.5-6.4)

2.3.38 Uric acid

Age	mg/dL (µmol/L)
1-3 yrs	1.8-5 (100-300)
4-6 yrs	2.2-4.7 (130-280)
7-9 yrs	2-5 (120-295)
10-11 yrs male	2.3-5.4 (135-320)
10-11 yrs female	3-4.7 (180-280)
12-13 yrs male	2.7-6.7 (160-400)
14-15 yrs male	2.4-7.8 (140-465)
12-15 yrs female	3-5.8 (180-345)
16-19 yrs male	4-8.6 (235-510)
16-19 yrs female	3-5.9 (180-350)

2.4 Urine

(see reference [13])

Normal Values	
Color	Clear, from almost colorless to dark yellow or amber
Turbidity	May be normal
Specific gravity	1.003-1.030
pH	4.6-8
Protein per 24 h	<4 mg/m^2/h
Sugars	None
Ketones	None or trace
RBCs and WBCs	<5/hpf on centrifuged specimen

2.5 Blood Gases (BG)

- Venous BG may assess acid-base status, not oxygenation; PCO_2 averages 6-8 mm >$PaCO_2$ and pH is slightly lower
- Capillary BG correlate best with arterial pH, moderately well with $PaCO_2$

Age	pH	PaO_2 (mm Hg)	$PaCO_2$ (mm Hg)	HCO_3 (mEq/L)
Newborn	7.26-7.29	60	55	19
1-28 days	7.37	70	33	20
1-24 months	7.40	90	34	20
7-19 yrs	7.39	96	37	22
>19 yrs	7.35-7.45	90-110	35-45	22-26

2.6 Water and Nutrient Supply

(see reference [12])

2.6.1 Maintenance water requirements[14]

- By body surface area: 1500 mL/m^2/24 h
- By body weight

Body weight	mL/kg/day	mL/kg/h
First 10 kg	100	4
Next 10 kg	50	2
Each additional kg	20	1

2.6.2 Maintenance electrolytes[13]

Electrolytes	mEq/100 mL H_2O (mEq/m^2/24 h)
Sodium	3 (30-50)
Chloride	2
Potassium	2 (20-40)

2.6.3 Estimated energy requirements for median weight and height

Age	Boy-sedentary (kcal/kg/d)	Boy-active (kcal/kg/d)	Boy-all (kcal/kg/d)	Girl-sedentary (kcal/kg/d)	Girl-active (kcal/kg/d)	Girl-all (kcal/kg/d)
0-2 months	-	-	107	-	-	104
3 months	-	-	95	-	-	95
4-35 months	-	-	82	-	-	82
3 yrs	80	104	-	76	100	-
4 yrs	74	97	-	70	93	-
5 yrs	68	90	-	65	87	-
6 yrs	63	84	-	61	81	-
7 yrs	59	80	-	56	75	-
8 yrs	56	75	-	52	71	-
9 yrs	53	71	-	48	65	-
10 yrs	49	67	-	44	60	-
11 yrs	46	63	-	41	56	-
12 yrs	44	60	-	38	52	-
13 yrs	42	57	-	36	50	-
14 yrs	40	55	-	34	47	-
15 yrs	39	54	-	33	45	-
16 yrs	38	52	-	32	44	-
17 yrs	36	50	-	31	43	-
18 yrs	35	49	-	30	42	-

2.7 Body Surface Area Nomogram

(see reference [15])

- Lay a straight edge on the corresponding height and weight points for the patient and read the intersecting point

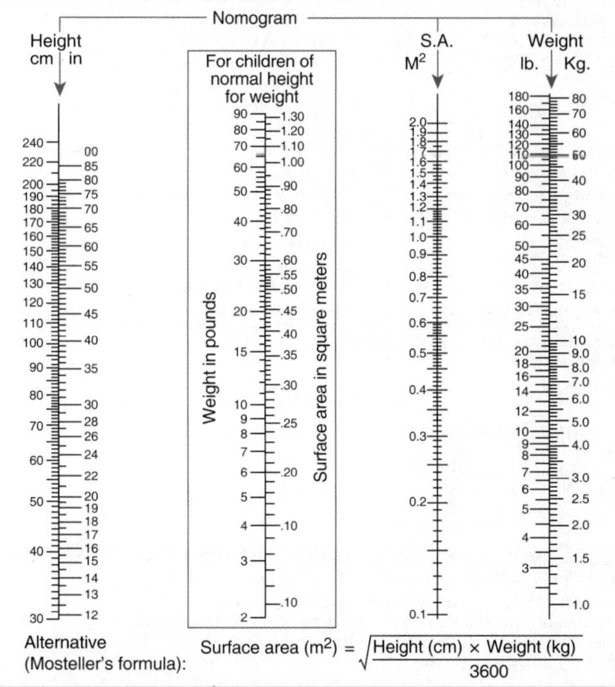

$$\text{Surface area (m}^2\text{)} = \sqrt{\frac{\text{Height (cm)} \times \text{Weight (kg)}}{3600}}$$

2.8 Other Formulae

(see reference [13])

Water and electrolytes	Formulae
Fluid deficit (L)	Pre-illness wt (kg) - illness wt (kg)
% dehydration	(Pre-illness wt - illness weight) / pre-illness wt x 100%
Na^+ deficit (mEq)	Fluid deficit (L) x proportion from ECF x Na^+ concentration (mEq/L) in ECF
K^+ deficit (mEq)	Fluid deficit (L) x proportion from ICF x K^+ concentration (mEq/L) in ICF
Electrolyte deficits in excess of ECF/ICF electrolyte losses: mEq required	(CD - CP) x fluid deficit x wt (kg pre-illness)
Serum osmolality (Normal: 275-295 mOsm/L)	$2[Na^+]$ + glucose (mg/dL)/18 + BUN (mg/dL)/2.8
Anion gap (Normal: 12 mEq/L ± 2 mEq/L)	$Na^+ - (Cl^- + HCO_3^-)$
CD: Concentration desired (mEq/L); CP: Concentration present (mEq/L)	

Respiratory	Formulae
Alveolar-arterial Oxygen Gradient (A-a gradient)	$P_AO_2 - P_aO_2$
Normal: 20-65 mm Hg on 100% O2 or 5-20 mm Hg on room air Larger gradient: More serious respiratory compromise	
Minute ventilation (V_E) (Normal VT: 10-15 mL/kg)	Respiratory Rate x Tidal Volume (V_T)
Endotracheal tube (ETT) • **Size** • **Depth in cm from lip/teeth**	 (Age in yrs + 16)/4 3 x ETT size

Creatinine clearance (Ccr)	Formulae
Ccr (ml/min/1.73 m^2)	(U x [V/P] x 1.73/BSA)
U (mg/dL): Urinary creatinine concentration V (mL/min): Total urine volume (mL)/duration of collection (min) P (mg/dL): Serum creatinine concentration BSA (m^2): Body surface area	

List of References

11 Hartman ME and Cheifetz IM. Pediatric Emergencies and Resuscitation. In Kliegman RM et al, eds. Nelson Textbook of Pediatrics, 19th edition, Philadelphia, Elsevier, 2011, p 280.

12 Ahsan S, Noether J. Hematology. In Tschudy MM, Arcara KM, eds, The Harriet Lane Handbook, 19th edition, Philadelphia, Mosby, 2012, p 260.

13 Arcara KM. Blood Chemistries and Body Fluids. In Tschudy MM, Arcara KM, eds, The Harriet Lane Handbook, 19th edition, Philadelphia, Mosby, 2012, p 678-687

14 Otten JJ et al, eds. Dietary Reference Intakes: The Essential Guide to Nutrient Requirements. Washington, DC, National Academies Press, 2006: 530-541

15 Nomogram modified from data of E. Boyd by C.D. West; from Behrman, R.E., Kliegman, R.M., & Jenson, H.B. (eds.). (2000). Nelson textbook of pediatrics (16th ed.). Philadelphia: W.B. Saunders

3 Critical and Emergency Care

(see reference [16])

3.1 Advanced Life Support

3.1.1 Pediatric bradycardia[17]

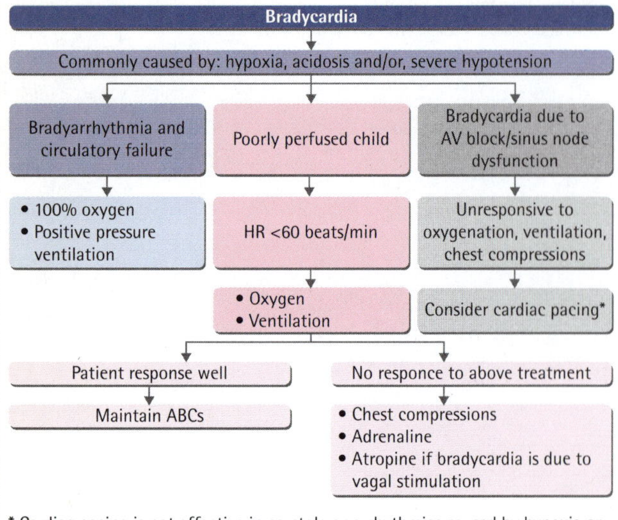

* Cardiac pacing is not effective in asystole or arrhythmias caused by hypoxia or ischemia

3.1.2 Pediatric tachycardia[18]

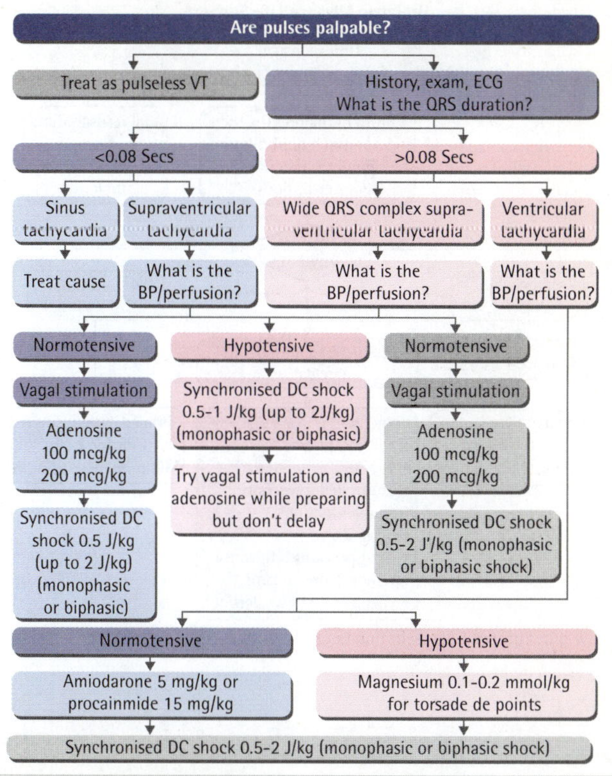

3.1.3 Pediatric cardiac arrest[17]

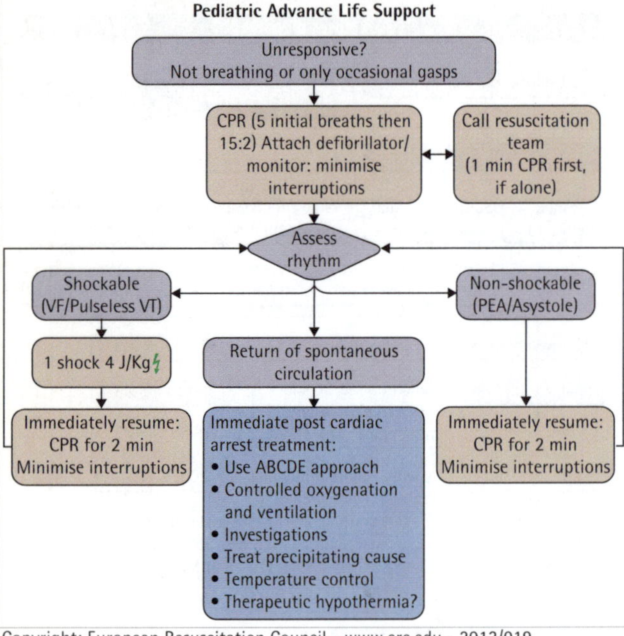

CPR quality
• Push hard (≥1/3 of anterior-posterior diameter of chest) and fast (at least 100/min) and allow complete chest recoil • Minimize interruption in compressions • Avoid excess ventilation • Rotate compressor every 2 min • If no advanced airway, 15:2 compression-ventilation ratio. If advanced airway, 8-10 breaths per min with continuous chest compressions

Reversible causes	
• Hypovolemia	• Tension pneumothorax
• Hypoxia	• Tamponade, cardiac
• Hydrogen ion (acidosis)	• Toxins
• Hypoglycemia	• Thrombosis, pulmonary
• Hypo-/hyperkalemia	• Thrombosis, coronary
• Hypothermia	

Management	
Shock energy for defibrillation	First shock 2 J/kg, second shock 4 J/kg, subsequent shocks ≥4 J/kg, maximum 10 J/kg or adult dose
Drug therapy	**Epinephrine IO/IV dose:** • 0.01 mg/kg (0.1 mL/kg of 1:1000 concentration) repeat every 3-5 min • If no IO/IV access, may give ET dose: 0.1 mg/kg (0.1 mL/kg of 1:1000 concentration)
	Amiodarone IO/IV dose: • 5 mg/kg bolus during cardiac arrest. May repeat up to 2 times for refractory VF/pulseless VT
Advanced airway	• Endotracheal intubation or supraglottic advanced airway • Waveform capnography or capnometry to confirm and monitor ET tube placement • Once advanced airway in place give 1 breath every 6-8 sec (8-10 breaths per min)
Return of spontaneous circulation (ROSC)	• Pulse and blood pressure • Spontaneous arterial pressure waves with intra-arterial monitoring

3.2 Glasgow Coma Scale (GCS)

→ Modified for infants and children[19]

	Child	Infant	Score
Eye opening	Spontaneous	Spontaneous	4
	To speech	To speech	3
	To pain only	To pain only	2
	No response	No response	1
Best verbal response	Oriented, appropriate	Coos and babbles	5
	Confused	Irritable cries	4
	Inappropriate words	Cries to pain	3
	Incomprehensible sounds	Moans to pain	2
	No response	No response	1
Best motor response*	Obeys commands	Moves spontaneously and purposefully	6
	Localizes painful stimulus	Withdraws to touch	5
	Withdraws in response to pain	Withdraws in response to pain	4
	Flexion in response to pain	Abnormal flexion posture to pain	3
	Extension in response to pain	Abnormal extension posture to pain	2
	No response	No response	1

*If patient is intubated, unconscious, or preverbal, the most important part is motor response

3.3 Pediatrics Equipment Tables

Equipment	Newborn/Small Infant (3-5 kg)	Infant (6-9 kg)	Toddler (10-11 kg)	Small Child (12-14 kg)
IV catheter (G)	22-24	22-24	20-24	20-24
Butterfly (G)	23-25	23-25	23-25	21
ETT size (mm) (uncuffed)	Preterm: 2.5; Term: 3.0-3.5	3-3.5	3-4	4-4.5
ETT length (cm at lip)	9-10	10-11	11-12	12-13.5
Stylet (F)	6	6	6	6
Laryngoscope blade size (miller)	0-1 straight	1 straight	1.5 straight	2 straight
Suction catheter (F)	6	8	8-10	10-12
Oxygen mask	Newborn	Newborn	Pediatric	Pediatric
Oral airway	Infant/Small child	Infant/ 50 mm	Small child	Child
Resuscitation bag	Child	Child	Child	Child
BP cuff (cm)	4x8	6x12	6x12	9x18
NG tube (Fr)	5-8	5-8	8-10	10
Urinary catheter (F)	6	6-8	8-10	10
Defibrillation/ cardioversion external paddles	Infant	Infant to 1 yr or 10 kg	Adult when > 1 yr or 10 kg	Adult
Chest tube (F)	8-12	10-14	20-24	20-24

Equipment (cont.)	Child (15–18 kg)	Child (19–22 kg)	Large Child (24–28 kg)	Teen/Adult (30–36 kg)
IV catheter (G)	20–24	16–18	16–18	16–18
Butterfly (G)	21–23	21–23	21–22	18–21
ETT size (mm) (uncuffed)	4.5-5	4.5-5	5-6	5-6.5
ETT length (cm at lip)	14–15	15.5-16.5	17–18	18.5-19.5
Stylet (F)	6	14	14	14
Laryngoscope blade size	2 straight or curved	2 straight or curved	2 straight or curved	3 straight or curved
Suction catheter (F)	10–12	10–12	10–12	12
Oxygen mask	Pediatric	Pediatric	Adult	Adult
Oral airway	Child	Child/small adult	Child/small adult	Medium adult
Resuscitation bag	Child	Child	Child/Adult	Adult
BP cuff	9x18	9x18	12x22	12x22
NG tube (F)	10–12	12–14	14–18	18
Urinary catheter (F)	10–12	12	12–14	12–14
Defibrillation/ cardioversion external paddles	Adult	Adult	Adult	Adult
Chest tube (F)	20–28	24–32	28–32	32–40

3.4 Shock

Definition	Tissue demands not adequately met by delivery of oxygen and nutrients
Compensated shock	Normal BP and perfusion of vital organs; possible tachycardia
Decompensated shock	Hypotension with poor perfusion and tachycardia

Type	Heart Rate	Preload	Contractility	Systemic Vascular Resistance	Treatment
Anaphylactic	↑	↓↓	↓	↓	Fluid, epinephrine
Cardiogenic	↑	↑	↓↓	↑	Fluid, dobutamine/ milrinone, epinephrine
Hypovolemic	↑	↓↓	+/–	↑	Fluid, dopamine, epinephrine
Neurogenic	↑	↓↓	+/–	↓↓	Fluid, norepinephrine
Septic (early warm)	↑	↓↓	+/–	↓	Fluid, dopamine, epinephrine
Septic (late cold)	↑	↓↓	↓	↑	Fluid, dopamine, epinephrine

Management[20]

0 Min

Recognition

- Give 100% oxygen, establish vascular access (IV/IO)

5 Min

Initial resuscitation

- Push bolus fluid 20 ml/kg. Continue until perfusion improves. If >40-60 ml/kg repeated bolus needed consider urgent tracheal intubation/ mechanical ventilation and inotropic support
- Give antibiotics. Correct hypoglycaemia, and electrolyte abnormalities
- Contact PICU

Shock not reversed

30 Min

Begin inotropes IV/IO

- Establish tracheal intubation/ mechanical ventilation, central venous and arterial access
- Consider central venous adrenaline for cold shock & noradrenaline for warm shock
- Continually reassess for fluid/electrolyte requirement/acid-base status Monitor urine output and CVP/$ScvO_2$

Low-dose (1 mg/kg) hydrocortisone if unresponsive to high-dose inotropes

Cold shock with normal BP	Cold shock with low BP	Warm shock with low BP
• 1° goal: Titrate adrenaline • $ScvO_2$ >70%, Hb >10 g/dl • Consider inodilator (eg, milrinone, dobutamine), with volume loading	• 1° goal: Titrate adrenaline • $ScvO_2$ >70%, Hb >10g/dl • Add noradrenaline • Consider inodilator if $ScvO_2$ >70%	• 1° goal: Titrate noradrenaline • $ScvO_2$ >70%, Hb >10 g/dl • Add noradrenaline • Consider vasopressin Add adrenaline or dobutamine if $ScvO_2$ >70%

Persistent resistant shock

60 Min

- Correct acidosis, monitor cardiac output to guide fluid/inotrope requirement
- Consider continuous veno-venous hemofiltration and ECMO

3.5 Pain Assessment

3.5.1 Neonatal infant pain scale (NIPS)[21]

- Range 0-7
- A falsely low score may be seen in an infant who is too ill to respond or who is receiving a paralyzing agent

Parameter	Finding	Points
Facial expression	Relaxed	0
	Grimace	1
Cry	None	0
	Whimper	1
	Vigorous	2
Breathing patterns	Relaxed	0
	Change in breathing	1
Arms	Restrained	0
	Relaxed	0
	Flexed	1
	Extended	1
Legs	Restrained	0
	Relaxed	0
	Flexed	1
	Extended	1
State of arousal	Sleeping	0
	Awake	0
	Fussy	1

3.5.2 FLACC pain assessment tool[22]

→ Age 0-3; Total score range 0-10

Categories	Score 0	Score 1	Score 2
Face	No smile or specific expression	Withdrawn, disinterested, occasional grimace or frown	Chin quivers, jaw clenched, frowns often
Legs	Normal relaxed position	Tense, uneasy, restless	Legs drawn up or kicking
Activity	Lays quietly, moves easily	Tense, squirms, shifts back and forth	Rigid, arched, or jerking
Cry	No cry	Whimpers or moans	Cries steadily, screams or sobs
Consolability	Relaxed, content	Distractible, easily comforted	Difficult to comfort or console

3.5.3 Wong-Baker faces pain rating scale[23]

→ Age 3 and over

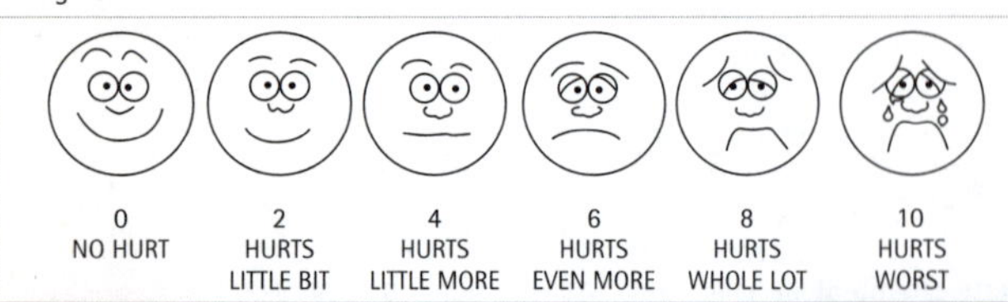

Wong-Baker faces pain rating scale		
Procedure	Explain that each face is of a person who feels happy because he has no pain, no hurt or sad because he has some or a lot of pain.	
	Face 0	Very happy, no hurt at all
	Face 1	Hurts just a tiny bit
	Face 2	Hurts a little more
	Face 3	Hurts even more
	Face 4	Hurts a whole lot
	Face 5	Hurts as much as you can imagine
Brief instructions	Point to each face using the words to describe the pain intensity. Ask the child to choose the face that best describes own pain and record the appropriate number.	

3.6 Pain Treatment

Nonpharmacologic	• Distraction • Hypnotherapy • Acupuncture	• Parental presence • Child life specialists • Sucrose for neonates
Nonopioid analgesics	• Aspirin • Acetaminophen	• NSAIDs: Ibuprofen, Ketorolac, Naproxen
Local anesthetic	• Topical local anesthetics: – EMLA: Lidocaine, prilocaine – LET: Lidocaine, epinephrine, tetracaine – TAC: Tetracaine, adrenaline (epinephrine), cocaine – Viscous lidocaine	• Injectable local anesthetics: – Lidocaine (with or without epinephrine) • Bupivacaine (with or without epinephrine)
Opiates	• Morphine • Fentanyl • Codeine • Meperidine	• Oxycodone • Methadone • Hydromorphone

3.7 Burns

(see reference [24])

3.7.1 Assessment of burn area in children[25]

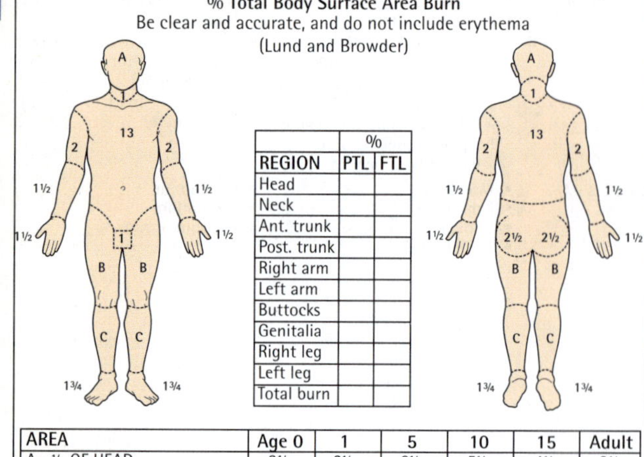

	%	
REGION	PTL	FTL
Head		
Neck		
Ant. trunk		
Post. trunk		
Right arm		
Left arm		
Buttocks		
Genitalia		
Right leg		
Left leg		
Total burn		

AREA	Age 0	1	5	10	15	Adult
A= ½ OF HEAD	9½	8½	6½	5½	4½	3½
B= ½ OF ONE THIGH	2¾	3¼	4	4½	4½	4¾
C= ½ OF ONE LOWER LEG	2½	2½	2¾	3	3¼	3½

3.7.2 Classification of burn depth[26]

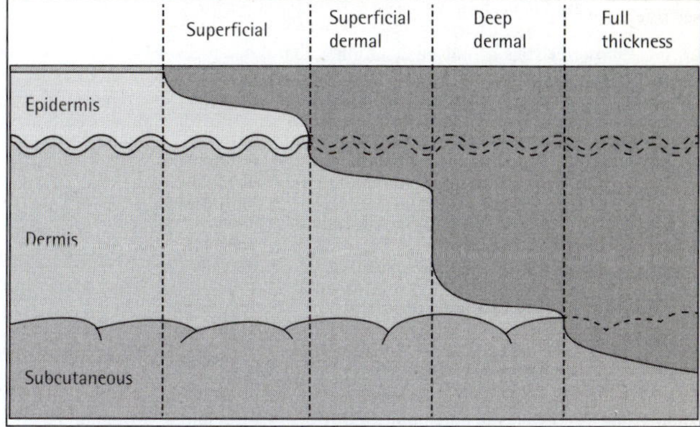

Burn degree	
First	Only epidermis involved
Second	Epidermis and dermis involved
Third	Epidermis and all of dermis destroyed
Fourth	Full-thickness destruction of skin and subcutaneous tissue

3.8 Poisoning

(see reference [27])

3.8.1 Characteristics of poison syndromes

Poison syndrome	Signs and symptoms	Possible toxins	Treatment
Anticholinergic (antihistamines, TCA)	Classic anticholinergic syndrome: • Mad as a hatter (delirium, hallucinations, mumbling speech, agitation) • Blind as a bat (mydriasis/dilated pupils) • Hot as Hades (hyperthermia) • Red as a beet (hyperthermia) • Dry as a bone (dry skin) Also: • Tachycardia • Urgency retention • Inhibited bowel sounds	• Antihistamines • Atropine • Jimson weed • Phenothiazines • Tricyclic antidepressants	Supportive
Cholinergic	The classic mnemonic **SLUDGE**: • **S**alivation • **L**acrimation • **U**rination • **D**iaphoresis and diarrhea • **G**astrointestinal upset • **E**xcessive bradycardia or tachycardia (muscarinic or nicotinic) Or **DUMBELS** • **D**iarrhea, diaphoresis • **U**rination • **M**iosis • **B**radycardia, bronchosecretions • **E**mesis • **L**acrimation • **S**alivation **3B**: Bronchorrhea-bronchospasm-bradycardia	• Alzheimer medications • Organophosphates • Nerve gases	Atropine 2 PAM, Decontaminate

Poison syndrome	Signs and symptoms (cont.)	Possible toxins	Treatment
Opioids	• Pinpoint pupil • Respiratory depression: Apnea, hypoxia • Unresponsiveness (CNS depression) • Flash pulmonary edema (rare) • Bradycardia • Hypotension • Hypothermia • Decreased intestinal motility	• Heroin • Methadone • Morphine • Oxycodone • Suboxone	Intubation Naloxone
Sympathomimetic	Fight or flight picture: • Tachycardia • Hypertension • Hyperthermia • Mydriasis • Diaphoresis • Dilated pupils • Hyperthermia • Agitation, psychosis, delirium • Seizures	• Amphetamines • Cocaine • Ecstasy • Pseudoephedrine • Caffeine • Theophylline	Sedation Hydration and treatment of complications
Withdrawal	• Hallucinations • Confusion • Delirium • Diarrhea • Diaphoretic • Mydriasis • Goose flesh • Tachycardia • Lacrimation • Yawning • HTN • Cramps • Seizures	• Opioids • Sedative-hypnotics • Ethanol	-

3.8.2 Screening laboratory clues in toxicologic diagnosis

Condition	Etiology
↑ Anion gap metabolic acidosis	**Mnemonic: MUDPILES** • Methanol or metformin • Uremia • DKA • Paraldehyde or phenformin • INH, iron, ibuprofen (massive) • Lactic acidosis (eg, cyanide, carbon monoxide) • Ethylene glycol, ethanol • Salicylates
Hypoglycemia	**Mnemonic: HOBBIES** • Hypoglycemics • Other (quinine, unripe ackee fruit) • Beta Blockers • Insulin excess • Ethanol (accidental ingestion) • Salicylates (late)
Rhabdomyolysis	**Mnemonic: MINDS** • Mushrooms (Tricholoma equestre) • Immobilization (eg, opioids) • Neuroleptic malignant syndrome • Diphenhydramine, doxylamine • Statins, sympathomimetics, seizures
Radiopaque substance on abdominal x-ray	**Mnemonic: CHIPPED** • Chloral hydrate, calcium carbonate • Heavy metals (lead, zinc, barium, arsenic, lithium, bismuth) • Iron • Phenothiazines • Play-doh, potassium chloride • Enteric-coated pills • Dental amalgam
↑ Osmolar gap	• Alcohols: – Ethanol – Isopropyl – Methanol – Ethylene glycol • Sugar • Lipids • Proteins

Condition	Etiology (cont.)
Hyperglycemia	• Salicylates (early) • Calcium channel blockers • Caffeine
Hypocalcemia	• Ethylene glycol • Fluoride • Sodium phosphate enemas

List of References

16 Hazinski MF, ed. Manual of Pediatric Critical Care. St. Louis, Mosby-Year Book, 1999.

17 D. Biarent et al. European Resuscitation Council. Guidlines. Volume 81, Issue 10 , Pages 1219-1276, October 2010

18 Guidlines 12.5; Management of specific dysrhythmias in pediatric advanced life suppot. Australian Resuscitation Council. December 2010, Pages 1-5

19 Adapted from Davis RJ et al: Head and spinal cord injury. In Textbook of Pediatric Intensive Care, edited by MC Rogers. Baltimore, Williams & Wilkins, 1987; James H, Anas N, Perkin RM: Brain Insults in Infants and Children. New York, Grune & Stratton, 1985; and Morray JP et al: Coma scale for use in brain-injured children. Critical Care Medicine 12:1018, 1984.

20 Modified from Anna Dehò, Simon Nadel, Understanding shock, Paediatrics and Child Health, Volume 19, Issue 3, March 2009, Pages 97-102

21 Lawrence J, Alcock D et al. The development of a tool to assess neonatal pain. Neonatal Network. 1993 Sep; 12 (6): 59-66.

22 Manworren R, Hyman L. Clinical validation of FLACC: Preverbal patient pain scale. Pediatr Nurs 2003; 29:140-146

23 From Hockenberry MJ, Wilson D: Wong's essentials of pediatric nursing, ed. 8, St. Louis, Mosby; 2009. Used with permission. Copyright Mosby.

24 Steffen KM. Trauma, Burns, and Common Critical Care Emergencies. In Tschudy MM, Arcara KM, eds. The Harriet Lane Handbook, 19th edition, Philadelphia, Mosby, 2012, p 109-116.

25 Lund CC, Browder NC. The estimation of areas of burns. Surg Gynecol Obstet 1944; 79: 352-358.

26 Hettiaratchy S, Papini R: Initial management of the major burn II: assessment and resuscitation, BMJ 329:101-103

27 O'Donnell KA, Ewald MB. Poisonings. In Kliegman RM et al, eds. Nelson Textbook of Pediatrics, 19th edition, Philadelphia, Elsevier, 2011, pp. 250-270

4 Neonatology and Genetics

(see reference [28])

4.1 Apgar Score

(see reference [29])

Sign	0	1	2
Heart rate	Absent	Below 100	Over 100
Respiratory effort	Absent	Slow, irregular	Good, crying
Muscle tone	Limp	Some flexion of extremities	Active motion
Reflex irritability	No response	Grimace	Cough or sneeze
Color	Blue, pale	Body pink, extremities blue	Completely pink

4.2 Maturity Assessment: New Ballard Score

(see reference [30])

→ Use this score sheet to assess the gestational maturity of your baby. At the end of the examination the total score determines the gestational maturity in weeks.

4.2.1 Neuromuscular maturity

SIGN	SCORE							SIGN SCORE
	-1	0	1	2	3	4	5	
Posture								
Square Window	>90°	90°	60°	45°	30°			
Arm Recoil		180°	140° - 180°	110° - 140°	90° - 110°	<90°		
Popliteal Angle	180°	160°	140°	120°	100°	90°	<90°	
Scarf Sign								
Heel To Ear								
TOTAL NEUROMUSCULAR SCORE								

4.2.2 Physical maturity

Sign	Score							Sign Score
	-1	0	1	2	3	4	5	
Skin	Sticky, friable, transparent	Gelatinous, red, translucent	Smooth pink, visible veins	Superficial peeling &/or rash, few veins	Cracking, pale areas, rare veins	Parchment, deep cracking, no vessels	Leathery, cracked, wrinkled	
Lanugo	None	Sparse	Abundant	Thinning	Bald area	Mostly bald	-	
Plantar surface	Heel-toe 40-50 mm: -1 <40 mm: -2	>50 mm no crease	Faint red marks	Anterior transverse crease only	Creases ant. 2/3	Creases over entire sole	-	
Breast	Imperceptible	Barely perceptible	Flat areola no bud	Stippled areola 1-2 mm bud	Raised areola 3-4 mm bud	Full areola 5-10 mm bud	-	
Eye/ear	Lids fused loosely: -1 tightly: -2	Lids open, pinna flat, stays folded	Sl. curved pinna; soft; slow recoil	Well-curved pinna; soft but ready recoil	Formed & firm instant recoil	Thick cartilage, ear stiff	-	
Genitals (male)	Scrotum flat, smooth	Scrotum empty, faint rugae	Testes in upper canal, rare rugae	Testes descending, few rugae	Testes down, good rugae	Testes pendulous, deep rugae	-	
Genital (female)	Clitoris prominent & labia flat	Prominent clitoris & small labia minora	Prominent clitoris & enlarging minora	Majora & minora equally prominent	Majora large, minora small	Majora cover clitoris & minora	-	
							Total physical maturity score	

4.2.3 Maturity rating

Total Score (Neuromuscular + Physical)	Weeks
-10	20
-5	22
0	24
5	26
10	28
15	30
20	32
25	34
30	36
35	38
40	40
45	42
50	44

4.3 Newborn Screening

Core conditions screened in all United States (as of 9/1/2011)[31]

- Hearing deficit
- Congenital hypothyroidism
- Congenital adrenal hyperplasia
- Cystic fibrosis
- Sickle cell disease, including sickle-C disease and sickle-β thalassemia
- Biotinidase deficiency
- Galactosemia
- Fatty acid disorder
- Organic acid disorder
- Amino acid disorder

4.4 Chromosomal Abnormalities

4.4.1 Clinical indications for karyotype analysis

- At least one major and two minor malformations
- At least two major malformations
- Developmental or growth retardation with ≥2 major or minor anomalies

4.4.2 Clinical findings with frequent chromosomal syndromes[32]

Syndrome	Clinical finding	
Trisomy		
T-21 Down	→76	
T-13 Patau	• Low-set or malformed ears • Ocular hypotelorism • Bulbous nose • Cleft lip often midline • Flexed fingers with postaxial polydactyly • Scalp defects • Early death	• Hypoplastic or absent ribs • Visceral and genital anomalies • Microcephaly • Cerebral malformation • Especially holoprosencephaly microphthalmia • Cardiac malformations
T-18 Edwards	• Prominent occiput • Micrognathia • Low birth weight • Closed fists with index finger overlapping 3rd digit and 5th digit overlapping 4th • Narrow hips with limited abduction	• Rocker-bottom feet • Short sternum • Microcephaly • Cardiac and renal malformations • Mental retardation • Early death
T-8 Mosaicism	• Dysmorphic facies • Expressionless face • Long face • High prominent forehead • Wide upturned nose • Thick everted lower lip • Microretrognathia • Low-set ears • High arched • Sometimes cleft palate	• Osteoarticular anomalies common (camptodactyly of 2nd to 5th digits, small patella) • Deep plantar and palmar creases • Moderate to severe mental retardation • Skeletal anomalies • Short or tall stature • Congenital heart defects
Sex Chromosomes		
Noonan	• Autosomal dominant with some phenotypic similarities to Turner syndrome • Distinctive facial features • Short stature • Low posterior hairline • Shield chest	• Congenital heart disease (but right sided) • Short or webbed neck • A flat nose bridge • Congenital heart disease • Affects both sexes
Fragile X	• Mental retardation • Autistic behavior • Macroorchidism	• Long face • Large ears • Prominent square jaw

Sex Chromosomes (cont.)		
45, X Turner	• Physical abnormalities • Webbed necks • Short stature • Congenital lymphedema • Orthopedic anomalies • Shield chest with wide-spaced nipples • Low posterior hairline • Congenital heart disease • Coarctation of aorta • Bicuspid aortic valve • Cardiac conduction abnormalities	• Horseshoe kidneys • Gonadal dysfunction • Nonverbal learning disabilities • Hypothyroidism • Insulin resistance • Visual impairments • Strabismus • Cataracts • Colorblindness • Recurrent otitis media • Sensorineural hearing loss • Inflammatory bowel disease
47, XXY 48, XXXy (rare other) Klinefelter	• Male hypogonadism and infertility • Small testicular size	• Mental impairment variable • Tall stature
47, XXY	• Learning disabilities • Delayed development of speech and language skills	• Normal intelligence
Deletion		
4p-Wolf-Hirschhorn	• "Greek helmet" facies described as microcephaly • Ocular hypertelorism • Prominent glabella • Frontal bossing • Microcephaly • Dolichocephaly • Hypoplasia of orbits • Ptosis	• Strabismus • Nystagmus • Epicanthic folds • Cleft lip and palate • Small chin • Hypospadias • Cardiac defects • Mental retardation
5p-Cri-du-chat	• Characteristic high-pitched monochromatic cry in first few weeks • Microcephaly with protruding metopic suture • Hypertelorism	• Epicanthic folds • High arched palate • Broad nasal bridge • Hypotonia • Short stature • Mental retardation

Deletion (cont.)		
9p–	• Craniofacial dysmorphology with trigonocephaly • Wide fontanelle • Slanted palpebral fissures • Discrete exophthalmos secondary to supraorbital hypoplasia • Arched eyebrows	• Flat and wide nasal bridge • Short neck with low hairline • Genital anomalies • Long fingers and toes with extra flexion creases • Cardiac malformations • Mental retardation
13q–	• Mental retardation • Low birth weight • Failure to thrive • Microcephaly • Broad prominent nasal bridge • Hypertelorism	• Ptosis • Retinoblastoma • Micrognathia • Foot and toe anomalies • Hypoplastic hands or absent thumbs and syndactyly
18p–	• Mostly minor malformations • Varying degrees of mental retardation • Some severe with holoprosencephaly	• Cleft lip and palate • Ptosis • Epicanthal folds • Hypotonia
18q–	• Growth deficiency • Hypotonia with "froglike" leg position • Broad nasal bridge • Depressed midface • Protrusion of mandible • Deep-set eyes • Epicanthal folds	• Short upper lip • Carp-shaped mouth • Antihelix of the ears is very prominent • Varying degrees of mental retardation and belligerent personality • Myelination abnormalities in CNS
Microdeletion and contiguous gene		
1p36	• Growth retardation • Straight thin eyebrows • Dysmorphic features with midface hypoplasia • Epicanthal folds • Pointy chin	• Sensorineural hearing loss • Congenital heart defects • Hypothyroidism • Seizures • Mental retardation
5q35 Sotos	• Overgrowth • Macrocephaly • Large hands and feet • Prominent forehead • Prominence of the pointed chin	• Prominence of extra-axial fluid spaces on brain imaging • Congenital hypotonia • Clumsiness • Mental disabilities

Microdeletion and contiguous gene (cont.)		
6p25 Axenfeld-Rieger	• Hearing loss • Dental anomalies • DD • Congenital heart defects	• Facial dysmorphism • Hypertelorism • Telecanthus • Flat nasal bridge
7q11.23 Williams	• Round face with full cheeks and lips • Flattened nasal bridge • Long philtrum • Stellate pattern in iris • Strabismus	• Varying degrees of mental retardation • Friendly personality • Supravalvular aortic stenosis • Other cardiac malformations
8p11 Kallmann syndrome 2	• Hypogonadotropic hypogonadism • Anosmia • Hyposmia	• Spherocytosis • Mental retardation • Multiple congenital anomalies
8q24.1-q24.13 Langer-Giedion	• Sparse hair • Cone shaped epiphyses • Multiple cartilaginous exostoses • Bulbous nasal tip • Upturned nares	• Prominent philtrum • Large protruding ears • Mild mental retardation • Thickened alar cartilage • Hypotonia
9q22 Gorlin	• Multiple basal cell carcinomas • Congenital cataracts • Odontogenic keratocysts	• Palmoplantar pits • Calcification falx cerebri
9q34	• Recognisable facial dysmorphism • Distinct face with synophrys • Prominent nasal bridge • Anteverted nares • Tented upper lip	• Protruding tongue • Midface hypoplasia • Conotruncal heart defects • Mental retardation
10p12-p13 DiGeorge 2	• Many of the DiGeorge 1 and velocardiofacial 1 features: conotruncal heart defects	• Immunodeficiency • Hypoparathyroidism • Hypocalcaemia • Dysmorphic features
11p11.2 Potocki-Shaffer	• Multiple exostoses • Parietal foramina • Craniosynostosis	• Facial dysmorphism • Syndactyly • Mental retardation
11q24.1-11qter Jacobsen	• Mental and growth retardation • Cardiac and digit anomalies	• Thrombocytopenia • Facial dysmorphism

Microdeletion and contiguous gene (cont.)		
11p13 WAGR	• Wilms tumor • Aniridia • Male genital hypoplasia of varying degrees • Gonadoblastoma • Cataract • Long Face	• Upward slanting palpebral fissures • Ptosis • Beaked nose • Low-set poorly formed auricles • Mental retardation
15q11-q13 (pat) Prader-Willi	• Mental retardation • Short stature • Voracious appetite and obesity in infancy • Severe hypotonia	• Feeding difficulties at birth • Scoliosis • Small hands and feet • Hypogonadism
15q11-q13 (mat) Angelman	• Severe mental retardation • Hypotonia • Feeding difficulties • GE reflux • Midface hypoplasia • Fair hair and skin	• Prognathism • Seizures • Tremors • Ataxia • Inappropriate laughter • Lack of speech • Sleep disturbances
16p13.3 Rubinstein-Taybi	• Mental retardation • Short stature • Microcephaly • Ptosis	• Broad thumbs and large toes • Prominent beaked nose • Low-lying philtrum
17p11.2 Smith-Magenis	• Mental retardation • Sleep disturbances • Severe behavioral problems • Short stature • Brachycephaly	• Midfacial hypoplasia • Prognathism • Myopia • Cleft lip and/or palate
17p13.3 Miller-Dieker	• Lissencephaly • Microcephaly • Pachygyria • Distinctive facial features • Narrow forehead	• Hypoplastic male external genitals • Seizures • Profound Mental retardation • Growth retardation
20p12 Alagille	• Ocular abnormalities (posterior embryotoxon) • Heart defects • Particularly pulmonary artery stenosis	• Skeletal defects such as butterfly vertebrae • Long nose • Bile duct paucity with cholestasis

Microdeletion and contiguous gene (cont.)		
22q11.2 Velocardio-facial-DiGeorge	• Congenital conotruncal cardiac anomalies • Learning disabilities • Cleft palate • Velopharyngeal incompetence	• Hypoplasia or agenesis of the thymus and parathyroid glands • Hypocalcemia • Hypoplasia of auricle • Psychiatric disorders
Xp21.2-p21.3	• Mental retardation • Duchenne muscular dystrophy • Adrenal hypoplasia	• Retinitis pigmentosa • Glycerol kinase deficiency
Xp22.2-p22.3	• Ichthyosis • Kallmann syndrome	• Chondrodysplasia punctata • Mental retardation
22q13.3	• Developmental delay • Hypotonia • Normal or accelerated growth	• Autistic behavior • Severe expressive language deficits
Xp22.3 MLS	• Microphthalmia • Linear skin defects • Poikiloderma	• Congenital heart defects • Seizures • Mental retardation
Micro-duplications		
1q21.1	• Macrocephaly • DD	• Learning disabilities
3q29	• Mild to moderate mental retardation	• Microcephaly
7q11.23 Williams	• DD and severe expressive language disorder	• Subtle dysmorphisms • Autistic features
15q13.3	• DD • Mental retardation	• Autistic features in duplications of maternal origin
15q24	• Growth retardation • DD • Microcephaly	• Connective tissue abnormalities • Digital anomalies • Hypospadias
16p11.2	• Short stature • GH deficiency • FTT	• Severe DD • Dysmorphic features
17q21.31	• Severe DD • Microcephaly	• Short and broad digits • Dysmorphic features
17p11.2 Potocki-Lupski	• Hypotonia • Cardiovascular anomalies • FTT • DD	• Autism • Anxiety • Learning disabilities • Failure to thrive
Xq28	• Immune deficiency • Dysmorphisms	• Autistic behavior • Regression in childhood

4.4.3 Down syndrome[33]

Clinical features in neonatal period	
Craniofacial	Upward slanted palpebral fissures, epicanthal folds, brachycephaly with flat occiput, flat face, frontal sinus and midface hypoplasia, mild microcephaly, short hard palate, small nose, flat nasal bridge, protruding tongue, open mouth, small, dysplastic ears, speckled irises (Brushfield spots), delayed fontanel closure, 3 fontanels
Musculoskeletal	Short neck, redundant skin, short metacarpals and phalanges, short 5th digit with clinodactyly, single transverse palmar creases, wide gap between 1st and 2nd toes, joint hyperflexibility, short sternum, two sternal manubrium ossification centers, pelvic dysplasia
CNS	Developmental delay, hypotonia, poor Moro reflex
Cutaneous	Cutis marmorata
Cardiovascular	Endocardial cushion defects, VSD, ASD, PDA, pulmonary hypertension, aberrant subclavian artery
Gastrointestinal	Duodenal atresia, tracheoesophageal fistula, Hirschsprung disease, imperforate anus, annular pancreas
Health supervision of children with Down syndrome: See AAP Committee on Genetics. Health Supervision for Children with Down syndrome. Pediatrics. 2011; 28(2):393-406. http://pediatrics.aappublications.org/content/128/2/393.abstract.	

4.5 Alcohol Embryopathy

- Short palpebral fissures
- Epicanthal folds
- Flat nasal bridge
- Long philtrum
- Variable mental deficiency
- Thin upper lip
- Small hypoplastic nails
- Small for gestational age
- May have cardiac defects

4.6 Neonatal Jaundice

(see reference [34])

→ Laboratory evaluation of the jaundiced infant of 35 or more weeks' gestation

When there is a finding of	Obtain
Jaundice in first 24 h	Total serum bilirubin (TSB)
Jaundice appears excessive for infant's age	TSB
An infant receiving phototherapy or having a TSB that is above the 75th percentile or rising rapidly (ie, crossing percentiles) and unexplained by history or findings on physical examination	• Blood type; also, perform a Coombs test, if not obtained with cord blood • Complete blood count, smear, and reticulocyte count • Direct (or conjugated) bilirubin. (Repeat TSB in 4 to 24 h, depending on infant's age and TSB level) • Consider the possibility of glucose-6-phosphate dehydrogenase (G6PD) deficiency, particularly in African American infants
A TSB approaching exchange level or not responding to phototherapy	Reticulocyte count, G6PD test, albumin
An elevated direct (or conjugated) bilirubin level	Urinalysis and urine culture; evaluate for sepsis if indicated by history and physical examination
Jaundice present at or beyond age 3 wk or the infant is sick	Total and direct bilirubin concentration; if direct bilirubin is elevated, evaluate for causes of cholestasis. (Also check results of newborn thyroid and galactosemia screen and evaluate infant for signs or symptoms of hypothyroidism)

Guidelines for phototherapy in hospitalized infants of ≥ 35 weeks' gestation[35]

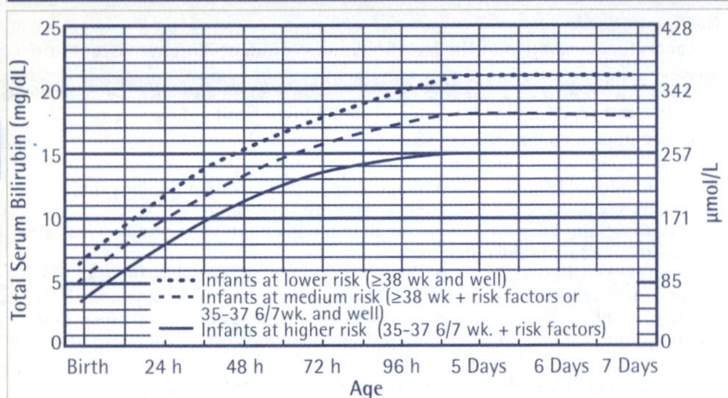

- Use total bilirubin. Do not subtract direct reacting or conjugated bilirubin.
- Risk factors = isoimmune hemolytic disease. G6PD deficiency, asphyxia, significant lethargy, temperature instability, sepsis, acidosis, or albumin < 3.0 g/dL (if measured)
- For well infants 35-37 6/7 wk can adjust TSB levels for intervention around the medium risk line. It is an option to intervene at lower TSB levels for infants closer to 35 wks and at higher TSB levels for those closer to 37 6/7 wk.
- It is an option to provide conventional phototherapy in hospital or at home at TSB levels 2-3 mg/dL (35-50 mmol/L) below those shown, but home phototherapy should not be used in any infant with risk factors.

Note: These guidelines are based on limited evidence and the levels shown are approximations. The guidelines refer to the use of intensive phototherapy which should be used when the TSB exceeds the line indicated for each category. Infants are designated as "higher risk" because of the potential negative effects of the conditions listed on albumin binding of bilirubin, the blood-brain barrier, and the susceptibility of the brain cells to damage by bilirubin.

→ Risk factors for development of severe hyperbilirubinemia in infants of 35 or more weeks' gestation.

Major risk factors	Minor risk factors	Decreased risk
Pre-discharge TSB or TcB level in high-risk zone	Pre-discharge TSB or TcB level in high intermediate-risk zone	TSB or TcB level in low-risk zone
Blood group incompatibility with positive direct antiglobulin test, other known hemolytic disease	Maternal age ≥25 yrs	Exclusive bottle feeding
Jaundice observed in first 24 h	Jaundice observed before discharge	Discharge from hospital >72 h
Cephalohematoma or significant bruising	LGA infant of a diabetic mother	Gestational age ≥41 weeks
Previous sibling received phototherapy	Previous sibling with jaundice	Black race
Gestational age 35-36 weeks	Gestational age 37-38 wk	-
Exclusive breastfeeding, particularly with nursing difficulty and excessive weight loss	Male gender	-
East Asian race	-	-
AAP. Management of hyperbilirubinemia in the newborn infant 35 or more weeks of gestation, PEDIATRICS July 1, 2004 vol. 114 no. 1 297-316		

Management

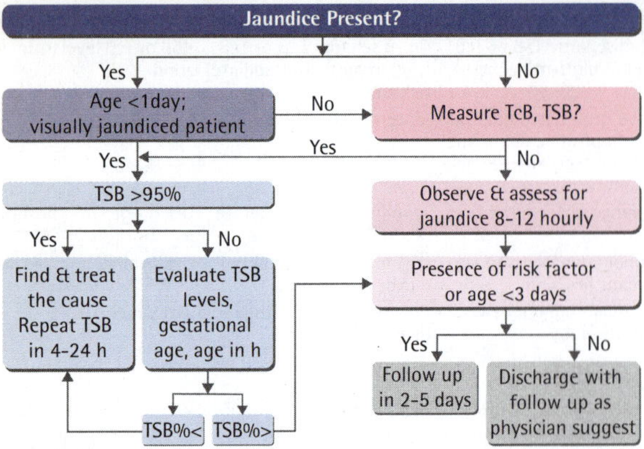

Jaundice Present?

Yes → Age <1day; visually jaundiced patient

No → Measure TcB, TSB?

Age <1day; visually jaundiced patient — No → Measure TcB, TSB?

Age <1day; visually jaundiced patient — Yes → TSB >95%

Measure TcB, TSB? — Yes → TSB >95%

Measure TcB, TSB? — No → Observe & assess for jaundice 8–12 hourly

TSB >95% — Yes → Find & treat the cause Repeat TSB in 4–24 h

TSB >95% — No → Evaluate TSB levels, gestational age, age in h

Evaluate TSB levels, gestational age, age in h → TSB%< → Find & treat the cause Repeat TSB in 4–24 h

Evaluate TSB levels, gestational age, age in h → TSB%> → Presence of risk factor or age <3 days

Observe & assess for jaundice 8–12 hourly → Presence of risk factor or age <3 days

Presence of risk factor or age <3 days — Yes → Follow up in 2–5 days

Presence of risk factor or age <3 days — No → Discharge with follow up as physician suggest

4.7 Respiratory Distress Syndrome

Respiratory Distress Syndrome (RDS)[36]	
Definition	Pulmonary surfactant insufficient, usually <32 weeks' gestation, in 60% of <30 weeks' gestation infants
Risk factors	Prematurity, perinatal asphyxia, cesarean section without labor, maternal diabetes, previous sibling with RDS, second twin
Protective factors (promote lung maturity)	Antenatal steroids, opiate addiction, maternal hypertension, or sickle cell disease; prolonged rupture of membranes, intrauterine growth retardation, or fetal stress
Clinical findings	**0–48 h**: Increased respiratory distress; **48–72 h**: symptom progression, then improvement. **CXR**: reticulogranular pattern
Prevention	Intrauterine steroids
Management	• Support ventilation, oxygenation • Surfactant therapy

Respiratory Distress Syndrome (RDS) (cont.)	
Prognosis	May develop bronchopulmonary dysplasia, oxygen requirement >28 days of age

4.8 Apnea of Prematurity

Brief discussion	
Definition	Respiratory pause >20 sec, or pause <20 sec with pallor, cyanosis, hypotonia, or bradycardia. May be central, obstructive or mixed; >50% incidence at <28 weeks' gestation, 50% at 30-32 weeks, <7% at 34-35 weeks
Clinical findings	Typical resolution by 34-36 weeks' postconceptual age; may last longer if <25 weeks' gestation
Causes	• CNS: IVH, seizures, hypoxic injury, herniation • Respiratory: Respiratory distress syndrome, pneumonia, obstructive lesion, atelectasis, phrenic nerve paralysis, pneumothorax, hypoxia • GI: GE reflux, Necrotizing entercolitis, aspiration, intestinal perforation • Cardiovascular: Heart failure, ↓/↑ BP, anemia, hypovolemia, vagal tone • Infectious: Sepsis, meningitis, RSV, HSV, pertussis • Metabolic: ↓ Glucose, ↓ calcium, ↑ magnesium, ↓/↑ sodium, ↑ ammonia, ↑ organic acids, ↑ ambient temperature, hypothermia • Other: Drugs, post-anesthesia, immaturity of respiratory center
DDx	• Hypoxemia • Infection (sepsis, meningitis, pneumonia) • Necrotizing enterocolitis • Intracranial hemorrhage • Hydrocephalus • Seizures • Patent ductus arteriosus • Hypoglycemia
Management	• Consider treatable causes above • Nonpharmacologic treatment: Tactile stimulation; repositioning of head, high-flow oxygen via nasal canula, CPAP • Pharmacotherapy: Methylxanthines (theophylline or caffeine) • Home monitoring

4.9 Neonatal Hypoglycemia

Brief discussion	
Definition	Serum glucose <40 mg/dL
Etiology	• Increased circulating insulin (Infant of diabetic mother, maternal drugs, tumors, Beckwith-Wiedemann syndrome) • Insufficient glucose delivery • Decreased glycogen stores • Endocrine & metabolic disorders • Hypothermia • Sepsis • Shock • Asphyxia • Polycythemia
Evaluation	Capillary glucose with venous confirmation, assess symptoms, confirm adequate glucose intake, sepsis evaluation, electrolytes, consider insulin and C-peptide levels
Management	Follow recommendations below and monitor glucose levels every 30-60 min until normal

Management of Neonatal Hypoglycemia

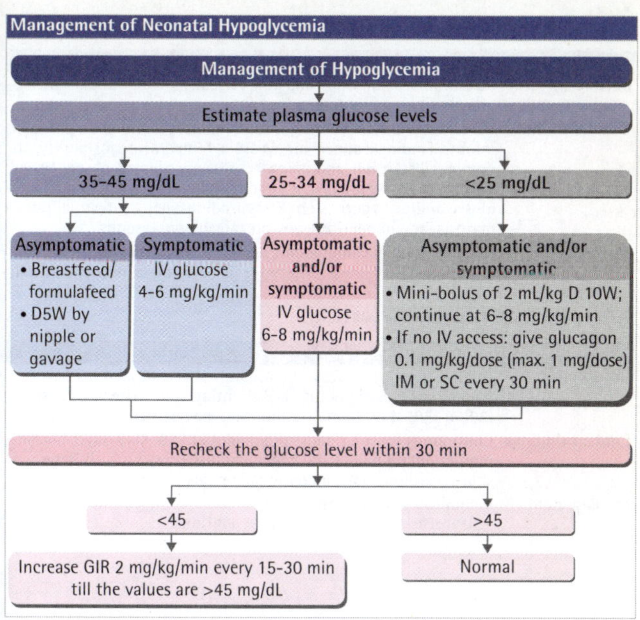

4.10 Necrotizing Enterocolitis

Brief discussion	
Definition	Intestinal inflammation and injury usually due to bowel ischemia, immaturity, and infection
Clinical findings	Usually starts after feeding initiation, more common in preterm infants. Findings: apnea, bradycardia, temperature instability, abdominal distension, abdominal tenderness or mass, absent bowel sounds, elevated pregavage residuals, bloody stool, metabolic acidosis, and/or hypotension. X-ray findings: ileus, intestinal pneumatosis, pneumoperitoneum, portal vein gas, ascites
Management	NPO, NG tube decompression, adequate hydration and perfusion, antibiotics 7-14 days, surgery for perforation or necrotic bowel

4.11 Patent Ductus Arteriosus

Patent Ductus Arteriosus (PDA)	
Definition	Ductus arteriosus does not close in first few days of life, or reopening of closed ductus. L-R shunting starts after decrease of PVR. If PVR stays high, R-L shunting may cause hypoxemia
Clinical findings	Continuous murmur, most prominent at LSB. May have: bounding peripheral pulses and widened pulse pressure with large shunt, cardiomegaly, increase pulmonary vascular markings
Management	• Ibuprofen, indomethacin • Transcatheter closure, surgical ligation

4.12 ICH and Periventricular Leukomalacia

Intracranial Hemorrhage (ICH) and Periventricular Leukomalacia (PVL)[37]	
Definition	• Neonatal ICH usually spontaneous; may also be due to asphyxia, trauma, primary hemorrhagic disturbance or congenital vascular anomaly • Intraventricular hemorrhage (IVH) occurs in prematures without apparent trauma • PVL may occur following IVH, with focal necrotic lesions in periventricular white matter
Clinical findings	IVH may be initially asymptomatic, or may have acute deterioration with apnea, hypotension, poor suck, seizures, metabolic acidosis, shock, and/or anemia. PVL presents later in infancy with spastic motor deficits. **Grades of IVH:** • I: Bleeding only in subependymal area • II: Ventricular bleeding in ventricle without dilatation • III: Ventricular dilatation • IV: Parenchymal hemorrhage **Grades of Ventriculomegaly:** • Mild: 0.5-1 cm • Moderate: 1-1.5 cm • Severe: >1.5 cm
Management	• Fluid and electrolyte management for shock and acidosis • Transfusion for anemia and coagulopathy • Anticonvulsants for seizures • Shunt insertion for post-hemorrhagic hydrocephalus • Early intervention referral in later infancy

4.13 Retinopathy of Prematurity

<table>
<tr><th colspan="3">Retinopathy of Prematurity (ROP)[38]</th></tr>
<tr><td>Definition</td><td colspan="2">Interruption of normal retinal vascularization in premature infants associated with exposure to high oxygen concentrations</td></tr>
<tr><td rowspan="9">Clinical findings</td><td colspan="2">Dilated funduscopic examination shows abnormal retinal findings
Classification of ROP:
• Stages:</td></tr>
<tr><td>Stage 1</td><td>Demarcation line separates avascular from vascularized retina</td></tr>
<tr><td>Stage 2</td><td>Ridge forms along demarcation line</td></tr>
<tr><td>Stage 3</td><td>Extraretinal fibrovascular proliferation tissue forms on ridge</td></tr>
<tr><td>Stage 4</td><td>Partial retinal detachment</td></tr>
<tr><td>Stage 5</td><td>Total retinal detachment</td></tr>
<tr><td colspan="2">• Zone: 1, 2, or 3, with Zone 1 including macula and optic nerve and Zone 3 most peripheral
• Plus disease: Arteriolar tortuosity of posterior retinal vessels with increased venous dilatation
• Number of 30-degree sectors involved
Types of ROP:</td></tr>
<tr><td>Type 1</td><td>Type 2</td></tr>
<tr><td>• Zone I, any stage with plus disease
• Zone I, stage 3
• Zone II, stage 2 or 3 with plus disase</td><td>• Zone I, stage 1 or 2 without plus disease
• Zone II, stage 3 without plus disase</td></tr>
<tr><td>Management</td><td>• Type I ROP: Consider peripheral retinal ablation</td><td>• Type 2 ROP: Serial examinations</td></tr>
</table>

4.14 Polycythemia

Polycythemia	
Definition	Central hematocrit >65%, confirmed consecutively on 2 samples
Clinical findings	Plethora, irritability, lethargy, respiratory distress, poor feeding, hypoglycemia, seizures, apnea, jitteriness, cardiac failure, jaundice, thrombocytopenia
Management	Partial exchange transfusion if symptomatic: replacing blood with 10-20 mL increments of isotonic fluid until hematocrit is <55. • Estimated blood volume: Use birth weight [kg] x 90 • Volume of exchange: Blood volume x (Observed - Desired hematocrit) ÷ Observed hematocrit

4.15 Neonatal Nutrition

4.15.1 Fluids requirement

Insensible water loss in preterm infants in first few days

Body weight (g)	Insensible water loss (mL/kg/day)
<1000	60-70
1000-1250	60-65
1251-1500	30-45
1501-1750	15-30
1751-2000	15-20

Newborn water requirements (mL/kg/24 h) by age			
Birth weight (g)	**1-2 days**	**3-7 days**	**7-30 days**
<750	100-250	150-300	120-180
750-1000	80-150	100-150	120-180
1000-1500	60-100	80-150	120-180
>1500	60-80	100-150	120-180

4.15.2 Glucose requirement

Age group	Requirements in mg/kg/min of glucose
Preterm	5-6 (40-100 mg/dL)
Term	3-5

4.15.3 Electrolyte requirements

Electrolytes	Before 48 h of life	After 48-72 h of life
Sodium	None, unless serum sodium <135 mEq/L without evidence of volume overload	• Term infants: 2-3 mEq/kg/day • Preterm infants: 3-5 mEq/kg/day
Potassium	None	1-2.5 mEq/kg/day if adequate urine output is established and serum level <4.5 mEq/L

4.15.4 Vitamin requirements, preterm infants

Infants <34 weeks' gestation have higher requirements of calcium, vitamin D, iron, phosphorus and sodium, and need breast-milk fortifier or special preterm formulas with iron

4.15.5 Mineral requirements, preterm infants

After age 4-8 weeks, enterally fed preterm infants require elemental iron supplementation of 2 mg/kg/day

List of References

28 Merves MH. Neonatology, in Tschudy MM, Arcara KM, eds, The Harriet Lane Handbook, 19th edition, Philadelphia, Mosby, 2012, p 481-505

29 Apgar V: A proposal for a new method of evaluation of the newborn infant, Res Anesth Analg 32:260-267, 1953.

30 Reproduced with permission, Ballard JL, Khoury JC, Wedig K, et al: New Ballard Score, expanded to include extremely premature infants. J Pediatrics 1991; 119:417-423.

31 http://www.cdc.gov/ncbddd/pediatricgenetics/newborn_screening.html

32 Bacino CA, Lee B. Abnormalities of Chromosome Structure, In Kliegman et al, eds. Nelson Textbook of Pediatrics, 19th edition, Philadelphia, Elsevier, 2011, p 394-414.

33 Summar K, Brendan Lee. Down Syndrome and Other Abnormalities of Chromosome Number. In Kliegman et al, eds. Nelson Textbook of Pediatrics, 19th edition, Philadelphia, Elsevier, 2011, p 399-404.

34 Bhutani VK, Johnson L, Sivieri EM. Predictive ability of a predischarge hour-specific serum bilirubin for subsequent significant hyperbilirubinemia in healthy term and near-term newborns. Pediatrics. 1999;103: 6 -14

35 Reproduced with permission from Pediatrics 2004;114(1):304, ©2004 by the AAP.

36 Taeusch HW, Ballard RA (eds): Schaeffer and Avery's diseases of the newborn, 7th ed. Philadelphia, WB Saunders, 1998, pp 1033-1046.

37 Carlo WA. Intracranial-Intraventricular Hemorrhage and Periventricular Leukomalacia. In Kliegman et al, eds. Nelson Textbook of Pediatrics, 19th edition, Philadelphia, Elsevier, 2011, 566-568.

38 AAP. Screening examination of premature infants for retinopathy of prematurity. Pediatrics 2006; 117:572-576

5 Cardiovascular Disorders

5.1 Congenital Heart Disease

(see reference [39])

5.1.1 Acyanotic congenital heart disease

Condition	Physical examination	ECG/Chest radiography	Management
Patent ductus arteriosus	1-4/6 continuous murmur, prominent at ULSB	**ECG**: Normal or LVH in small-moderate PDA; BVH in large PDA **CXR**: Possible cardiomegaly and increased PVM	Surgical or transcatheter closure
Atrial septal defect	2-3/6 SEM, prominent at ULSB, with wide, fixed split S2, may have mid-diastolic rumble at LLSB	**ECG**: Normal in small ASD; RAD with mild RVH or RBBB in hemodynamically significant ASD **CXR**: Possible cardiomegaly with increased PVM with significant ASD	Spontaneous, surgical, or transcatheter closure
Ventricular septal defect	2-5/6 holosystolic murmur, prominent at LLSB	**ECG**: Normal in small VSD; LVH or BVH with possible LAE in medium-large VSD **CXR**: Possible cardiomegaly with increased PVM	Spontaneous or surgical closure; treatment of CHF with large VSDs
Atrioventricular septal defect	Systolic thrill at LLSB with hyperactive precordium & loud S2. May have 3-4/6 holosystolic murmur along LLSB	**ECG**: Superior QRS axis; possible BVH **CXR**: Cardiomegaly with increased PVM	Surgical closure

Condition (cont.)	Physical examination	ECG/Chest radiography	Management
Aortic stenosis	2-4/6 harsh SEM at 2nd RICS or 3rd LICS radiating to neck and apex. Systolic thrill at URSB, suprasternal notch or over carotids **Valvular AS**: Ejection click, not varying with respiration	**ECG**: Normal in mild AS; LVH in moderate-severe AS **CXR**: Normal	Balloon valvuloplasty or surgical valvulotomy
Pulmonic stenosis	**Valvular:** Ejection click at ULSB, more intense with expiration. 2-5/6 SEM at ULSB radiating to back and sides	**ECG**: Normal in mild PS; RAD and RVH in moderate PS; RAE and RVH with strain in severe PS **CXR**: Normal to decreased PVMs	Balloon valvuloplasty or surgical valvulotomy
Coarctation of the aorta	BP in lower extremities < upper extremities. 2-3/6 SEM at ULSB with radiation to left interscapular area. May have systolic ejection click at apex & URSB if associated bicuspid valve	**ECG**: Infants: RVH or RBBB: Older: LVH **CXR**: Marked cardiomegaly and pulmonary venous congestion. After age 5, rib notching from collateral circulation.	Surgery (various techniques)

5.1.2 Cyanotic congenital heart disease

Condition	Physical examination	ECG/Chest radiography	Management
Transposition of great arteries	Single, loud S2, extreme cyanosis	**ECG**: RAD, RVH, upright T in V1 after 3 days of age **CXR**: Egg on string with cardiomegaly, possible increased PVMs	Metabolic stabilization; possible balloon atrial (Rashkind) septostomy; arterial switch (Jatene) procedure (d-TGA with intact ventricular septum) by 2 weeks of life
Tetralogy of Fallot: **1.Large VSD** **2.RV outlet obstruction** **3.RVH** **4.Overriding aorta**	Loud SEM at LMSB and LUSB, may have thrill; loud, single S2	**ECG**: RAD, RVH **CXR**: Boot-shaped heart, possible decreased PVM	Metabolic stabilization; early total repair with open heart surgery vs. stabilization with palliative systemic-to-pulmonary artery shunt (Blalock-Taussig shunt) and later primary repair
Tricuspid atresia	2-3/6 systolic murmur at LLSB if VSD; single S2	**ECG**: Superior QRS axis; RAE or BAE, LVH **CXR**: Normal or slight cardiomegaly; may be boot-shaped	Metabolic stabilization; possible systemic-to-pulmonary artery shunt; bidirectional Glenn shunt at 3-6 months, modified Fontan operation at 1.5-3 yrs
Total anomalous pulmonary venous return	2-3/6 SEM at ULSB, S2 fixed and widely split, mid-diastolic rumble at LLSB, hyperactive RV	**ECG**: RAD, RVH, may be RAE **CXR**: Cardiomegaly with increased PVMs	Urgent total repair or extracorporeal membrane oxygenation until repair performed

5.2 Dysrhythmias

Type	ECG Findings	Cause	Management
Atrial flutter	Atrial rate 250-400/ min; sawtooth pattern rising gradually and falling abruptly with variable ventricular response and normal QRS	Idiopathic in newborns, dilated atria, previous intra-atrial surgery, valvular or ischemic heart disease	Synchronized cardioversion or pacing, medication, treat cause, radiofrequency catheter ablation, or surgical procedures
Atrial fibrillation	Irregular atrial rate 350-600/min, absence of P waves, irregular ventricular response (irregular R-R intervals) with normal QRS	HTN, Familial, WPW, alcohol, dilated atria, previous intra-atrial surgery, valvular or ischemic heart disease, hyperthyroidism	Anticoagulation, synchronized cardioversion, rate control
Sinus bradycardia	NSR, HR <60 beats/ min	Athletic conditioning, vagal stimulation, hypoxia, hyperkalemia, hypothyroidism, hypothermia, drugs, long QT syndrome, increased ICP, seizure	Treat the cause; if symptomatic, see bradycardia algorithm →48
Sinus tachycardia	NSR, HR >100	Hypovolemia, CHF, myocardial disease, dehydration, drugs, shock, anemia, sepsis, fever, anxiety, hypoxia	Treat underlying causes if present
Supraventricular tachycardia	Run of >3 premature supraventricular beats >230/min; narrow QRS, abnormal P wave	Idiopathic; can also occur with congenital heart disease	**Stable:** Vagal maneuvers, adenosine **Unstable:** Synchronized cardioversion

Type (cont.)	ECG Findings	Cause	Management
Premature atrial contraction	Abnormal P waves, Narrow QRS, ectopic atrial focus	Medications or normal variant	Treat digitalis toxicity; for other causes reassurance
Premature ventricular contraction	Abnormally wide QRS appears prematurely, unifocal or bifocal	Anxiety, congenital and acquired heart disease, drugs, hypokalemia, hypoxia, hypomagnesemia, stress, alcohol	Treat cause, elimination of triggers
Ventricular tachycardia	>3 PVCs at 120-250/min, wide QRS, dissociated, retrograde or no P wave	Congenital/acquired heart disease, drugs, electrolyte disturbance, hypoxia	See tachycardia algorithm →49
Ventricular fibrillation	Abnormal QRS of varying size and morphology with irregular, rapid rate	Myocarditis, postcardiac surgery, drugs, severe hypoxia, electrolyte disturbance, long QT	See asystole and pulseless arrest algorithm →50 needs immediate defibrillation

List of References

[39] Tschudy MM, Arcara KM, eds, The Harriet Lane Handbook, 19th edition, Philadelphia, Mosby, 2012, p 204-207.

6 Neurology and Development

6.1 Primitive Reflexes

Reflex	How to elicit	Response	Timeline
Moro	When supine, allow head to fall back ~3 cm	Extension, adduction, then abduction of UEs with semiflexion	Birth to 3-6 months
Galant	In prone suspension, stroke paravertebral area from thoracic to sacral region	Truncal incurvature with concavity to stimulated side	Birth to 4-9 months
Asymmetric tonic neck reflex	When supine, rotate head laterally 45-90°	Extension of limbs on chin side & flexion on occiput side	Birth to 4-9 months
Tonic labyrinthine supine	When supine, extend neck	Tonic extension of trunk & LEs, shoulder retraction & adduction	Birth to 6-9 months
Tonic labyrinthine prone	When prone, flex neck	Active flexion of trunk with protraction of shoulders	Birth to 6-9 months
Positive support	Suspend vertically and bounce large toes on firm surface	Early: Momentary LE extension followed by flexion	Birth to 2-4 months
		Mature: Extension of LEs to support body weight	By 6 months
Stepping	Suspend vertically, stimulating large toes	Stepping gait	Birth to 2-3 months
Crossed extension	When prone, stimulate large toe of one LE in full extension	Initial flexion, adduction, then extension of contralateral limb	Birth to 9 months
Plantar grasp	Stimulate large toes	Plantar flexion grasp	Birth to 9 months
Palmar grasp	Stimulate palm	Palmar grasp	Birth to 9 months

Reflex (cont.)	How to elicit	Response	Timeline
Lower extremity placing	Suspend vertically, rub tibia or dorsal foot against table edge	Initial flexion, then extension, then placing of LE on tabletop	At 1 day
Upper extremity placing	Rub lateral surface of forearm along edge of table from elbow to wrist to dorsal hand	Flexion, extension, then placing of hand on tabletop	At 3 months
Downward thrust	Vertical suspension, thrust LEs downward	Full extension of LEs	At 3 months

6.2 Neurodevelopmental Milestones

Social/ Emotional	Language/ Communication	Cognitive (learning, thinking, problem-solving)	Movement/ Physical development
2 months			
• Begins to smile at people • Can briefly calm himself (may bring hands to mouth and suck on hand) • Tries to look at parent	• Coos, makes gurgling sounds • Turns head toward sounds	• Pays attention to face • Begins to follow things with eyes and recognize people at a distance • Begins to act bored (cries, fussy) if activity doesn't change	• Can hold head up and begins to push up when lying on tummy • Makes smoother movements with arms and legs

Social/ Emotional (cont.)	Language/ Communication	Cognitive (learning, thinking, problem-solving)	Movement/ Physical development
4 months			
• Smiles spontaneously, especially at people • Likes to play with people and might cry when playing stops • Copies some movements and facial expressions, like smiling or frowning	• Begins to babble • Babbles with expression and copies sounds he hears • Cries in different ways to show hunger, pain, or being tired	• Lets you know if she is happy or sad • Responds to affection • Reaches for toy with one hand • Uses hands and eyes together, such as seeing a toy and reaching for it • Follows moving things with eyes from side to side • Watches faces closely • Recognizes familiar people and things at a distance	• Holds head steady, unsupported • Pushes down on legs when feet are on a hard surface • May be able to roll over from tummy to back • Can hold a toy and shake it and swing at dangling toys • Brings hands to mouth • When lying on stomach, pushes up to elbows

Social/ Emotional (cont.)	Language/ Communication	Cognitive (learning, thinking, problem-solving)	Movement/ Physical development
6 months			
• Knows familiar faces and begins to know if someone is a stranger • Likes to play with others, especially parents • Responds to other people's emotions and often seems happy • Likes to look at self in a mirror	• Responds to sounds by making sounds • Strings vowels together when babbling ("ah," "eh," "oh") and likes taking turns with parent while making sounds • Responds to own name • Makes sounds to show joy and displeasure • Begins to say consonant sounds (jabbering with "m", "b")	• Looks around at things nearby • Brings things to mouth • Shows curiosity about things and tries to get things that are out of reach • Begins to pass things from one hand to the other	• Rolls over in both directions (front to back, back to front) • Begins to sit without support • When standing, supports weight on legs and might bounce • Rocks back and forth, sometimes crawling backward before moving forward
9 months			
• May be afraid of strangers • May be clingy with familiar adults • Has favorite toys	• Understands "no" • Makes a lot of different sounds like "mamamama" and "bababababa" • Copies sounds and gestures of others • Uses fingers to point at things	• Watches the path of something as it falls • Looks for things he sees you hide • Plays peek-a-boo • Puts things in her mouth • Moves things smoothly from one hand to the other • Picks up things like cereal o's between thumb and index finger	• Stands, holding on • Can get into sitting position • Sits without support • Pulls to stand • Crawls

Social/ Emotional (cont.)	Language/ Communication	Cognitive (learning, thinking, problem-solving)	Movement/ Physical development
1 yr			
• Is shy or nervous with strangers • Cries when mom or dad leaves • Has favorite things and people • Shows fear in some situations • Hands you a book when he wants to hear a story • Repeats sounds or actions to get attention • Puts out arm or leg to help with dressing • Plays games such as "peek-a-boo" and "pat-a-cake"	• Responds to simple spoken requests • Uses simple gestures, like shaking head "no" or waving "bye-bye" • Makes sounds with changes in tone (sounds more like speech) • Says "mama" and "dada" and exclamations like "uh-oh!" • Tries to say words you say	• Explores things in different ways, like shaking, banging, throwing • Finds hidden things easily • Looks at the right picture or thing when it's named • Copies gestures • Starts to use things correctly; for example, drinks from a cup, brushes hair • Bangs two things together • Puts things in a container, takes things out of a container • Lets things go without help • Pokes with index (pointer) finger • Follows simple directions like "pick up the toy"	• Gets to a sitting position without help • Pulls up to stand, walks holding on to furniture ("cruising") • May take a few steps without holding on • May stand alone

Social/ Emotional (cont.)	Language/ Communication	Cognitive (learning, thinking, problem-solving)	Movement/ Physical development
18 months (1½ years)			
• Likes to hand things to others as play • May have temper tantrums • May be afraid of strangers • Shows affection to familiar people • Plays simple pretend, such as feeding a doll • May cling to caregivers in new situations • Points to show others something interesting • Explores alone but with parent close by	• Says several single words • Says and shakes head "no" • Points to show someone what he wants	• Knows what ordinary things are for; for example, telephone, brush, spoon • Points to get the attention of others • Shows interest in a doll or stuffed animal by pretending to feed • Points to one body part • Scribbles on his own • Can follow 1-step verbal commands without any gestures; • for example, sits when you say "sit down"	• Walks alone • May walk up steps and run • Pulls toys while walking • Can help undress herself • Drinks from a cup • Eats with a spoon

Social/ Emotional (cont.)	Language/ Communication	Cognitive (learning, thinking, problem-solving)	Movement/ Physical development
2 yrs			
• Copies others, especially adults and older children • Gets excited when with other children • Shows more and more independence • Shows defiant behavior (doing what he has been told not to) • Plays mainly beside other children, but is beginning to include other children, such as in chase games	• Points to things or pictures when they are named • Knows names of familiar people and body parts • Says sentences with 2 to 4 words • Follows simple instructions • Repeats words overheard in conversation • Points to things in a book	• Finds things even when hidden under two or three covers • Begins to sort shapes and colors • Completes sentences and rhymes in familiar books • Plays simple make-believe games • Builds towers of 4 or more blocks • Might use one hand more than the other • Follows two-step instructions such as "Pick up your shoes and put them in the closet" • Names items in a picture book such as a cat, bird, or dog	• Stands on tiptoe • Kicks a ball • Begins to run • Climbs onto and down from furniture without help • Walks up and down stairs holding on • Throws ball overhand • Makes or copies straight lines and circles

Social/ Emotional (cont.)	Language/ Communication	Cognitive (learning, thinking, problem-solving)	Movement/ Physical development
3 yrs			
• Copies adults and friends • Shows affection for friends without prompting • Takes turns in games • Shows concern for a crying friend • Understands the idea of "mine" and "his" or "hers" • Shows a wide range of emotions • Separates easily from mom and dad • May get upset with major changes in routine • Dresses and undresses self	• Follows instructions with 2 or 3 steps • Can name most familiar things • Understands words like "in", "on" and "under" • Says first name, age, and sex • Names a friend • Says words like "I", "me", "we" and "you" and some plurals (cars, dogs, cats) • Talks well enough for strangers to understand most of the time • Carries on a conversation using 2 to 3 sentences	• Can work toys with buttons, levers, and moving parts • Plays make-believe with dolls, animals, and people • Does puzzles with 3 or 4 pieces • Understands what "two" means • Copies a circle with pencil or crayon • Turns book pages one at a time • Builds towers of more than 6 blocks • Screws and unscrews jar lids or turns door handle	• Climbs well • Runs easily • Pedals a tricycle (3-wheel bike) • Walks up and down stairs, one foot on each step

Social/ Emotional (cont.)	Language/ Communication	Cognitive (learning, thinking, problem-solving)	Movement/ Physical development
4 yrs			
• Enjoys doing new things • Plays "Mom" and "Dad" • Is more and more creative with make-believe play • Would rather play with other children than by himself • Cooperates with other children • Often can't tell what's real and what's make-believe • Talks about what she likes and what she is interested in	• Knows some basic rules of grammar, such as correctly using "he" and "she" • Sings a song or says a poem from memory such as the "Itsy Bitsy Spider" or the "Wheels on the Bus" • Tells stories • Can say first and last name	• Names some colors and some numbers • Understands the idea of counting • Starts to understand time • Remembers parts of a story • Understands the idea of "same" and "different" • Draws a person with 2 to 4 body parts • Uses scissors • Starts to copy some capital letters • Names four colors • Plays board or card games • Tells you what he thinks is going to happen next in a book	• Hops and stands on one foot up to 2 sec • Catches a bounced ball most of the time • Pours, cuts with supervision, and mashes own food

Social/ Emotional (cont.)	Language/ Communication	Cognitive (learning, thinking, problem-solving)	Movement/ Physical development
5 yrs			
• Wants to please friends • Wants to be like friends • More likely to agree with rules • Likes to sing, dance, and act • Is aware of gender • Can tell what's real and what's make-believe • Shows more independence (for example, may visit a next-door neighbor by himself [adult supervision is still needed]) • Is sometimes demanding and sometimes very cooperative	• Speaks very clearly • Tells a simple story using full sentences • Uses future tense; eg, "Grandma will be here." • Says name and address	• Counts 10 or more things • Can draw a person with at least 6 body parts • Can print some letters or numbers • Copies a triangle and other geometric shapes • Knows about things used every day, like money and food	• Stands on one foot for 10 sec or longer • Hops; may be able to skip • Can do a somersault • Uses a fork and spoon and sometimes a table knife • Can use the toilet on her own • Swings and climbs

6.3 Epilepsy

(see reference [40])

Definitions
• A seizure is a transient incident with signs and/or symptoms due to abnormal excessive or synchronous neuronal brain activity • Epilepsy is a brain disorder in individuals who have had at least one seizure and are predisposed to further seizures, with biologic and psychosocial consequences

Classification of seizures		
Seizure class/type		**Clinical features**
Generalized	**Absence**	Abrupt onset, no aura, brief duration, prompt recovery, starts at 4-12 yrs
	Atonic	Drop attacks
	Tonic-clonic	Stiffening (tonic phase), followed by jerking (clonic phase)
	Myoclonic	Sudden, brief, involuntary muscle jerks
Partial	**Simple**	Sudden episodic change in movement, sensation, emotions; no LOC
	Complex	Sudden episodic change in movement, sensation, emotions; with LOC

6.4 Status Epilepticus

(see reference [41])

Brief discussion
Definition
Seizures lasting 30 min or more, or two or more sequential seizures without full recovery of consciousness between them of 30 min or longer duration
Diagnostic assessment
• In child with treated epilepsy, antiepileptic drug levels should be considered • When there is clinical suspicion or when the initial evaluation reveals no etiology, toxicology studies and metabolic studies for inborn errors of metabolism may be considered • An EEG may be considered to determine focal or generalized epileptiform abnormalities to guide further testing, and to assess for nonepileptic or nonconvulsive status epilepticus • Neuroimaging may be considered after stabilization for clinical indications or when the etiology is unknown • There are insufficient data to support or refute recommendations for routine blood cultures, lumbar puncture, or neuroimaging

Treatment [42]
• Stabilize patient, administer basic life support measures, obtain IV or IO access • Begin anticonvulsant therapy with lorazepam or diazepam; may repeat in 5-10 min • If seizure persists by 15-25 min, load with fosphenytoin, phenytoin, or Phenobarbital • If seizure persists in 25-40 min, begin drip of levetiracetam or valproate – May give Phenobarbital if still seizing after 5 min and fosphenytoin or phenytoin previously used – May give additional fosphenytoin or phenytoin to achieve serum level of 10 mg/L – May give additional Phenobarbital every 15-30 min to max dose 30 mg/kg • At 40-60 min, if seizure persists, consider pentobarbital, midazolam, or general anesthesia in intensive care

6.5 Febrile Seizures

(see reference [43])

Simple Febrile Seizure	Complex Febrile Seizure
Definitions	
• Duration ≤15 min • Generalized, nonfocal; and • Occur once per 24 h period	• Duration ≥15 min • Focal; or • Occur ≥ once per 24 h period
Diagnostic assessment[44]	
• Consider lumbar puncture if: clinical symptoms or signs of meningitis • Option of LP if: – "Infant 6-12 months of age with seizure and fever when deficient in Hib or PCV immunizations, or with unknown immunization status – Children with seizures and fever who are pretreated with antibiotics • EEG, blood chemistry testing, or neuroimaging are not required after simple febrile seizures	Consider EEG & neuroimaging

Treatment[45]	
• Anticonvulsant therapy not recommended • Antipyretic therapy not recommended to prevent recurrence of seizures, but may improve child comfort	• Consider intermittent oral diazepam • Consider continuous anticonvulsant therapy in exceptional, recurrent cases

List of References

40 Fisher RS, Boas WE, Blume W et al. Epileptic seizures and epilepsy: Definitions proposed by the International League Against Epilepsy and the International Bureau for Epilepsy. Epilepsia 2005; 46:470-472.

41 Riviello JJ, Ashwal S, Hirtz D et al. Practice Parameter: Diagnostic assessment of the child with status epilepticus (an evidence-based review). Neurology 2006; 67:1542-1550.

42 Valente C. Emergence Management. In Tschudy MM, Arcara KM, eds, The Harriet Lane Handbook, 19th edition, Philadelphia, Mosby, 2012, p 16.

43 Micati MA. Febrile seizures. In Kliegman RMet al, eds. Nelson Textbook of Pediatrics, 19th edition, Philadelphia, Elsevier, 2011, p 2017-2018.

44 Subcommittee on Febrile Seizures, American Academy of Pediatrics. Clinical Practice Guideline - Febrile Seizures: Guideline for the neurodiagnostic evaluation of the child with a simple febrile seizure. Pediatrics 2011; 127:389-394.

45 Subcommittee on Febrile Seizures, American Academy of Pediatrics. Clinical Practice Guideline for the long-term management of the child with simple febrile seizures. Pediatrics 2008; 121:1281-1286.

7 Gastroenterology and Nutrition

7.1 Inflammatory Bowel Disease (IBD)

(see reference [46])

Definitions	
Ulcerative colitis (UC)	Characterized by diffuse mucosal inflammation limited to the colon
Crohn's disease (CD)	Characterized by patchy, transmural inflammation, which may affect any part of the GI tract

Evaluation

- The diagnosis is confirmed by clinical evaluation and a combination of biochemical, endoscopic, radiological, histological, or nuclear medicine investigations
- A full history should include recent travel, medication, dietary and family history, and a detailed bowel history
- Physical examination includes appearance, weight and height percentiles, pubertal status using Tanner staging, pulse rate, blood pressure, temperature, and detailed abdominal examination
- Laboratory investigations should include CBC, CRP, ESR, and LFTs (especially albumin), stool cultures, and additional tests if recent international travel
- Imaging should include abdominal x-ray, small bowel series and follow-through, upper GI endoscopy and colonoscopy

7.1.1 Treatment of Crohn's disease[46]

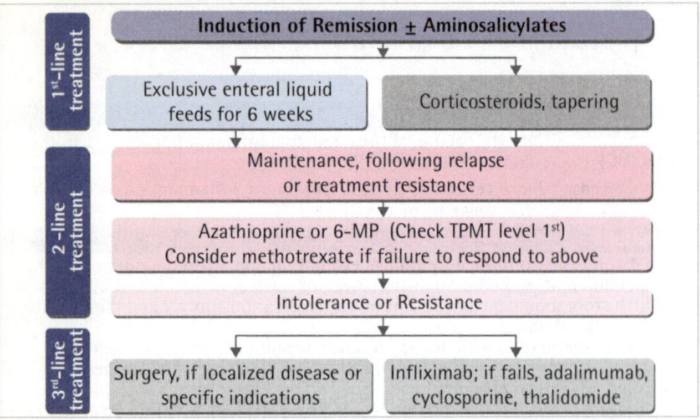

1st-line treatment
Induction of Remission ± Aminosalicylates
Exclusive enteral liquid feeds for 6 weeks
Corticosteroids, tapering
2-line treatment
Maintenance, following relapse or treatment resistance
Azathioprine or 6-MP (Check TPMT level 1st)
Consider methotrexate if failure to respond to above
Intolerance or Resistance
3rd-line treatment
Surgery, if localized disease or specific indications
Infliximab; if fails, adalimumab, cyclosporine, thalidomide

7.1.2 Treatment of ulcerative colitis[46]

Induction of Remission
1st-line treatment
Mild disease: ASA/sulfasalazine
Moderate to severe disease: Corticosteroids
Maintenance
Aminosalicylates
Recurrent relapse or treatment resistance
2nd-line treatment
Azathioprine or 6-MP

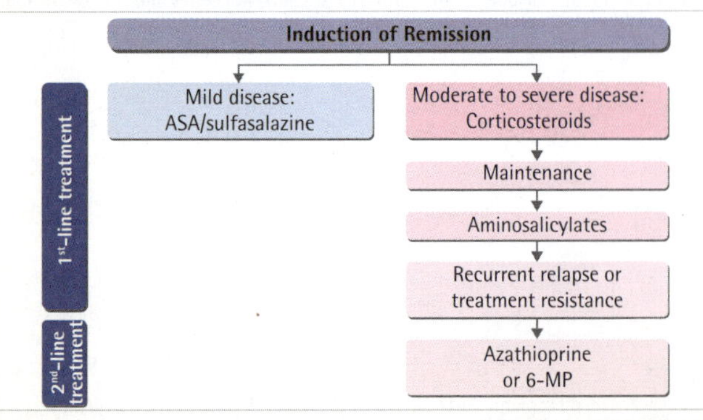

Reference: Sandhu BK, Fell J, Beattie RM et al. Guidelines for the Management of Inflammatory Bowel Disease in Children in the United Kingdom. Journal of Pediatric Gastroenterology & Nutrition 2010; 50: S1-S13

Specific conditions	Treatment
Acute toxic megacolon	• Resistance to medical therapy • Surgery (consider cyclosporine)
Left-sided/ distal colitis	• Oral aminosalicylates +/- topical treatment, ie, enemas (aminosalicylates or steroid)

7.2 Cow Milk Protein Allergy (CMPA)

(see reference [47])

Definition	
• Adverse reactions after ingesting cow milk can occur from birth onward, even among infants exclusively breast fed, but not all such reactions are allergic • Most children with CMPA have IgE-mediated (typically immediate) hypersensitivity and may also have other atopic symptoms • A subset of patients have non-IgE-mediated, probably cell-mediated allergy, and present mainly with typically delayed-onset GI symptoms	
Clinical features	
Immediate-onset CMPA	• Anaphylaxis (in severe cases) • Lip swelling, oral pruritus, tongue swelling, and a sensation of tightness in the throat • Nausea, vomiting and colicky abdominal pain • Abdominal pain, diarrhea, and occasionally bloody stools • Urticaria, generalized maculopapular rashes, flushing, angioedema • Nasal pruritus and congestion, rhinorrhea, and sneezing • Wheezing, dyspnea, and chest tightness
Delayed-onset CMPA	• Atopic dermatitis • Nausea, vomiting, abdominal pain, diarrhea • Malabsorption, failure to thrive, weight loss • Dysphagia, chest pain
Non-allergic-associated symptoms	• Constipation • Colic

Evaluation	
• Period of tentative avoidance, followed by open reintroduction schedule • The use of milk-symptom diaries • Skin testing • Evaluation of serum food-specific IgE • Formal oral food challenges	
Treatment	
General treatment principles	• The elimination diet must be effective and complete. Some children may tolerate some baked products • Inhalation and skin contact should also be prevented • Consumers' rights as to ingredients awareness should be reflected in adequate labeling legislation • Beef allergy usually implies milk allergy but the reverse is not generally true • All elimination diets should be nutritionally safe • Dietary compliance should be closely monitored • Periodical review through diagnostic challenge should be carried out to prevent unnecessarily prolonged elimination diets
Treatment strategies	• Avoid cow's milk proteins until 2 yrs of age • For breast-fed infants, mothers should continue breast-feeding, avoid dairy products, and supplement with calcium • For non-breastfed infants, available substitutes include extensively hydrolyzed cow's milk whey and/or casein formula and amino acid-based formula

7.3 Gluten Enteropathy (Celiac Disease)

(see reference [48])

Definition	
Celiac disease is an immune-mediated enteropathy caused by a permanent sensitivity to gluten in genetically susceptible individuals	
Clinical features	
• Gastrointestinal symptoms • Short stature • Delayed puberty • Persistent iron deficiency anemia • Dermatitis herpetiformis • Dental enamel defects • Osteoporosis	• In symptomatic individuals with: – Type 1 diabetes – Down syndrome – Turner syndrome – Williams syndrome – Selective Ig A deficiency – First-degree relatives

Diagnosis

- Those with symptoms of or increased risk for celiac disease should have a blood test for antibody to tissue transglutaminase (TTG)
- If TTG elevated, refer to pediatric gastroenterologist for intestinal biopsy

Treatment

Patients with celiac disease on intestinal histopathology should be treated with strict gluten-free diet

7.4 Intussusception

(see reference [49])

Definition and epidemiology

- Portion of intestine telescoped into an adjacent segment. Upper portion is intussusceptum, which invaginates into lower portion: intussuscipiens
- Most common cause of intestinal obstruction from 3 mo- 6 yrs
- Most common abdominal emergency under 2 yrs
- Incidence 1 - 4/1,000 live births
- Male:female→ 3:1

Clinical features

- Sudden onset paroxysmal colicky pain in previously well child, recurring frequently, accompanied by straining with legs and knees flexed and loud cries
- Though initially playful between paroxysms, child becomes progressively weaker and lethargic
- Lethargy may be disproportional to abdominal signs
- Eventual shock-like state with fever
- Vomiting is usual
- Bloody stool; 60% currant jelly appearance with red blood and mucus
- Palpable sausage-shaped abdominal mass may be present

Diagnosis

- Ultrasound has 98-100% sensitivity and 88% specificity
- Contrast enema may be diagnostic and therapeutic. Air reduction is associated with fewer complications and less radiation exposure than traditional hydrostatic contrast enema

Treatment

- Hydrostatic reduction is effective in 80-95% of patients, but should not be attempted in unstable patients
- Bowel perforation occurs in 0.5-2.5% of attempted barium and saline reductions, and in 0.1-0.2% of air reductions
- Surgical resection may be required

7.5 Constipation

(see reference [50])

Definition	
Delay or difficulty in defecation, present for 2 or more weeks	
Diagnosis	
History	• Age, sex, chief complaint • Constipation history, including stool description, age of onset, toilet training, change in appetite, weight loss, perianal symptoms, diet, medications • Family history: GI, endocrine, CF • Past medical history: Birth, injuries, illnesses, hospitalizations, surgeries, growth and development, urinary symptoms and infections, sensitivity to cold, coarse hair, dry skin • Developmental history • Psychosocial history
Physical examination	• General appearance, vital signs • HEENT, neck • Cardiovascular, lungs and chest • Abdominal distension, organomegaly, fecal mass • Anal position, perianal or clothes soiling, skin tags, fissures • Rectal exam: Anal wink, tone, fecal mass, stool presence, explosive stool on withdrawal of finger, occult blood • Back: Sacral dimple, tuft of hair • Neurological
Differential diagnosis	**Nonorganic:** • Developmental/behavioral problems: cognitive, ADD, depression • Situational: Coercive toilet training, school bathroom avoidance, sexual abuse, other • Constitutional: Colonic inertia, genetic predisposition • Reduced stool volume and dryness: low fiber diet, dehydration, malnutrition

Differential diagnosis (cont.)	**Organic:** • Anatomic malformations to anus or sacral mass • Metabolic/GI: Hypothyroidism, hypercalcemia, hypokalemia, CF, DM, multiple endocrine neoplasia type 2B, celiac disease • Neuropathic: Spinal cord anomalies or trauma, neurofibromatosis, static encephalopathy • Intestinal nerve or muscle disorders: Hirschsprung disease, intestinal neuronal dysplasia, visceral myopathies or neuropathies • Abnormal abdominal musculature: Prune belly, gastroschisis, Down syndrome • Connective tissue disorders: Scleroderma, SLE, Ehlers-Danlos syndrome • Drugs: Opiates, Phenobarbital, sucralfate, antacids, antihypertensives, anticholinergics, antidepressants, sympathomimetics • Other: Lead toxicity, vitamin D intoxication, botulism, cow milk protein allergy/intolerance
Physical findings supporting organic cause of constipation	• Failure to thrive • Abdominal distension • Lack of lumbosacral curve • Pilonidal dimple with tuft of hair • Midline pigmentary abnormalities of lower spine • Sacral agenesis • Flat buttocks • Anteriorly displaced or patulous anus • Tight, empty rectum with palpable fecal mass • Gush of liquid stool and air from rectum on finger withdrawal • Occult fecal blood • Absent anal wink • Absent cremasteric reflex • Decreased lower extremity tone and/or strength • Absence or delay in relaxation phase of lower extremity deep tendon reflexes

Treatment

Age birth–1 yr

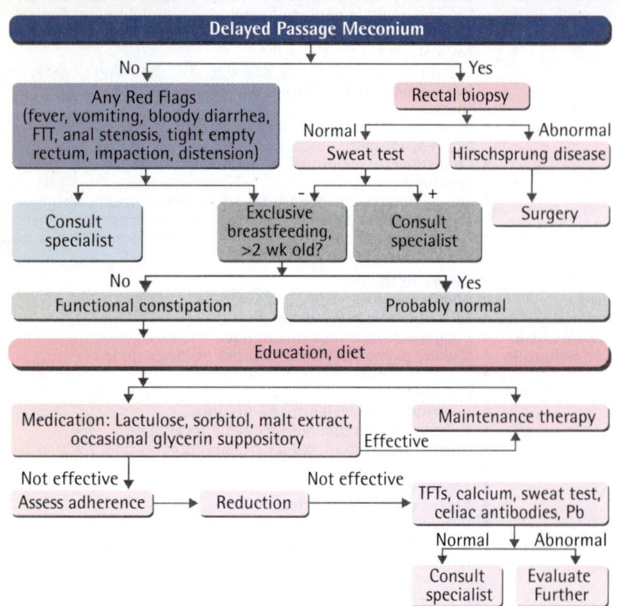

Age over 1 yr

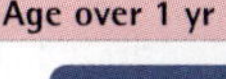

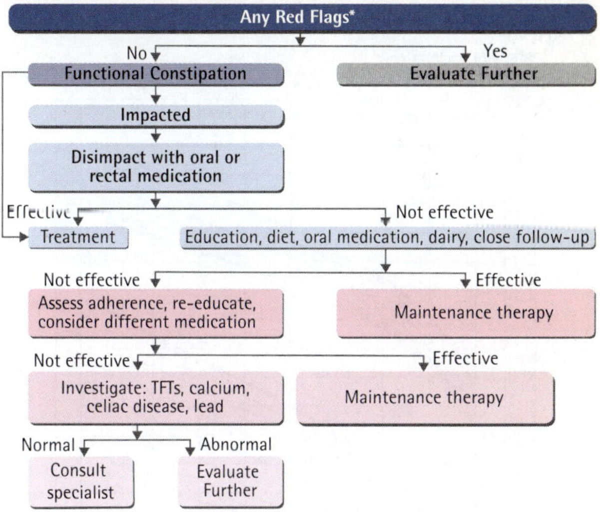

- **Any Red Flags***
  - No → **Functional Constipation**
    - → Impacted
      - → Disimpact with oral or rectal medication
        - Effective → Treatment
        - Not effective → Education, diet, oral medication, dairy, close follow-up
          - Effective → Maintenance therapy
          - Not effective → Assess adherence, re-educate, consider different medication
            - Effective → Maintenance therapy
            - Not effective → Investigate: TFTs, calcium, celiac disease, lead
              - Normal → Consult specialist
              - Abnormal → Evaluate Further
    - → Treatment
  - Yes → **Evaluate Further**

(* Fever, vomiting, bloody diarrhea, FTT, anal stenosis, tight empty rectum)

7.6 Normal Nutrition

7.6.1 Growth charts

(see reference [51])

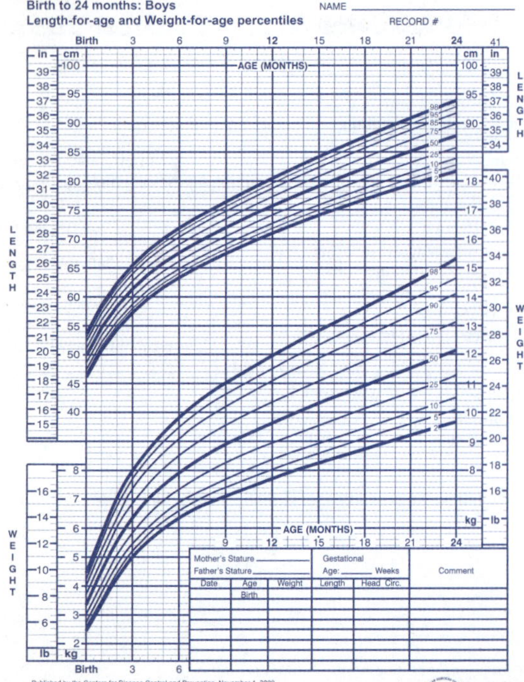

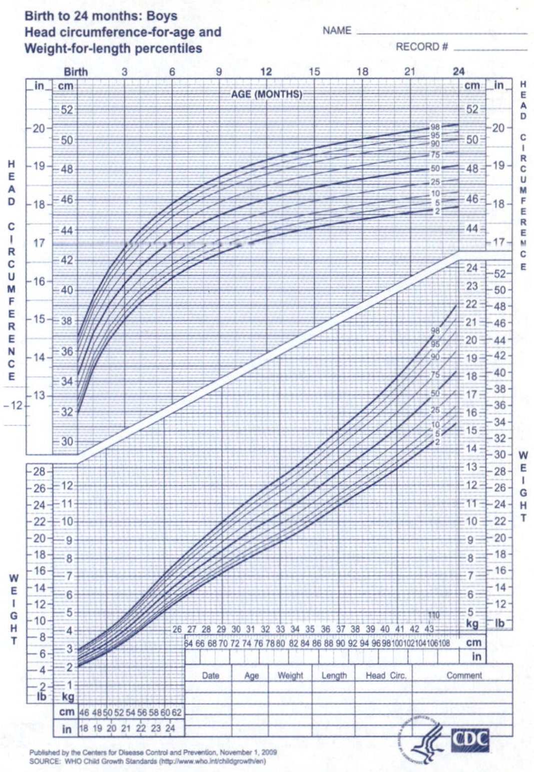
Birth to 24 months: Boys
Head circumference-for-age and
Weight-for-length percentiles
NAME
RECORD #
AGE (MONTHS)
HEAD CIRCUMFERENCE
WEIGHT
Date
Age
Weight
Length
Head Circ.
Comment
CDC
Published by the Centers for Disease Control and Prevention, November 1, 2009
SOURCE: WHO Child Growth Standards (http://www.who.int/childgrowth/en)

2 to 20 years: Boys
Body mass index-for-age percentiles

NAME ______________________

RECORD # ______________

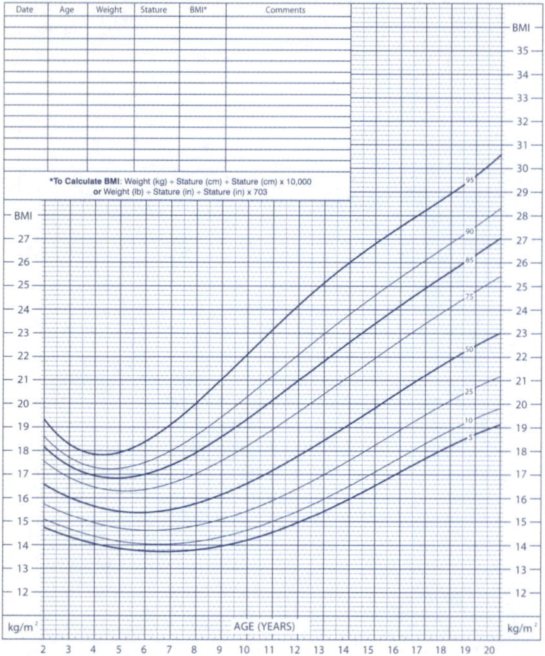
Date
Age
Weight
Stature
BMI*
Comments
*To Calculate BMI: Weight (kg) ÷ Stature (cm) ÷ Stature (cm) x 10,000
or Weight (lb) ÷ Stature (in) ÷ Stature (in) x 703
BMI
35
34
33
32
31
30
29
28
27
26
25
24
23
22
21
20
19
18
17
16
15
14
13
12
95
90
85
75
50
25
10
5
kg/m²
AGE (YEARS)
2
3
4
5
6
7
8
9
10
11
12
13
14
15
16
17
18
19
20

Published May 30, 2000 (modified 10/16/00).
SOURCE: Developed by the National Center for Health Statistics in collaboration with the National Center for Chronic Disease Prevention and Health Promotion (2000).
http://www.cdc.gov/growthcharts

CDC
SAFER · HEALTHIER · PEOPLE™

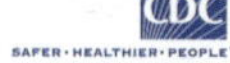

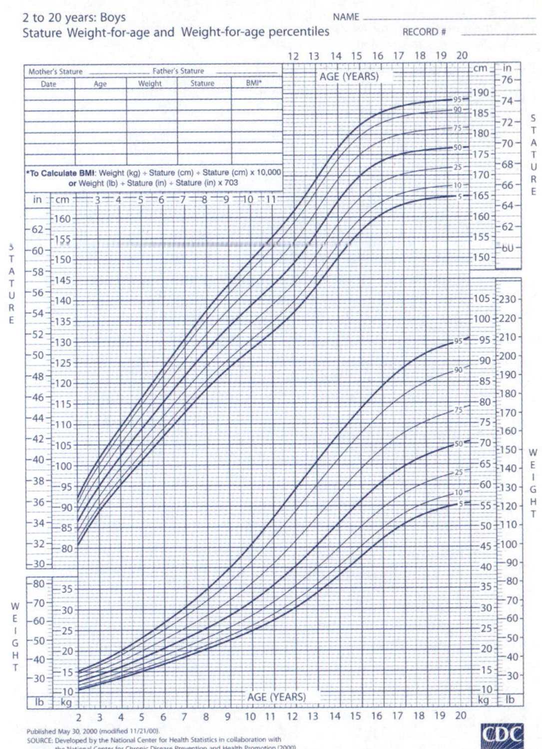

2 to 20 years: Boys
Stature Weight-for-age and Weight-for-age percentiles
NAME
RECORD #
Mother's Stature
Father's Stature
Date
Age
Weight
Stature
BMI*
*To Calculate BMI: Weight (kg) ÷ Stature (cm) ÷ Stature (cm) x 10,000
or Weight (lb) ÷ Stature (in) ÷ Stature (in) x 703
AGE (YEARS)
STATURE
WEIGHT
Published May 30, 2000 (modified 11/21/00).
SOURCE: Developed by the National Center for Health Statistics in collaboration with
the National Center for Chronic Disease Prevention and Health Promotion (2000).
http://www.cdc.gov/growthcharts
CDC
SAFER · HEALTHIER · PEOPLE™

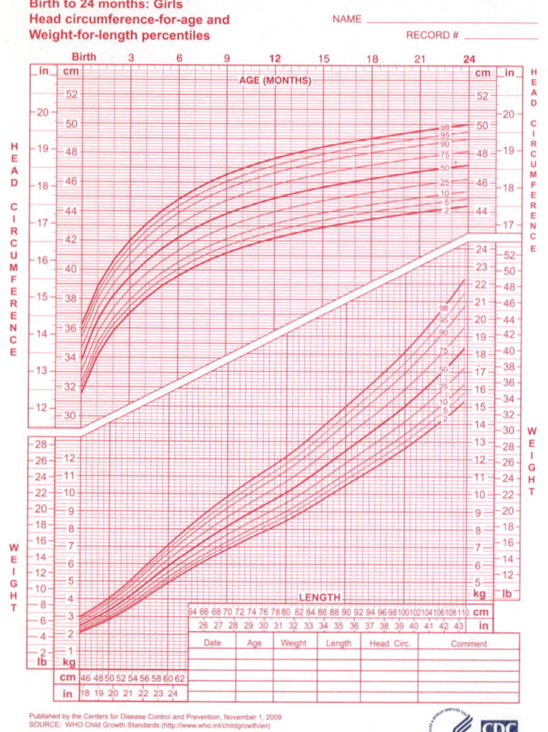
Birth to 24 months: Girls
Head circumference-for-age and
Weight-for-length percentiles
NAME
RECORD #
Birth 3 6 9 12 15 18 21 24
AGE (MONTHS)
HEAD CIRCUMFERENCE
WEIGHT
LENGTH
in
cm
kg
lb
Date
Age
Weight
Length
Head Circ.
Comment
Published by the Centers for Disease Control and Prevention, November 1, 2009
SOURCE: WHO Child Growth Standards (http://www.who.int/childgrowth/en)
CDC

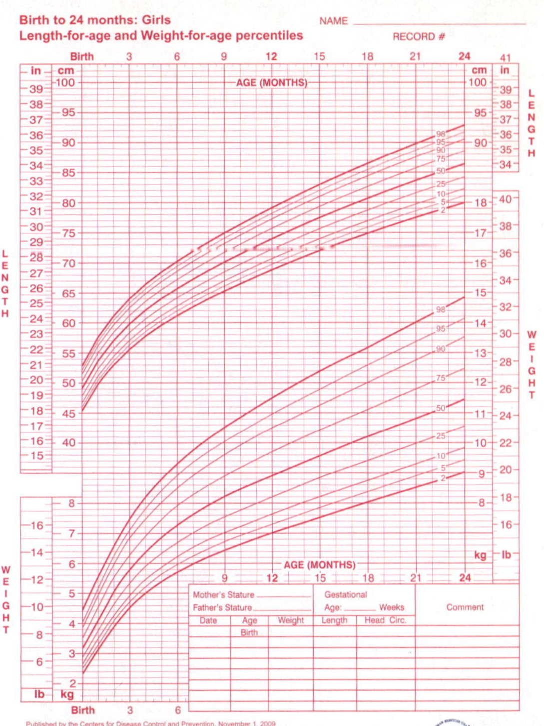

Birth to 24 months: Girls
Length-for-age and Weight-for-age percentiles
NAME
RECORD #
AGE (MONTHS)
LENGTH
WEIGHT
Mother's Stature
Father's Stature
Gestational Age: Weeks
Comment
Date
Age
Weight
Length
Head Circ.
Birth
Published by the Centers for Disease Control and Prevention, November 1, 2009
SOURCE: WHO Child Growth Standards (http://www.who.int/childgrowth/en)
CDC

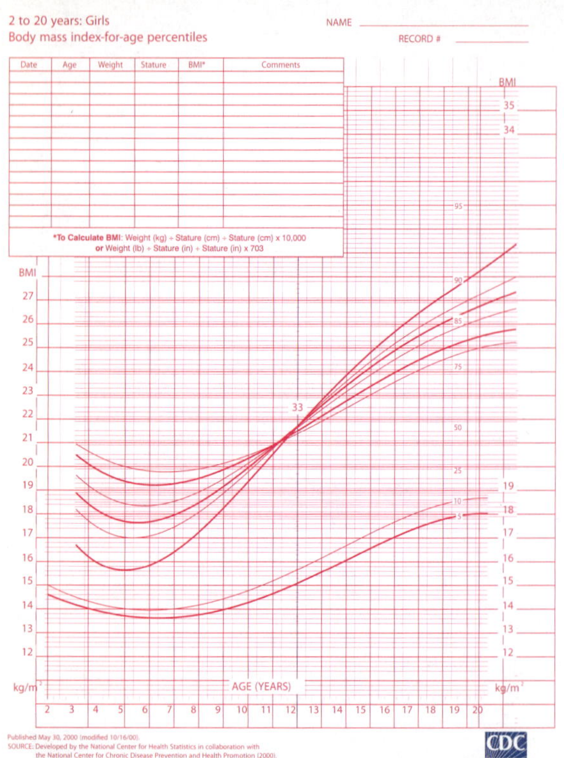
2 to 20 years: Girls
Body mass index-for-age percentiles
NAME
RECORD #
Date
Age
Weight
Stature
BMI*
Comments
*To Calculate BMI: Weight (kg) ÷ Stature (cm) ÷ Stature (cm) x 10,000
or Weight (lb) ÷ Stature (in) ÷ Stature (in) x 703
BMI
95
90
85
75
50
25
10
5
AGE (YEARS)
kg/m²
Published May 30, 2000 (modified 10/16/00).
SOURCE: Developed by the National Center for Health Statistics in collaboration with the National Center for Chronic Disease Prevention and Health Promotion (2000).
http://www.cdc.gov/growthcharts
CDC
SAFER · HEALTHIER · PEOPLE™

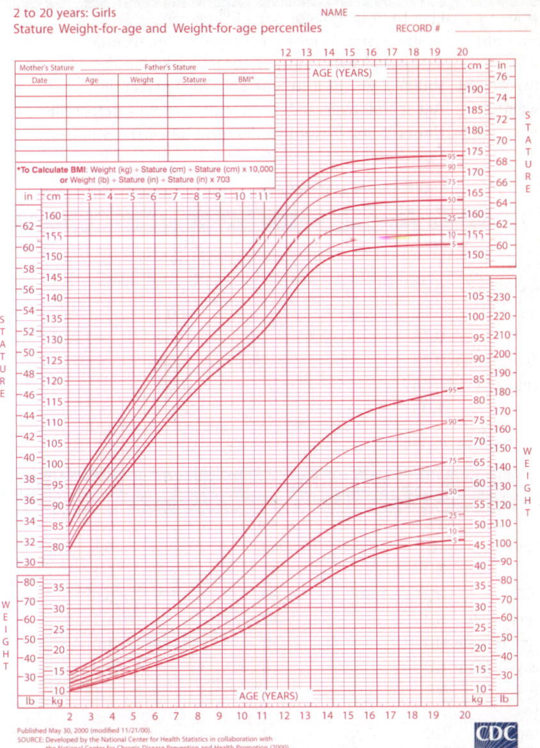
2 to 20 years: Girls
Stature Weight-for-age and Weight-for-age percentiles
NAME
RECORD #
Mother's Stature
Father's Stature
Date
Age
Weight
Stature
BMI*
*To Calculate BMI: Weight (kg) ÷ Stature (cm) ÷ Stature (cm) x 10,000
or Weight (lb) ÷ Stature (in) ÷ Stature (in) x 703
AGE (YEARS)
STATURE
WEIGHT
Published May 30, 2000 (modified 11/21/00).
SOURCE: Developed by the National Center for Health Statistics in collaboration with
the National Center for Chronic Disease Prevention and Health Promotion (2000).
http://www.cdc.gov/growthcharts
CDC
SAFER · HEALTHIER · PEOPLE™

Body pattern	
Stunting	Length or height for age <5th percentile
Underweight	**Under 2 yrs:** Weight for length <5th percentile **Age 2 and over:** BMI for age <5th percentile
Healthy weight	**Under 2 yrs**: BMI for age 5th - 85th percentile
Overweight	**Age 2 and over:** BMI for age 85th - <95th percentile
Obese	**Under 2 yrs:** Weight for length >95th percentile **Age 2 and over:** BMI for age >95th percentile

7.6.2 Protein & calcium requirements[52]

Age	Protein(g/kg/d)	Calcium (mg/d)
0-6 mo	-	ND
6-12 mo	1.0	ND
1-3 yrs	0.87	500
4-8 yrs	0.76	800
9-13 yrs	0.76	1100
14-18 yrs	0.73	1000
Pregnancy	0.88	1000
Lactation	1.05	ND

7.6.3 Fat requirement[52]

Age	Total fat (g/day)	Linoleic acid (g/day)	α-Linolenic Acid (g/day)
0-6 mo	31	4.4	0.5
6-12 mo	30	4.6	0.5
1-3 yrs	ND	7	0.7
4-8 yrs	ND	10	0.9
9-13 yrs, male	ND	12	1.2
9-13 yrs,female	ND	10	1.0
14-18 yrs, male	ND	16	1.6
14-18 yrs, female	ND	11	1.1
Pregnancy	ND	13	1.4
Lactation	ND	13	1.3

7.6.4 Vitamin requirements[52]

Age	A (µg/d)	C (mg/d)	D (µg/d)	E (mg/d)	K (µg/d)	Thiamin (mg/d)	Riboflavin (mg/d)
0–6 mo	400	40	10	4	2.0	0.2	0.3
6–12 mo	500	50	10	5	2.5	0.3	0.4
1–3 yrs	300	15	15	6	30	0.5	0.5
4–8 yrs	400	25	15	7	55	0.6	0.6
9–13 yrs	600	45	15	11	60	0.9	0.9
14–18 yrs (M)	900	75	15	15	95	1.2	1.3
14–18 yrs (F)	700	65	15	15	75	1.0	1.0
Pregnancy 14–18 yrs	750	80	15	15	75	1.4	1.4
Lactation 14–18 yrs	1200	115	15	19	75	1.4	1.6

Age	Niacin (mg/d)	B6 (mg/d)	Folate (µg/d)	B12 (µg/d)	Pantothenic acid (mg/d)	Biotin (µg/d)	Choline (mg/d)
0–6 mo	2	0.1	65	0.4	1.7	5	125
7–12 mo	4	0.3	80	0.5	1.8	6	150
1–3 yrs	6	0.5	150	0.9	2	8	200
4–8 yrs	8	0.6	200	1.2	3	12	250
9–13 yrs	12	1.0	300	1.8	4	20	375
14–18 yrs (M)	16	1.3	400	2.4	5	25	550
14–18 yrs (F)	14	1.2	400	2.4	5	25	400
Pregnancy 14–18 yrs	18	1.9	600	2.6	6	30	450
Lactation 14–18 yrs	17	2.0	500	2.8	7	35	550

7.6.5 Fiber requirements[52]

Age	Total fiber (g/day)
0–12 mo	ND
1–3 yrs	19
4–8 yrs	25
9–13 yrs, male	31
9–13 yrs, female	26
14–18 yrs, male	38
14–18 yrs, female	26
Pregnancy	28
Lactation	29

7.6.6 Vitamin-mineral supplementation

Fluoride	• 0-6 mo: Not necessary • >6 mo (exclusively breast-fed): 0.5 mg/day • Also think of supplementation if bottled or filtered water does not contain adequate fluoride • Fluoridated toothpaste: avoided until 2 yrs, and then only pea size until 6 yrs
Vitamin D	• For infants consuming less than 1,000 mL per day of vitamin D-fortified formula or cow milk: 400 IU/d • For children and adolescents who get less sunlight exposure, ingest less than 1,000 mL/day of vitamin D-fortified milk, or do not take a daily multivitamin: 600 IU/d
Iron	**Full-term:** • Breast-fed: 1 mg/kg/d after 4-6 mo, preferably from iron-fortified cereal • Formula-fed: Iron fortified formula with 4-12 mg/L or iron from birth to 12 mos **Preterm or low-birth-weight:** • Breast-fed: 2 mg/kg/d from 2-12 mos • Formula fed: Additional 1 mg/kg/d via iron drops or multivitamin with iron drops • All infants under 12 months: Only formula fortified with iron for weaning or supplementing breast milk

7.7 Failure to Thrive (FTT)

(see reference [53])

Definition	
Even though there is no standard definition, FTT occurs when a child's physical growth over time is inadequate when compared to a standard growth chart.	
Causes of FTT	
• Can be endogenous or exogenous • Increased metabolic demands • Failure of a caregiver to offer adequate calories or child to take in sufficient calories • Child can't retain and use sufficient calories	
Common causes of FTT by age	
0–6 mo	• Congenital disorders • Breastfeeding difficulties • Recurrent infections • Improper formula preparation • Impaired parent-child interaction, child neglect • Prenatal infections or teratogenic exposures • Poor feeding (sucking, swallowing) or feeding aversion • Maternal psychological disorder • Congenital heart disease • CF • Neurologic abnormalities
6–12 mo	• Recurrent infections • Child neglect • Celiac disease • Food intolerance or allergy • Delayed introduction of age-appropriate foods or poor transition to food
After infancy	• Recurrent infections • Acquired chronic diseases • Highly distractible child • Inappropriate mealtime environment • Inappropriate diet (eg, excessive juice, avoidance of high-calorie foods)

Differential diagnosis of FTT	
Psychosocial/ behavioral	• Food refusal • Child-parent interaction problems • Inadequate diet due to poverty/food insufficiency, errors in food preparation • Poor parenting skills • Rumination • Parental cognitive or mental health problems • Child abuse or neglect; emotional deprivation
Neurologic	• Cerebral palsy • Hypothalamic and other CNS tumors • Neuromuscular disorders • Neurodegenerative disorders
Renal	• Recurrent UTI • Renal tubular acidosis, renal failure
Endocrine	• Hypothyroidism /hyperthyroidism • DM • Diabetes insipidus • Growth hormone deficiency • Adrenal insufficiency
Genetic/ metabolic/ congenital	• Chromosomal disorders • Sickle cell disease • Inborn errors of metabolism • Fetal alcohol syndrome • Multiple congenital anomaly syndromes (VATER, CHARGE) • Skeletal dysplasias
Gastrointestinal	• GERD • Repair of tracheoesophageal fistula • Malrotation • Food allergy • Malabsorption syndromes • Celiac disease • Milk intolerance • Pancreatic insufficiency syndromes • Chronic cholestasis • Pyloric stenosis • Inflammatory bowel disease • Chronic congenital diarrhea states • Short bowel syndrome • Pseudo-obstruction • Hirschsprung disease

Differential diagnosis of FTT (cont.)	
Cardiac	• CHF • Cyanotic heart disease • Vascular rings
Pulmonary/ respiratory	• Adenoid/tonsillar hypertrophy • Bronchopulmonary dysplasia • Chronic respiratory failure • Cystic fibrosis, bronchiectasis • Obstructive sleep apnea • Severe asthma
Miscellaneous	• Collagen-vascular disease • Malignancy • Primary immunodeficiency • Transplantation
Infections	• HIV • TB • Perinatal infection • Occult/chronic infections • Parasitic infestation

Diagnostic Approach to FTT	
History/physical examination	**Diagnostic consideration**
Mouth breathing, enlarged tonsils, snoring	Adenoid hypertrophy, obstructive sleep apnea
Vomiting, food refusal	Chronic tonsillitis, gastroesophageal reflux, food allergies
Diarrhea, fatty stools	Malabsorption, intestinal parasites, milk protein intolerance
Recurrent wheezing, pulmonary infections	Asthma, aspiration, food allergy
Recurrent infections	HIV or congenital immunodeficiency diseases
Travel to/from developing countries	Parasitic or bacterial infections of the gastrointestinal tract

Treatment of FTT

- Requires multidisciplinary approach: Dietician, psychologist, social work
- Appropriate feeding environment in home
- Indications for hospitalization:
  - Severe malnutrition
  - Failure of outpatient management
- Children with severe malnutrition must be re-feed carefully with an incremental increase in calories to avoid re-feeding syndrome
- Type of caloric supplementation based on severity of FTT and underlying medical condition
- Multivitamin supplement needed

7.8 Obesity

7.8.1 Identification and assessment[54]

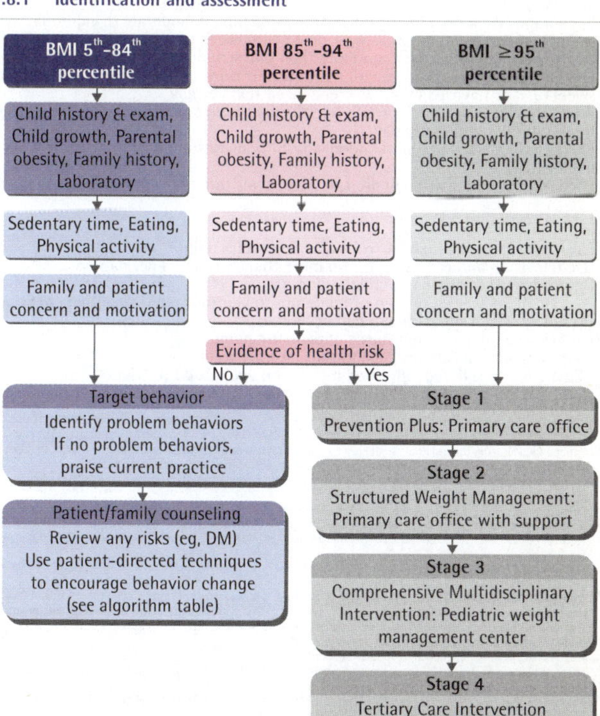

7.8.2 Recommendations for prevention

- Measure height and weight and calculate BMI plus BMI percentile for all children at least once a year
- Encourage all children to engage in at least 60 min of moderate to vigorous physical activity on most, preferably all, days of the week to achieve a healthy weight
- Advise patients to consume no more than one serving of sweetened beverages (eg, fruit juice, fruit drink, regular-calorie soft drink, sports drink, energy drink, sweetened or flavored milk, sweetened iced tea) per day
- Advise families to limit children's television viewing and other screen time to no more than two hours per day
- Encourage families to limit children's fast-food consumption to no more than once per week
- Encourage families with children to have meals together as often as possible

7.8.3 Prevention and protocol

- Eat five or more servings of fruits and vegetables daily
- Use television and computer for no more than two hours per day
- Do not keep a television in child's bedroom
- Participate in at least 60 min of moderate to vigorous physical activity per day
- Do not consume sugar-sweetened beverages
- Eat breakfast daily & limit meals outside the home
- Have family meals at least five to six times per week
- Allow child to self-regulate food intake and avoid food restriction (eg, a child should be permitted to eat portions of food until satiated, no more or less)

List of References

46 Sandhu BK, Fell J, Beattie RM et al. Guidelines for the Management of Inflammatory Bowel Disease in Children in the United Kingdom. Journal of Pediatric Gastroenterology & Nutrition 2010; 50: S1-S13

47 Fiocchi A, Schünemann H, Brozek J, et al. Diagnosis and rationale for action against cow's milk allergy: A summary report. J All Clin Immunol 2010; 126:1119-1128

48 Celiac Disease Guidelines Committee of the North American Society for Pediatric Gastroenterology, Hepatology and Nutrition. Guideline for the Diagnosis and Treatment of Celiac Disease in Children: Recommendations of the North American Society for Pediatric Gastroenterology, Hepatology and Nutrition. Journal of Pediatric Gastroenterology and Nutrition 2005; 40:1-19.

49 Kennedy M, Liacouras CA. Intussusception. In Kliegman RM et al, eds. Nelson Textbook of Pediatrics, 19th edition, Philadelphia, Elsevier, 2011, p 1287-1289

50 NASPGHAN Constipation Guideline Committee. Evaluation and Treatment of Constipation in Infants and Children: Recommendations of the North American Society for Pediatric Gastroenterology, Hepatology and Nutrition. Journal of Pediatric Gastroenterology and Nutrition 2006; 43:e1-e13

51 2000 CDC Growth Charts for the United States: Methods and Development. http://www.cdc.gov/growthcharts/2000growthchart-us.pdf.

52 Otten JJ, Hellwig JP, Meyers LD (eds): Dietary reference intakes: the essential guide to nutrient requirements. Washington, DC, National Academies Press, 2006.

53 McLean HS, Price DT. Failure to thrive. In Kliegman RM et al, eds. Nelson Textbook of Pediatrics, 19th edition, Philadelphia, Elsevier, 2011, p 147-149

54 Barlow SE; Expert Committee: Expert Committee recommendations regarding the prevention, assessment, and treatment of child and adolescent overweight and obesity: summary report. Pediatrics: 2007;120:S164-S192

8 Infectious Diseases

(see infectious exanthems →28)

8.1 Immunization Schedule

(see reference 55,56)

8.1.1 Recommended immunization schedule (aged 0-6 yrs)

Vaccine \ Age	Birth	1 month	2 month	4 month	6 month	12 month	15 month	18 month	19–23 months	2–3 years	4–6 years
Hepatitis B	HepB1	HepB2 →			HepB3 →						
Rotavirus			RV1	RV2	RV3						
Diphtheria, Tetanus, Pertussis			DTaP1	DTaP2	DTaP3		DTaP4 →				DTaP5
Haemophilus influenzae type b			Hib1	Hib2	Hib3	Hib4 →					
Pneumococcus			PCV1	PCV2	PCV3	PCV4 →					
Inactivated Poliovirus			IPV1	IPV2	IPV3 →						IPV4
Influenza					Annual Influenza →						
Measles, Mumps, Rubella						MMR1 →					MMR2
Varicella						Varicella1 →					Varicella2
Hepatitis A						HepA1 →				HepA2 →	
Meningococcal (high risk)										MCV4 →	

8.1.2 Recommended immunization schedule (aged 7-18 yrs)

Vaccine \ Age	7-10 years	11-12 years	13-18 years
Tetanus, Diphtheria, Pertussis		Tdap →	→
Human Papillomavirus		HPV 3 dose series (0,2,6 mos) →	→
Meningococcal	MCV4 (high risk)	MCV4 (booster 5 y later) →	→
Influenza (annual)	Annual Influenza →	→	→
Pnenumococcus[1]	PPV (high risk) →	→	→
Hepatitis A[1]	HepA 2 dose series →	→	→
Hepatitis B[1]	HepA 3 dose series →	→	→
Inactivated Poliovirus[1]	IPV 4 dose series →	→	→
Measles, Mumps, Rubella[1]	MMR 2 dose series →	→	→
Varicella[1]	Varicella 2 dose series →	→	→

[1]If not previously completed

8.2 Infectious Mononucleosis

(see reference [57])

Etiology

Caused by Epstein-Barr virus

Clinical Findings

- Symptoms of fatigue, malaise, fever, sore throat, and generalized lymphadenopathy; usually caused by Epstein-Barr virus (EBV).
- Incubation period: 30-50 days in adolescents; may be shorter in younger children, whose cases are usually clinically silent.
- Splenomegaly may occur rapidly, and may cause left upper quadrant abdominal pain and tenderness.
- Physical findings: generalized lymphadenopathy (90% of cases), splenomegaly (50% of cases), and hepatomegaly (10% of cases).
- Elevated liver enzyme values are frequent.
- Throat: findings resemble streptococcal pharyngitis.
- Skin: possible maculopapular rashes and edema of eyelids.
- Up to 80% of patients have a rash after treatment with ampicillin or amoxicillin.
- May develop Gianotti-Crosti syndrome: Asymmetric rash on cheeks and sometimes on extremities and buttocks with multiple erythematous papules, coalescing into plaques, lasting 15-50 days.

Diagnosis

Presumptive diagnosis may be made from typical clinical symptoms with atypical lymphocytosis on CBC. The diagnosis may be confirmed by serologic testing.

Clinical Status and EBV-specific Antibody

	IgM-VCA	IgG-VCA	EA-D	EA-R	EBNA
Negative reaction	<1:8	<1:10	<1:10	<1:10	<1:2.5
Acute primary infection: Infectious mononucleosis	1:32-1:256	1:160-1:640	1:40-1:160	-	- to 1:2.5
Recent primary infection: infectious mononucleosis	- to 1:32	1:320-1:1,280	1:40-1:160	-	1:5-1:10
Remote infection	-	1:40-1:160	-	- to 1:40	1:10-1:40
Reactivation: Immunosuppressed or immunocompromised	-	1:320-1:1,280	-	1:80-1:320	- to 1:160

EA-D, diffuse staining component of early antigen; EA-R, cytoplasmic-restricted component of early antigen; EBNA, EBV-determined nuclear antigens; EBV, Epstein-Barr virus; Ig, immunoglobulin; VCA, viral capsid antigen; - negative; +, positive.

Treatment

There is no specific treatment for infectious mononucleosis.

Complications

Most serious complication: Subcapsular splenic hemorrhage or splenic rupture, usually during the second week of the disease. Rupture is frequently related to mild trauma and is rarely fatal.

8.3 Epiglottitis vs. Croup

(see reference [58])

Feature	Epiglottitis	Croup
Age (most common)	2-7 yrs	6-36 months
Clinical findings	Fever, drooling, anxious, respiratory distress, tachypnea, stridor, toxic appearing	Fever, stridor, barking cough (seal's bark), rarely toxic appearing
Management	**Unstable**: Intubate STAT **Stable**: Intubation under general anesthesia Reduce agitation until airway secure Begin antibiotics	• Cool mist, hydration, oxygen, antipyretics • Consider racemic epinephrine, dexamethasone • Consider another etiology if not improving

8.4 Diphtheria

(see reference [59])

Definition
Diphtheria: Acute toxic infection typically caused by Corynebacterium diphtheriae. Most infections are in the tonsils and pharynx, followed by the nose and larynx.
Clinical findings
• Clinical findings are influenced by anatomic site of infection, host immune status, and production and systemic spread of toxin. • Mild pharyngeal injection is followed by tonsillar membrane formation, which can extend to nearby areas. • "Bull-neck" appearance: Due to soft-tissue edema and enlarged lymph nodes • Death may occur from airway compromise or toxin-mediated complications. • Cutaneous diphtheria: an indolent, nonprogressive infection with a superficial, ecthymic, nonhealing ulcer with a gray-brown membrane.

Management

- Establish artificial airway and resect pseudomembrane
- Respiratory tract obstruction by pseudomembranes may require bronchoscopy or intubation and mechanical ventilation
- Culture specimens from nose, throat and any other mucocutaneous lesion. The laboratory must be notified to use selective medium.
- Administer diphtheria specific antitoxin (available in the United States only from CDC) on the basis of clinical diagnosis. If suspected diphtheria in United States, contact CDC diphtheria duty officer (770-488-7100 at all times).

8.5 Respiratory Syncytial Virus (RSV)

Clinical findings

- Symptom appear 4-6 days after coming in contact with the virus.
- In infants lower respiratory tract infection is common, such as pneumonia or bronchiolitis, with acute inflammation of the small airway passages entering the lungs, edema, and necrosis of airway epithelium leading to increased mucus production and bronchospasm
- Variable course ranging from transient apnea, breathing may be short, shallow, and rapid and mucus plugging to progressive lower airway disease
- Initial symptoms: Clear rhinorrhea, nasal obstruction, diminished appetite, fever
- Later symptoms: Tachypnea, wheezing, dyspnea, irritability
- Radiographic findings: Hyperinflation, patchy atelectasis

Management[60]

- Supportive care
- Hospitalization based on clinical presentation, with strong consideration for patients <12 weeks, history of prematurity, underlying cardiopulmonary disease, or immunodeficiency
- Oxygen therapy if low oxygen saturation
- A trial of bronchodilators should be continued only if there is documented improved clinical response to trial dose
- Corticosteroids and antibiotics (unless signs of bacterial co-infection) should not be used routinely in bronchiolitis
- Fluid support is often needed due to increased losses from tachypnea, fever, and poor oral intake
- Hold oral feedings in hospitalized tachypneic infants to minimize risk of aspiration.

Immunoprophylaxis with palivizumab for high-risk infants[61]

- Infants and children <2 yrs with chronic lung disease (CLD) who have required medical therapy (oxygen, bronchodilators, diuretics, or corticosteroids) within the 6 months before the RSV season. These children should receive a maximum of five doses. Data are limited, but these patients may also benefit from prophylaxis during a second RSV season
- Infants ≤32 weeks estimated gestational age (EGA) at birth who do not have CLD: May benefit from prophylaxis. These children should receive a maximum of five doses
  - EGA ≤28 weeks: Consider during RSV season until age 12 months
  - EGA 29-32 weeks: Consider if <6 months at the start of RSV season
- Infants 32 to <35 weeks EGA: Palivizumab should be limited to those at greatest risk of hospitalization due to RSV. This includes those infants <3 months at the start of the RSV season or born during the RSV season and who are likely to have increased RSV exposure including at least one risk factor (child care attendance or siblings younger than 5 yrs). These children should receive a maximum of three doses, none being after 3 months of age.
- Infants with congenital abnormalities of the airway or neuromuscular disease born before 35 weeks EGA should be considered for prophylaxis and should receive a maximum of 5 doses during the first year of life
- Infants with hemodynamically significant cyanotic or acyanotic congenital heart disease who are 24 months of age or less should be considered for prophylaxis, including children who:
  - Are receiving medication for congestive heart failure
  - Have moderate to severe pulmonary hypertension
  - Have a cyanotic heart lesion
  - Have undergone surgery where bypass was used (should receive a postoperative dose of palivizumab as soon as clinically stable)
- There are no specific recommendations for severely immunocompromised children, who may benefit from prophylaxis

8.6 Lyme Disease

(see reference [62])

Etiology
It is a zoonosis caused by the transmission of Borrelia burgdorferi to humans through the bite of an infected tick of the Ixodes genus.

Clinical findings

- The initial lesion, at the site of the bite, erythema migrans (EM) can be uniformly erythematous or a target lesion with central clearing. The rash may be itchy or painful, though usually it is asymptomatic.
- Clinical stages:

Lyme disease stage	Timing after tick bite	Usual clinical manifestations
Early localized	3-30 days	EM (single), may have headache, fever, myalgia, arthralgia, fatigue
Early disseminated	3-12 weeks	EM (single or multiple), worse constitutional symptoms, cranial neuritis, meningitis, ocular disease, carditis
Late	>2 months	Arthritis

Diagnosis
ELISA is most common method to detect IgG and IgM antibodies . This test is sensitive but not specific, with false-positive results due to antibodies cross-reacting with other spirochetal or viral infections or autoimmune diseases.

Treatment		
Drug	**Pediatric dosing**	
Amoxicillin	Oral	50 mg/kg/day in 3 divided doses (max 1,500 mg/day)
Doxycycline	Oral	4 mg/kg/day in 2 divided doses (max 200 mg/day) (see text regarding doxycycline use in children)
Cefuroxime axetil	Oral	30 mg/kg/day in 2 divided doses (max 1,000 mg/day)
Ceftriaxone	IV	50-75 mg/kg/day once daily (max 2,000 mg/day)
Recommended Therapy Based on Clinical Manifestation		
Erythema migrans	Oral regimen, 14-21 days	
Meningitis	IV ceftriaxone, 10-28 days	
Cranial nerve palsy	Oral regimen, 14-21 days (see text regarding possible need for lumbar puncture)	
Cardiac disease	Oral regimen or ceftriaxone, 14-21 days (see text for specifics)	
Arthritis	Oral regimen, 28 days	
Late neurologic disease	Ceftriaxone, 14-28 days	

8.7 Tuberculosis

(see reference [63,64])

Clinical Findings

- Latent tuberculosis infection (LTBI): begins after inhaling infected droplets containing Mycobacterium tuberculosis. Diagnosis: reactive tuberculin skin test (TST) with absent clinical and radiographic manifestations.
- Tuberculosis (TB): Reactive TST with signs and symptoms or radiographic changes.
- Untreated infants with LTBI have up to a 40% likelihood of developing TB
- The greatest risk for progression from LTBI to TB is in first 2 yrs after infection.
- Scrofula: TB of the superficial lymph nodes; most common form of extrapulmonary TB in children.
- TB of central nervous system: most serious complication in children; fatal without prompt and appropriate treatment.
- Congenital TB: may be present at birth but more commonly begin by the 2nd or 3rd week of life. Most common signs and symptoms: respiratory distress, fever, poor feeding, lethargy or irritability, failure to thrive, hepatic or splenic enlargement, lymphadenopathy, abdominal distention, ear drainage, and skin lesions.

High-risk groups for TB in low-incidence countries:
• Children exposed to high-risk adults • Foreign-born persons from high-prevalence countries • Homeless persons • Injection drug users • Present and former residents or employees of correctional institutions, homeless shelters, and nursing homes • Health care workers caring for high-risk patients (if inadequate infection control)
Risk factors for progression of LTBI to TB:
• Infants and children ≤4 yrs of age, especially those <2 yrs of age • Adolescents and young adults: - Co-infected with HIV - Skin test conversion in the past 1-2 yrs • Persons who are immunocompromised
Risk factors for drug-resistant TB:
• Personal or contact history of treatment for TB • Contacts of patients with drug-resistant TB • Birth or residence in country with high rate of drug resistance • Poor response to standard therapy • Positive sputum smears (acid-fast bacilli) or culture ≥2 month after initiating appropriate therapy

Diagnosis

- Mantoux TST: intradermal injection of 0.1 mL purified protein derivative (PPD)
- The amount of induration in response to the test should be measured by a trained person 48-72 h after administration. Onset of induration >72 h after placement is also a positive result.
- Immediate hypersensitivity reactions to tuberculin or other constituents of the preparation are short lived (<24 h) and not considered a positive result.
- Tuberculin sensitivity develops 3-13 weeks (usually 4-8 weeks) after inhalation of organisms.
- Host-related factors depressing skin test reaction in TB-infected child: very young age, malnutrition, immunosuppression by disease or drugs, viral infections (measles, mumps, varicella, influenza), vaccination with live-virus vaccines, and overwhelming tuberculosis.
- Corticosteroid therapy: variable decrease TST reaction, but TST done upon initiating corticosteroid therapy is usually reliable.
- Approximately 10% of immunocompetent children with TB (up to 50% with meningitis or disseminated disease) do not initially react to PPD; most react after several months of antituberculosis therapy.
- A common reason for a false-negative TST is poor technique and misreading of the results.
- False-positive reactions to TST can be caused by cross sensitization to antigens of nontuberculous mycobacteria
- Previous vaccination with Bacille Calmette-Guérin (BCG) also can cause a TST reaction. Approximately 50% of infants receiving BCG vaccine never develop a reactive TST, and reactivity usually wanes in 2-3 yrs in those with initially positive skin test results.
- In adults and children with highest risk for infection progression to disease, a reactive area of ≥5 mm is classified as a positive result.
- In other high-risk groups, a reaction of ≥10 mm is considered positive.
- For low-risk persons, especially in communities with low TB prevalence, the cutoff point for a positive reaction is ≥15 mm.
- An increase of induration of ≥10 mm within 2-3 yrs is considered a TST conversion at any age.

TST or interferon-γ release assay (IGRA) recommendations:

- Children who should have immediate TST or IGRA:
- Contacts with confirmed or suspected contagious tuberculosis
- Radiographic or clinical findings suggesting TB
- International adoptees and other immigrants from countries with endemic infection
- Travel to countries with endemic infection with substantial contact with indigenous people
- Children who should have annual TST or IGRA:
- Children infected with HIV
- Incarcerated adolescents
- The most specific confirmation of pulmonary tuberculosis is isolation of M. tuberculosis via sputum collection for culture from adolescents and older children who can expectorate. Sputum induction with a jet nebulizer and chest percussion followed by nasopharyngeal suctioning is effective in children >1 month. Sputum samples should be sent for both culture and smear staining; gastric aspirates are usually cultured.

Treatment

- Ethambutol: See →230
- Isoniazid: See →250
- Pyrazinamide: See →252
- Rifampin: See →252

Four recommended drug regimens for treating TB patients caused by drug-susceptible organism. Each regimen has an **initial phase** of 2 months, followed by several options for **continuation phase** of therapy for 4 or 7 months.

Recommended regimens	Initial phase (2 months)	Continuation phase (4 or 7 months)
Option 1	INH + RIF + PZA + EMB[2] daily x 8 wks	INH + RIF daily or 2 x/wk x 18 wks (DOT) or INH + RPT[1] once/wk x 18 wks
Option 2	INH + RIF + PZA + EMB[2] daily x 2 wks, then 2 x/wk, then 2 x/wk x 6 wks	INH + RIF 2 x/week x 18 wks (DOT) or INH + RPT[1] once/wk x 18 wks
Option 3	INH + RIF + PZA + EMB[2] 3 x/wk x 8 wks	INH + RIF 3x/wk x 18 wks (DOT)
Option 4	INH + RIF + EMB[2] daily x 8 wks or 5 x/wk x 8 wks	INH + RIF daily x 31 weeks or INH + RIF 5 d/wk for 31 wks or INH + RIF 2 x/wk x 31 wks (DOT)

EMB = ethambutol; INH = isoniazid; PZA = pyrazinamide; RIF = rifampin; RPT = rifapentine; DOT = directly observed therapy (for continuation phase when given 2–3 x/week).

[1] Used only for HIV-negative patient with negative sputum smears after 2 months of therapy without cavitation on initial CXR.
[2] If (when) drug susceptibility test results are known and organism is susceptible, discontinue EMB.

Blumberg HM, Burman WJ, Chaisson RE, et al. American Thoracic Society/Centers for Disease Control and Prevention/Infectious Diseases Society of America: treatment of tuberculosis. *Am J Respir Crit Care Med.* 2003;167:603–662.

Doses (1st Line Therapy for Adults)

Drug	Daily	2 x/week (DOT)	3 x/week (DOT)
INH	5 mg/kg (300 mg)	15 mg/kg (900 mg)	15 mg/kg (900 mg)
RIF	10 mg/kg (600 mg)	10 mg/kg (600 mg)	10 mg/kg (600 mg)
PZA	18–26 mg/kg (1–2 g)	36–53 mg/kg (2–4 g)	27–40 mg/kg (1.5–3 g)
EMB	14–21 mg/kg (0.8–1.6 g)	36–53 mg/kg (2–4 g)	22–36 mg/kg (1.2–2.4 g)
RPT	10 mg/kg (600 mg) once/week for continuation phase		

Blumberg HM, Burman WJ, Chaisson RE, et al. American Thoracic Society/Centers for Disease Control and Prevention/Infectious Diseases Society of America: Treatment of Tuberculosis. *Am J Respir Crit Care Med.* 2003;167:603–662.

8.8 Pertussis

(see reference [65])

Clinical findings	
Pertussis is classically divided into 3 stages.	
Catarrhal stage (1-2 weeks)	• Begins after 3-12 day incubation period with congestion & rhinorrhea; can have low-grade fever, sneezing, lacrimation, conjunctival suffusion. • Leukocytosis (15,000-100,000 cells/mm^3) with absolute lymphocytosis.
Paroxysmal stage (2-6 weeks)	• After initial symptoms wane, a dry, intermittent, irritating hacking cough evolves into paroxysms. • After coughing ceases a loud whoop follows (from inspired air traversing partially closed airway). • Exhaustion & frequent posttussive emesis • Frequency & severity of paroxysms escalate up to 7 days & stay at that level for days to weeks.
Convalescent state (≥2 weeks)	Diminishing number, severity, & duration of episodes.
• Infants <3 months of age do not show classic stages. The catarrhal phase can be unobserved or lasts only a few days. Then, after an insignificant startle, a previously well-appearing infant begins to choke, gasp, gag, and flail extremities, with face reddened. Cough may not be significant, especially in the early phase, and whooping is uncommon. Apnea and cyanosis can follow a coughing paroxysm, but apnea can occur without a cough and may be the only symptom. • Adolescents and previously immunized children have briefer stages. Adults have no distinct stages. Adolescents and adults typically describe a sudden feeling of strangulation or suffocation with uninterrupted coughs, bursting headache, diminished awareness, and then a gasping breath, usually without a whoop. Posttussive emesis and intermittent paroxysms may be separated by hours of well-being. At least 30% of older individuals with pertussis have nonspecific cough lasting >21 days.	

Diagnosis

- All current methods for confirmation of infection due to B. pertussis have limitations in sensitivity, specificity, or practicality.
- Isolation of B. pertussis in culture is the gold standard for diagnosis. The specimen is obtained with deep nasopharyngeal aspiration or by using a flexible swab, preferably a Dacron or calcium alginate-tipped swab, held in the posterior nasopharynx for 15-30 sec (or until cough occurs).
- Direct fluorescent antibody (DFA) testing (reliable only in laboratories with continuous experience)using specific antibody for B. pertussis and B. parapertussis maximizes recovery rates.
- Polymerase chain reaction (PCR) analysis to test nasopharyngeal wash specimens has a sensitivity similar culture and avoids difficulties of isolation, but a standardized validated test is not universally available.
- Results of DFA, culture, and PCR are all expected to be positive in unimmunized, untreated children during the catarrhal and early paroxysmal stages of disease.

Treatment

- Erythromycin: →249 , recommended agent <1 month
- Azithromycin →246
- Clarithromycin →249
- TMP-SMZ: →253 , CI in infants <2 months due to kernicterus risk

(See Drug chapter for specific dosing)

8.9 HIV and AIDS

(see reference [66,67])

Since the implementation of recommendations for universal prenatal HIV counseling and testing, antiretroviral prophylaxis, scheduled cesarean delivery, and avoiding breastfeeding, perinatal HIV transmission has decreased to less than 2% in the United States and Europe.

Counseling and Testing

The US Centers for Disease Control (CDC) recommends that HIV screening be universally included in the routine prenatal panel with an opt-out consent provision. Repeat HIV antibody testing should be done in the third trimester, preferably < 36 weeks' gestation for the following high-risk women:

- Living in states with high HIV prevalence
- In hospitals with prenatal HIV prevalence ≥1:1,000
- Women with increased risk of acquiring HIV:
  - Current signs/symptoms of acute HIV infection
  - IV drug user (self or sex partner)
  - Exchanges sex or money for drugs
  - Had another STI diagnosed during pregnancy
  - Sex partner is HIV infected
  - New or > one sex partner during pregnancy

Perinatal and newborn testing

Women with undocumented HIV-infection status during the pregnancy should have maternal testing done at delivery with opt-out consent, using a rapid HIV antibody test. If the mother refuses the test, the newborn should have rapid HIV antibody testing.

Adolescent testing

Universal HIV-1 screening should be part of routine care for patients beginning at age 13 yrs with opt-out consent. Repeat HIV-1 antibody testing should be performed on a regular basis for adolescents who remain at risk.

Management

Management of Perinatal HIV Exposure and Prevention of Mother to Child Transmission

- Combination of antepartum, intrapartum, and infant anti-retroviral (ARV) prophylaxis is recommended to prevent perinatal transmission of HIV. Combination antenatal ARV prophylaxis taken over a longer duration is more effective than a short-course single-drug regimen in reducing perinatal transmission. ARV drugs are highly effective in preventing transmission, even in HIV-infected women with advanced disease, so all HIV-infected pregnant women should be counseled about and administered ARV drugs during pregnancy for prevention of perinatal transmission, regardless of their HIV RNA levels. When mothers have not received antenatal ARV drugs, combination infant ARV prophylaxis is recommended in the United States
- Scheduled cesarean delivery is recommended for HIV-infected pregnant women who have HIV RNA levels >1,000/mL near the time of delivery.
- Breastfeeding by HIV-infected women is not recommended in the United States
- When mothers have unknown HIV status, rapid HIV antibody testing of mothers and/or infants should be done as soon as possible after birth, with immediate initiation of infant ARV prophylaxis if the rapid test is positive.
  - When the rapid test is positive, standard antibody confirmatory testing such as a Western blot also should be performed on mothers (or their infants) as soon as possible. Confirmatory test results should not delay initiation of postnatal prophylaxis. If the confirmatory test is negative, ARV prophylaxis can be discontinued.
  - If the HIV antibody confirmatory test is positive, a newborn HIV DNA polymerase chain reaction (PCR) assay should be performed.
  - If the newborn HIV DNA PCR is positive, ARV prophylaxis should be discontinued and the infant promptly referred to a pediatric HIV specialist to confirm the diagnosis and treatment of HIV infection with standard combination ARV therapy.
- A 6-week course of zidovudine chemoprophylaxis (see Drug chapter for dosing), starting within 6-12 h of delivery, is recommended for HIV-exposed newborns to reduce perinatal HIV transmission.
- Infants of HIV-infected women who have not received antepartum ARV drugs should receive prophylaxis with zidovudine for 6 weeks combined with 3 doses of nevirapine in the first week of life (at birth, 48 h later, and 96 h after the second dose), begun as soon after birth as possible.
- The National Perinatal HIV Hotline (1-888-448-8765) is available for free clinical consultation.

Monitoring HIV-exposed newborns

- CBC and differential should be performed as a baseline evaluation.
- Decisions about subsequent hematologic monitoring of hematologic parameters depend on baseline values, gestational age at birth, clinical condition of the infants, the zidovudine dose being administered, receipt of other ARV drugs and concomitant medications, and maternal antepartum ARV therapy.
- If hematologic abnormalities are identified in infants receiving prophylaxis, decisions on whether to continue infant ARV prophylaxis need to be individualized in consultation with a pediatric HIV expert.
- Virologic tests are required to diagnose HIV infection in infants <18 months of age and should be performed within the first 14-21 days of life, at 1-2 months, and at 4-6 months of age.
- To prevent Pneumocystis jirovecii pneumonia (PCP), all infants born to HIV infected women should begin PCP prophylaxis at ages 4-6 weeks, after completing their ARV prophylaxis regimen, unless HIV infection is presumptively excluded by adequate test information.
- Health care providers should routinely instruct HIV-infected caregivers to avoid premastication of foods fed to infants, and advise on safer feeding options.

List of References

55 Casasanta KS. Immunoprophylaxis. In Tschudy MM, Arcara KM, eds, The Harriet Lane Handbook, 19th edition, Philadelphia, Mosby, 2012, p 401-436.

56 Centers for Disease Control and Prevention. Recommended immunization schedules for persons aged 0-18 yrs-United States, 2011. MMWR 2011;60

57 Jenson HB. Epstein-Barr virus. In Kliegman RM et al, eds. Nelson Textbook of Pediatrics, 19th edition, Philadelphia, Elsevier, 2011, p 1110-1115.

58 Valenti C. Emergency management. In Tschudy MM, Arcara KM, eds, The Harriet Lane Handbook, 19th edition, Philadelphia, Mosby, 2012, p 3-18.

59 Buescher S. Diphtheria. In Kliegman RM et al, eds. Nelson Textbook of Pediatrics, 19th edition, Philadelphia, Elsevier, 2011, p 929.

60 AAP Subcommittee on Diagnosis and Management of Bronchiolitis. Diagnosis and Management of Bronchiolitis. Pediatrics 2006 118: 1774-1793.

61 AAP Committee on Infectious Diseases. Modified Recommendations for Use of Palivizumab for Prevention of Respiratory Syncytial Virus Infections. Pediatrics 2009 124: 1694-1701

62 Wormser GP, Dattwyler RJ, Shapiro ED, et al: The clinical assessment, treatment, and prevention of Lyme disease, human granulocytic anaplasmosis, and babesiosis: clinical practice guidelines by the Infectious Diseases Society of America. Clin Infect Dis 43:1089-1134, 2006

63 American Academy of Pediatrics. Tuberculosis. In: Pickering LK, Baker CJ, Kimberlin DW, Long SS, eds. Red Book: 2009 Report of the Committee on Infectious Diseases. 28th ed. Elk Grove Village, IL: American Academy of Pediatrics; 2009: 680-701.

64 Starke JR. Tuberculosis. In Kliegman RM et al, eds. Nelson Textbook of Pediatrics, 19th edition, Philadelphia, Elsevier, 2011, p 996-1011.

65 Long SS. Pertussis. In Kliegman RM et al, eds. Nelson Textbook of Pediatrics, 19th edition, Philadelphia, Elsevier, 2011

66 Branson BM, Handsfield HH, Lampe MA et al. Revised Recommendations for HIV Testing of Adults, Adolescents, and Pregnant Women in Health-Care Settings. MMWR 2006 (Sept 22); 55 (RR14): 1-17.

67 Panel on Treatment of HIV-Infected Pregnant Women and Prevention of Perinatal Transmission. Recommendations for Use of Antiretroviral Drugs in Pregnant HIV-1-Infected Women for Maternal Health and Interventions to Reduce Perinatal HIV Transmission in the United States. Available at http://aidsinfo.nih.gov/contentfiles/lvguidelines/PerinatalGL.pdf. Accessed 12/1/2012.

150 9 Respiratory Disorders and SIDS

9 Respiratory Disorders and SIDS

9.1 Pulmonary Function Test (PFT)

(see reference [68])

9.1.1 Peak expiratory flow rate (PEFR)

- During forced expiration, maximal flow rate generated
- Useful to follow course of asthma and response to therapy
- "Personal best" determined when asymptomatic may be more accurate standard than normal predicted value
- Measurement is effort dependent
- Normal predicted PEFR
  - Highest flow rate during forced expiration
  - Trace course of asthma and therapy response
- Highest asymptomatic PEFR may be more accurate standard than normal predicted PEFR
  - PEFR depends on patient's effort
  - Predicted PEFR

Formula for calculating PEFR in Children	[(Height in cm - 100)× 5] + 100

Predicted PEFR		Home Asthma Management Plans		
Height in Inches	**Predicted PEFR Boys and Girls**	**Red Zone <50% Predicted PEFR**	**Yellow Zone 50-80% Predicted PEFR**	**Yellow Zone 50-80%**
72	540	<270	270-430	>430
71	525	<265	265-420	>420
70	510	<255	255-410	>410
69	500	<250	250-400	>400
68	485	<245	245-390	>390
67	470	<235	235-375	>375
66	455	<230	230-365	>365
65	440	<220	220-350	>350
64	430	<215	215-345	>345
63	415	<210	210-330	>330
62	40	<200	200-320	>320
61	390	<195	195-310	>310
60	375	<190	190-300	>300

Predicted PEFR (cont.)		Home Asthma Management Plans		
Height in Inches	Predicted PEFR Boys and Girls	Red Zone <50% Predicted PEFR	Yellow Zone 50-80% Predicted PEFR	Yellow Zone 50-80%
59	360	<180	180-290	>290
58	350	<175	175-280	>280
57	335	<170	170-270	>270
56	320	<160	160-260	>260
55	310	<155	155-250	>250
54	295	<150	150-235	>235
53	280	<140	140-225	>225
52	265	<130	130-210	>210
51	255	<130	130-205	>205
50	245	<125	125-195	>195
49	230	<115	115-185	>185
48	215	<110	110-170	>170
47	200	<100	100-160	>160
46	185	<95	95-150	>150
45	175	<90	90-140	>140
44	160	<80	80-130	>130
43	150	<75	75-120	>120
42	140	<70	70-110	>110
41	130	<65	65-105	>105

9.1.2 Spirometry

Terminology

- Forced vital capacity (FVC): Maximum air volume exhaled after maximum inspiration
- Forced expiratory volume in 1 second (FEV1): Volume exhaled during first second of FVC
- Forced expiratory flow (FEF25-75): Mean airflow rate over middle half of FVC

Interpretation of spirometry		
Spirometry measure	Restrictive (interstitial fibrosis, scoliosis, neuromuscular disorder)	Obstructive (asthma, CF)
FVC	↓	Normal or ↓
FEV1	Normal or ↓	↓
FEV_1/FVC ratio	Normal or ↑	↓
FEF25-75%	Normal or ↓	↓
PEFR	Normal or ↓	Normal or ↓

9.2 Asthma

9.2.1 Definition

Chronic, inflammatory airway disorder with recurrent wheezing, dyspnea, chest tightness, and cough, especially at night and in early morning.

9.2.2 Clinical findings

- Cough, tachypnea, retractions, accessory muscle use, wheezing, hypoxia, and hypoventilation
- Lack of audible wheezing may be due to poor air movement and severe bronchospasm
- Chest x-ray often shows peribronchial thickening, hyperinflation, and/or atelectasis

9.2.3 Classification of severity[69]

Age 0-4 yrs	Intermittent	Mild persistent	Moderate persistent	Severe persistent
Symptoms	≤2 days/wk	>2 days/wk, not daily	Daily	Throughout day
Wake at night	0	1-2x/mo	3-4x/mo	>1x/wk
Rescue medication use	≤2 days/wk	>2 days/wk, not daily	Daily	Several times each day
Interrupt normal activity	None	Minor limitation	Some limitation	Extremely limited
Step below to start treatment	Step 1	Step 2	Step 3	Step 3

Age 5-11 yrs	Intermittent	Mild persistent	Moderate persistent	Severe persistent
Symptoms	≤2 days/wk	>2 days/wk, not daily	Daily	Throughout day
Wake at night	≤2x/mo	3-4x/mo	>1x/wk, not nightly	Often daily
Rescue medication use	≤2 days/wk	>2 days/wk, not daily	Daily	Several times each day
Interrupt normal activity	None	Minor limitation	Some limitation	Extremely limited
Lung function	Normal FEV1 between exacerbations FEV1 >80% predicted FEV1/FVC >85%	FEV1 >80% predicted FEV1/FVC >80%	FEV1= 60-80% predicted FEV1/FVC = 75-80%	FEV1 <60% predicted FEV1/FVC <75%
Step below to start treatment	Step 1	Step 2	Step 3	Step 3 or 4

Age >11 yrs	Intermittent	Mild persistent	Moderate persistent	Severe persistent
Symptoms	≤2 days/wk	>2 days/wk, not daily	Daily	Throughout day
Wake at night	≤2x/mo	3-4x/mo	>1x/wk, not nightly	Often daily
Rescue medication use	≤2 days/wk	>2 days/wk, not daily	Daily	Several times each day
Interrupt normal activity	None	Minor limitation	Some limitation	Extremely limited
Lung function	Normal FEV1 between exacerbations; FEV1 >80% predicted FEV1/FVC normal	FEV1 >80% predicted; FEV1/FVC normal	FEV1 = 60-80% predicted; FEV1/FVC reduced 5%	FEV1 <60% predicted; FEV1/FVC reduced >5%
Step below to start treatment	Step 1	Step 2	Step 3	Step 4 or 5

9.2.4 Management[70]

Age & treatment type	Step 1	Step 2	Step 3 Consult specialist	Step 4 Consult specialist	Step 5 Consult specialist	Step 6 Consult specialist
0–4 yrs, preferred	SABA	Low-dose ICS	Medium-dose ICS	Medium-dose ICS + LABA or montelukast	High-dose ICS + LABA or montelukast	High-dose ICS + oral CS + LABA or montelukast
0–4 yrs, alternative	-	Cromolyn or montelukast	-	-	-	-
5–11 yrs, preferred	SABA	Low-dose ICS	Low-dose ICS + LABA, LTRA or theophylline, OR Medium-dose ICS	Medium-dose ICS + LABA	High-dose ICS + LABA	High-dose ICS + oral CS + LABA
5–11 yrs, alternative	–	Cromolyn, LTRA, nedocromil, or theophylline	–	Medium-dose ICS + LTRA or theophylline	High-dose ICS + LTRA or theophylline	High-dose ICS + oral CS + LTRA or theophylline
>12 yrs, preferred	SABA	Low-dose ICS	Low-dose ICS + LABA OR Medium-dose ICS	Medium-dose ICS + LABA	High-dose ICS + LABA	High-dose ICS + oral CS + LABA
>12 yrs, alternative	-	Cromolyn, LTRA, nedocromil, or theophylline	Low-dose ICS + LTRA, theophylline OR zileuton	Medium-dose ICS + LTRA, theophylline or zileuton	Consider omalizumab with allergic asthma	Consider omalizumab with allergic asthma

9.3 Sudden Infant Death Syndrome (SIDS)

Definition

Sudden unexpected death of an infant younger than 1 yr, which is unexplained after a thorough case investigation, including complete autopsy, examination of death scene, and review of clinical history.

Risk factors

- Prematurity
- Pre- and postnatal tobacco exposure
- Side and prone sleeping
- Sleeping on soft bedding
- Overbundling
- Co-sleeping on same bed with caregiver
- Recent infection
- Siblings with SIDS
- Low socioeconomic status

Protective factors

- Sleeping in prone position
- Sleeping on firm mattress
- Pacifier use during sleep
- Sleeping in same room as caregiver
- Tobacco smoke-free environment

List of References

68 Kirk A. Pulmonology. In Tschudy MM, Arcara KM, eds, The Harriet Lane Handbook, 19th edition, Philadelphia, Mosby, 2012, p 623-638.

69 National Asthma Education and Prevention Program. Expert Panel Report 3: Guidelines for the Diagnosis and Management of Asthma. National Heart, Lung, and Blood Institute, 2007, p 29

70 Wood PR, Hill VL. Practical management of asthma. Pediatrics in Review 2009; 30:375-385.

10 Renal Disorders

(see reference [71])

10.1 Renal Tubular Disorders

10.1.1 Renal tubular acidosis [72,73]

	Type 1	Type 2	Type 4
Etiology	• Hereditary • Toxins/drugs • Sickle cell • Obstructive uropathy • Connective tissue disorder • Cirrhosis	• Hereditary • Prematurity • Fanconi Syndrome • Metabolic disease • Toxins/Heavy Metals • Amyloidosis • PNH	• Adrenal failure • CAH • Absolute mineralocorticoid deficiency • DM • Pseudohypoaldosteronism • Interstitial nephritis
Minimal urine pH	>5.5	<5.5	<5.5
Urinary citrate excretion	↓	↑	?
Plasma K^+ concentration	Normal or ↓	Usually ↓	↑
Urine anion gap	+	+ or -	+
Nephrocalcinosis/ Nephrolithiasis	Common	Rare	Rare
Treatment	HCO_3 1-3 mEq/kg/day (5-10 mEq/kg/day if bicarb wasting)	HCO_3 5-20 mEq/kg/day	HCO_3 1-5 mEq/kg/day May add fludrocortisone & potassium binders

10.1.2 Fanconi syndrome

Clinical manifestations
• A generalized dysfunction of proximal tubule • Bicarbonate loss • Variable wasting of phosphate, glucose, and amino acids • May be hereditary, as in cystinosis and galactosemia, or • Acquired from toxin injury and other immunologic factors • Characterized by rickets and impaired growth

10.2 Glomerular Disorders

Nephrotic syndrome[74]	
Clinical characteristics	• Initially facial and pretibial edema • Abdominal pain from decreased oncotic pressure and reduced splanchnic flow • Proteinuria (<40 mg/m^2/h), hypercholesterolemia (>200 mg/dL), and hypoproteinemia (<2 g/dL)
Etiology	**Primary (90%):** Idiopathic (most common): • MCNS (most common) • FSGS • Membranous nephropathy **Secondary**: Infections, SLE, DM, IgA nephropathy, drugs, malignancy
MCNS suggested by age 1-11, no family history, no extrarenal or chronic disease, normal BP, no casts or renal failure.	

Nephrotic syndrome (cont.)	
Management of MCNS	• Aim: Restore intravascular volume, encourage diuresis, avoid fluid overload • If no atypical features, try course of steroid without renal biopsy • Hospitalize if overwhelming edema or infection • Steroid-responsive: – Remission after 8 weeks course of prednisone – 95% of MCNS and 20% of FSGS patients – Response is best prognostic factor • Frequently relapsing: ≥2 relapses within 6 months of initial response, or ≥4 relapses in any 12 months • Steroid-dependent – ≥2 relapses during tapering or within 14 days of steroid cessation. • Some may be managed with alternate day low-dose steroids • 2nd line treatment for frequently relapsing and steroid-dependent NS: Cyclophosphamide, chlorambucil, cyclosporine, levamisole • Steroid-resistant: – Often requires continued high-dose steroid >8 weeks – 2nd line agents: Calcineurin inhibitors, high-dose pulse methylprednisolone, mainly combined with alkylating agent • Renal biopsy for macroscopic hematuria, severe high blood pressure, persistent renal insufficiency, low complement levels, and persistent proteinuria after 4 weeks of adequate steroids
Complications	Acute kidney injury, thromboembolic disease, infections, steroid adverse effects

Post-streptococcal glomerulonephritis					
Clinical characteristics	Edema, hematuria, proteinuria and hypertension of sudden onset after skin or throat infection due to nephritogenic strain of group A β-hemolytic streptococci				
Laboratory investigation	• CBC • Complement profile • Streptococcal antibodies • Comprehensive metabolic panel • Complete urinalysis • Imaging and renal biopsy not generally indicated				
Long-term follow-up and prognosis	**0–6 wks**	**8–10 wks**	**3, 6, 9 months**	**12 months**	**2, 5, 10 yrs**
	• BP control • Resolving edema • Resolving hematuria & azotemia	Resolving azotemia, ↑ BP, anemia, C3 & C4	• Resolving hematuria & proteinuria • Normal BP	Resolving proteinuria & hematuria	Check urine, BP, serum creatinine
Indications for consulting pediatric nephrologist	• Severe hypertension, oliguria, proteinuria, or edema • Moderate to marked azotemia • Recurrent gross hematuria • ≥8 weeks of depressed C3				

10.3 Acute Kidney Injury

Acute Kidney Injury (Acute Renal Failure)[75,76]	
Definition	Sudden decrease in renal function with increasing BUN/Cr
Etiology	• Prerenal: Most common type in children, usually due to dehydration • Renal: From parenchymal disease: Arterial or glomerular lesions • Postrenal: Due to obstruction of urinary tract; especially in neonates with anatomic anomalies
Clinical features	• Oliguria, pallor, decreased urinary output, edema, hypertension, vomiting, lethargy • ATN: Diagnosis of exclusion – Oliguric phase: severe oliguria lasting ~ 10 days – Diuretic phase: begins with ↑ urine output, with urine sodium 80-150 mEq/L – Recovery phase: Usually resolves rapidly, polyuria may persist for weeks
Treatment concerns	• Place indwelling catheter to monitor urine output • Exclude prerenal and postrenal factors • Maintain intravascular volume • Consult pediatric nephrologist • Complications include: – Fluid overload, with hypertension, CHF, pulmonary edema – Electrolyte disturbances, with hyperkalemia, metabolic acidosis, hyperphosphatemia, and uremia

Management

Acute Kidney Injury
Prerenal
Renal
Postrenal
Most common type in children
• Burns
• Blood loss
• Diarrhea, vomiting
• Shock
• Drugs
• Cardiac diseases with low cardiac output
From parenchymal disease: Arterial or glomerular lesion
From obstruction of urinary tract; specially in neonates with anatomic anomalies
• Vascular
• Vasculitis
• HTN
• Kawasaki disease
• Scleroderma
Acute glomerulonephritis
Acute interstitial nephritis
Acute tubular necrosis

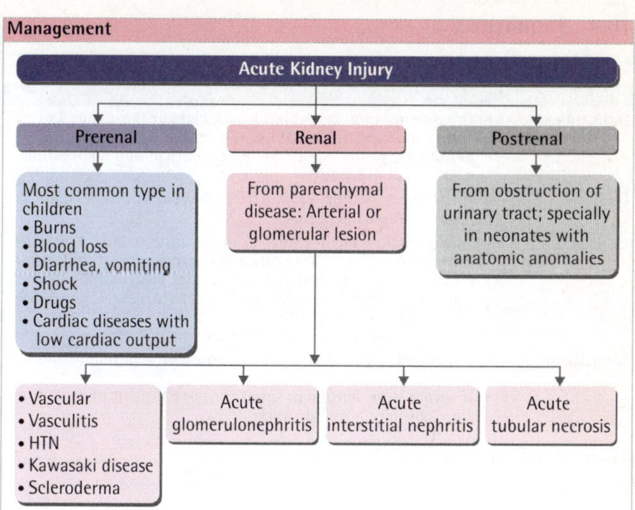

10.4 Hematuria

(see reference [77])

Brief discussion	
Definitions	• Gross hematuria: Bright red blood, clots or tea-colored urine • Microscopic: >5 RBCs/hpf on >2 occasions • Significant or persistent: 3+ urine dipsticks and microscopic exams over 2-3 weeks
Etiology	Kidney stones, trauma, AVM, ATN, renal vein thrombosis, IgA nephropathy, Alport nephritis
Evaluation	• Family history, medications, examine urine sediment, dipstick for protein, urine culture, sickle cell screen, urine Ca/Cr, serum electrolytes, BUN, serum Cr, serum total protein and albumin, CBC with smear, immunoglobulins, hepatitis serologies, ASO, C3, C4, ANA, consider HIV • Renal ultrasonography, consider audiology screen
Management	• Depending on evaluation above, consider nephrology and/or urology referral • If severe hypertension or significant impairment of renal function, consider hospitalization

10.5 Proteinuria

(see reference [78])

Brief discussion	
Diagnosis	• Normal upper limit 150 mg/24 h (4 mg/m^2/h) • Urine dip: – 1+ ~ 30 mg/dL – 2+ ~ 100 mg/dL – 3+ ~ 300 mg/dL – 4+ ~ >2000 mg/dL • Quantify persistent proteinuria with 24 h urine collection
Etiology, non-nephrotic (rarely associated with edema)	• Transient proteinuria (exercise, stress, fever, seizures, drugs), orthostatic proteinuria, glomerulopathies, overload proteinuria, tubular disorders, acute inflammation of urinary tract, uroepithelial tumors
Evaluation	• Check if present in supine and standing positions; if not in supine, patient has benign orthostatic proteinuria

Evaluation (cont)	• If present both supine and standing and non-nephrotic: – CMP, C3, C4, ANA – Hepatitis B and C – Renal sonogram, 24 h urine protein and creatinine – Renal biopsy if protein persistently >4 $mg/m^2/h$ or worsening proteinuria

Management

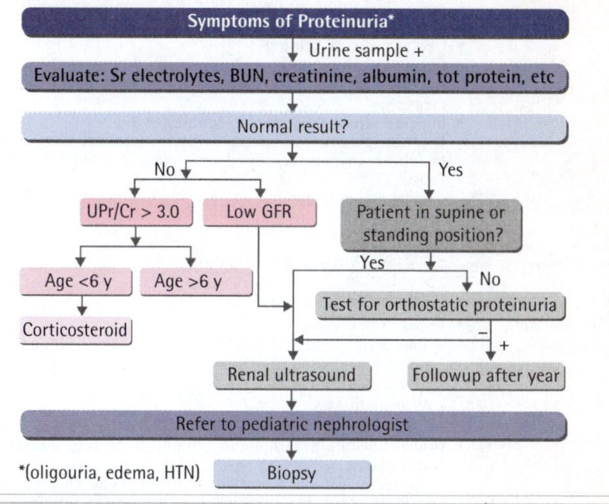

List of References

71 Cooper S. Nephrology. In Tschudy MM, Arcara KM, eds, The Harriet Lane Handbook, 19th edition, Philadelphia, Mosby, 201, p 507-536.

72 Holliday MA et al. Pediatric Nephrology. Baltimore: Williams & Wilkins, 1994, p 650

73 Soriano JR. Renal tubular acidosis: the clinical entity. J Am Soc Nephrol. 2002;13:2160-2170

74 Gordillo R, Spitzer A. The nephrotic syndrome. Pediatr Rev. 2009;30(3): 94-104

75 Whyte DA, Fine RN. Acute renal failure in children. Pediatr Rev. 2008;29(9): 299-306.

76 14. Andreoli SP. Acute kidney injury in children. Pediatr Nephrol. 2009;24(2): 253-263.

77 Massengill SF. Hematuria. Pediatr Rev. 2008;29(10):342-348

78 Cruz C, Spitzer A. When you find protein or blood in urine. Contemp Pediatr. 1998;15(9):89.

11 Allergic & Rheumatic Disorders

11.1 Allergic Rhinitis

Clinical findings	• Nasal congestion • Rhinorrhea (watery discharge), pruritus (itchy nose), red eyes • Blocked nose and sneezing • Family history of pruritus • Postnasal drip, sore throat, cough • Ocular pruritus, tearing • Coexisting atopic diseases • Allergic facies: Shiners, mouth breathing, transverse nasal crease • Injected sclera, conjunctival cobblestoning • There are two types of allergic rhinitis: seasonal allergic rhinitis (also known as hay fever) and perennial allergic rhinitis • Labs: – Peripheral eosinophilia – Nasal smear for eosinophils – Total IgE: Nonspecific – Radioallergosorbent testing (RAST) – Skin testing • May consider PFTs and sleep study
Treatment	• Avoid of allergens – There are two types of allergic rhinitis: seasonal allergic rhinitis (also known as hay fever) and perennial allergic rhinitis – Do not mow the grass – Wear sunglasses – Keep windows closed both at home and in the car • Oral antihistamines: Diphenhydramine, cetirizine, loratadine, fexofenadine • Nasal spray/intranasal corticosteroids (in children over age 6 yrs): Fluticasone, mometasone, budesonide, flunisolide, triamcinolone • LTRI: Montelukast • Mast cell stabilizers: Cromolyn • Intranasal antihistamines: Azelastine, olopatadine • Anticholinergics: Ipratropium • Immunotherapy • Nasal rinsing with hypertonic saline

11.2 Food Allergies

Clinical findings	• Anaphylaxis or other systemic allergic reaction • Skin symptoms: – Pruritus – Erythema • Respiratory syndromes: – Rhinitis, nasal itching, sneezing, nasal congestion – Asthma – Heiner syndrome: Pulmonary infiltrates, hemosiderosis, anemia, recurrent pneumonia, and FTT from cow milk IgG precipitates • GI syndromes: – Angioedema of the lips, tongue, & palate – Nausea – Vomiting – Diarrhoea – Colicky pain
Diagnosis	• History: – Timing and type of reaction – Fresh vs. cooked food – Food diary helpful • RAST • Skin testing • Food challenges • Trial elimination diet
Treatment	• Learn to read product labels • Allergen avoidance • Treat angioedema and urticaria with antihistamines, corticosteroids • Treat atopic dermatitis with symptomatic control, topical corticosteroids (hydrocortisone, triamcinolone, mometasone)

11.3 Juvenile Idiopathic Arthritis

→JIA, formerly JRA, (see reference[79,80])

Classification	• Oligoarticular • Polyarticular • Systemic
Clinical findings	• Minimum duration 6 weeks • Age of onset <6 yrs • Oligoarticular JIA: – <4 joints in 1st 6 months after presentation – Persistent <4 joints for course of disease – Extended >4 joints after 6 months • Polyarticular JIA – >5 joints in 1st 5 months after presentation – It is divided in to two groups: Rheumatoid factor (RF) negative & RF positive • Systemic JIA – Fever, rash, arthritis • Psoriatic JIA • Enthesitis related • Undifferentiated arthritis
Investigations	• ESR, CRP, FBE • Synovial fluid culture if septic arthritis is considered
Treatment	• Pharmacologic – Short-term analgesics – NSAIDS – Disease-modifying antirheumatic drugs (DMARDs) – Biologic agents – Steroids: Intra-articular and oral • Psychological/educational • Nutrition, re. anemia and osteoporosis • Physical and occupational therapy

List of References

79 Callender MA. Rheumatology. In Tschudy MM, Arcara KM, eds, The Harriet Lane Handbook, 19th edition, Philadelphia, Mosby, 2012, p 653-676.

80 Sherry DD. Juvenile idiopathic arthritis. In Tschudy MM, Arcara KM, eds, The Harriet Lane Handbook, 19th edition, Philadelphia, Mosby, 2012, p 658-662.

12 Blood and Neoplastic Disorders

(see reference [81])

12.1 Anemia

(see reference [82])

12.1.1 Evaluation of anemia

Brief discussion	
History	Fatigue, slow growth/development, diet (low iron, high milk), blood loss, ethnicity, medications, family history
Physical examination	Vital signs, pallor, jaundice, murmur, hepatosplenomegaly, signs of systemic illness
Laboratory	CBC, reticulocyte count, peripheral smear, stool for occult blood, serum bilirubin, iron studies, hemoglobin electrophoresis

12.1.2 Classification of anemia

Reticulocyte count	Low	Normal	High
Normocytic anemia	• Transient erythroblastopenia • Chronic disease • Aplastic anemia • Leukemia • Endocrinopathies • Juvenile idiopathic arthritis • Renal failure	• Hypersplenism • Acute hemorrhage • Dyserythropoietic anemia II	• Hypersplenism • Hemoglobinopathies • Acute blood loss • Microangiopathy • Membranopathies • Enzyme disorders • Antibody-mediated hemolysis • G6PD deficiency
Microcytic anemia	• Iron deficiency • Copper deficiency • Protein malnutrition • Lead poisoning • Aluminum toxicity • Chronic disease	• Thalassemia trait • Sideroblastic anemia	• Iron deficiency • Thalassemia syndromes • Hemoglobin C disorders

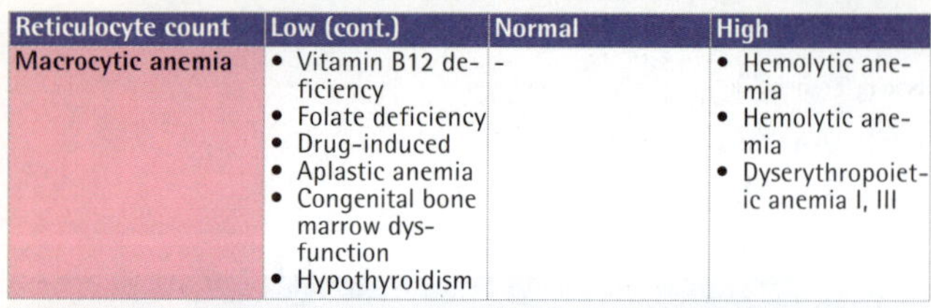

Reticulocyte count	Low (cont.)	Normal	High
Macrocytic anemia	• Vitamin B12 deficiency • Folate deficiency • Drug-induced • Aplastic anemia • Congenital bone marrow dysfunction • Hypothyroidism	-	• Hemolytic anemia • Hemolytic anemia • Dyserythropoietic anemia I, III

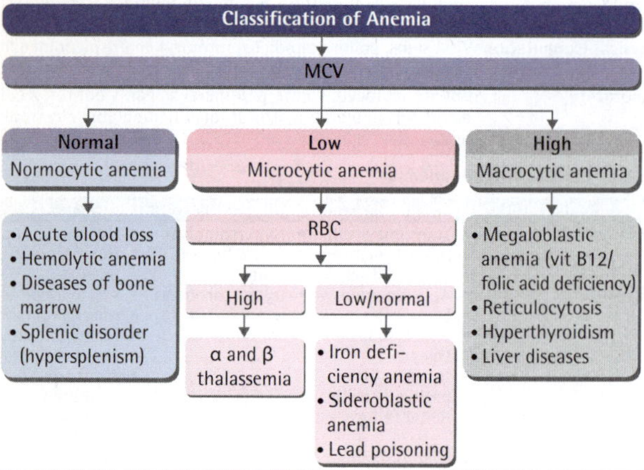

Classification of Anemia

- **MCV**
  - **Normal** – Normocytic anemia
    - Acute blood loss
    - Hemolytic anemia
    - Diseases of bone marrow
    - Splenic disorder (hypersplenism)
  - **Low** – Microcytic anemia
    - RBC
      - High
        - α and β thalassemia
      - Low/normal
        - Iron deficiency anemia
        - Sideroblastic anemia
        - Lead poisoning
  - **High** – Macrocytic anemia
    - Megaloblastic anemia (vit B12/folic acid deficiency)
    - Reticulocytosis
    - Hyperthyroidism
    - Liver diseases

12.1.3 Iron deficiency

Brief discussion	
Clinical features	• Hypochromic, microcytic anemia • Elevated red cell distribution width (RDW) • Low reticulocyte count • Serum ferritin low – 1st value to fall in iron deficiency – False elevation with inflammation/infection • Other labs: Low MCHC, low serum iron, elevated total iron-binding capacity (TIBC), low reticulocyte Hb • Mentzer index = MCV/RBC; – >13.5 suggests iron deficiency <11.5 suggests of thalassemia trait, especially if RDW normal
Treatment effects	• After adequate iron therapy (4-6 mg/Kg/day elemental iron): – Increased reticulocyte count in 2-3 days – Increased HCT in 1-4 weeks – Iron stores restored in 3 months

12.1.4 Sickle cell disease

Brief discussion	
Etiology	Genetic defect in β-globin
Diagnosis	• May be made on newborn screen with Hb electrophoresis • Rapid tests, eg, sickleprep or Sickledex, are positive with all sickle hemoglobinopathies & trait. False-negative results may occur with high fetal Hb concentrations.

Complications	Clinical presentation	Evaluation	Treatment
Fever	High temperature (fever) of 38°C (100.4°F) or above	• History, and Physical examination • CBC, differential reticulocyte count • Blood cultures • Chest x-ray	• IV antibiotics • Admit if <3, ill appearing, complications, concerning labs

Complications (cont.)	Clinical presentation	Evaluation	Treatment
Splenic sequestration	• Sudden weakness • Fast breathing • Splenomegaly	Blood type/ screen	• Serial abdominal exams • IV fluids, • RBC transfusion or exchange transfusion for cardiovascular compromise and Hb <4.5 g/dL
Vaso-occlusive crisis	• Ischaemia • Pain • Necrosis	Blood type/ screen	• Aggressive early pain treatment • Oral analgesics if outpatient • Parenteral analgesics & fluids if failure of outpatient treatment
Aplastic crisis	• Pallor • Tachycardia • Fatigue	• Blood type/ screen • Parvovirus serology and PCR	• Admit, IV fluids, PRBCs for symptomatic anemia • Isolation to protect susceptible individuals & women of child-bearing age until parvovirus excluded
Acute chest syndrome	• Chest pain • Difficulty breathing • Fever	• Blood cultures • Blood type/ screen • Chest x-ray	• Admit, O_2, incentive spirometry, bronchodilators • IV analgesia, antibiotics, fluids • Simple transfusion or partial exchange for moderately severe illness, double packed cell volume exchange transfusion for severe or rapidly progressing illness

Health care maintenance in sickle cell disease	
Immunizations	**Pneumococcal**: 23-valent polysaccharide vaccine at 2 yrs, booster at 5 yrs and every 5-7 yrs thereafter
	Meningococcal: At 2 yrs and booster every 10 yrs
	Influenza: Annual from 6 months
Medications	**Penicillin**: Begin at diagnosis, 125 mg BID; increase to 250 mg BID at 3 yrs
	Folic acid: Supplement starting at 1 yr
	Hydroxyurea: Consider with frequent crises or severe disease
Transcranial Doppler	Annual from 2-16 yrs to evaluate risk of CVA
Ophthalmology	Annual from 10 yrs for sickle retinopathy

12.2 Coagulation Disorders

Factor VIII deficiency (Hemophilia A)	
Characteristics	Prolonged aPTT, normal PT, normal BT, reduced factor VIII activity, X-linked recessive
Treatment	• Factor VIII concentrate, preferably recombinant Factor VIII to reduce risk of infection • Factor level recovers by 2% per 1 unit of factor VIII per kg of body weight • 1st dose has shorter T1/2, so if additional needed, 2nd dose should be given after 4-8 h. Subsequent doses can be given every 12 h • Continuous infusion may be preferred for surgical • patients or prolonged therapy: 50 U/kg loading dose, followed by 3-5 U/kg/h • Replace to 100% before diagnostic procedure (eg, CT scan) if intracranial bleeding is suspected
Factor IX deficiency (Hemophilia B, Christmas disease)	
Characteristics:	X-linked recessive, prolonged aPTT, reduced factor IX activity
Treatment	• Factor IX concentrate, optimally recombinant to reduce risk of infection • Factor level usually recovers by 1% for each unit of factor IX concentrate per kg of body weight • If 2nd dose is needed, it should be given at shorter interval than T1/2 of factor IX (18-24 h) • Recombinant factor IX has shorter T1/2; consider • Evaluation of in vivo factor IX survival • Replace to 100% before diagnostic procedure if intracranial bleeding is suspected

Von Willebrand disease	
Characteristics	vWF binds platelets to subendothelial surfaces, carries and stabilized factor VIII
Types	**Type 1:** Decreased vWF and ristocetin cofactor activity, may have identifiable gene mutation, mild-moderate bleeding, prolonged BT, normal platelet count, mild-moderate prolongation of aPTT
	Type 2: 4 subtypes, all with functional abnormalities of vWF, marked decrease in ristocetin cofactor activity compared to decrease in vWF, and moderate-severe bleeding
	Type 3: More severe decrease in vWF and factor VIII secondary to genetic mutations; severe bleeding
Treatment	• DDAVP • Severe or Type 2: Humate P (heat inactivated vWF-enriched concentrate), a similar product containing active vWF, or cryoprecipitate • Aminocaproic acid for oral bleeding or dental prophylaxis

12.3 Thrombocytopenia

Definition
Platelet count <150,000. In absence of other complicating factors clinically significant bleeding unlikely with platelet counts >20,000.

Causes	
Neonatal thrombocytopenia	**Caused by:** • Decreased production: Congenital malignancy (eg, leukemia) aplastic disorders, and viral infections • Increased consumption: Usually from disseminated intravascular coagulation (DIC) from infection or asphyxia • Immune mediated: IgG or complement attach to platelets & cause destruction. Specific causes: Pre-eclampsia, maternal ITP, sepsis, and platelet alloimmunization • Neonatal alloimmune thrombocytopenia: Transplacental antibodies produced by the mother in the second trimester cause fetal platelet destruction. If severe, maternal platelet transfusion is more effective in raising the platelet count than random donor platelets
	Evaluation/diagnosis • Check maternal platelet count (should be normal) & platelet-associated IgG (usually negative) • Absence of maternal PLA-1 antigen/HPA-1a or other specific antigens • Study of mother's or infant's plasma with panel of known minor platelet antigens • Mixing study of maternal or neonatal plasma and paternal platelets • Bone marrow biopsy to quantify megakaryocytes is the only direct way to determine the pathophysiologic mechanism
Idiopathic thrombocytopenic purpura (ITP)	• Diagnosis of exclusion; can be acute or chronic • WBC count, Hb levels, & peripheral smear are normal • Indications for treatment of patients without significant bleeding not well established
	• Treatment: – Rh (D) immune globulin (in Rh-positive, nonsplenectomized patients) – Intravenous immune globulin – Corticosteroids – Thrombopoietin receptor agonists – Chronic ITP: May consider splenectomy or chemotherapy – Platelet transfusions is necessary in life-threatening bleeding

Other causes of thrombocytopenia	• Drug-induced • Malignancy • Infection causing marrow suppression • HIV • Marrow infiltration • Microangiopathic hemolytic anemias • Cavernous hemangiomas (Kasabach-Merritt syndrome) • Thrombocytopenia with absent radii syndrome • Thrombosis • Hypersplenism • Other rare inherited disorders (eg, Wiskott-Aldrich, Paris-Trousseau, Noonan, and DiGeorge syndromes, myosin-9 associated mega-platelet disorders, chromosomal abnormalities)

12.4 Clinical Presentation of Pediatric Tumors

(see reference [83])

Type of Malignancy	Risk Factors/Patient Characteristics	Signs/Symptoms	Initial Workup
Leukemia	• ALL: White race, radiation exposure • AML: Familial monosomy 7 • Both: NF type 1, Down syndrome	Hepatomegaly, splenomegaly, lymphadenopathy, Limp, bone and joint pain, anemia, thrombocytopenia, petechiae, easy bruising, fatigue	Bone marrow examination, BMA, LP, laboratory studies including morphology and flow cytometry
Lymphoma	• Hodgkin's and Burkitt's lymphoma: EBV, more common in adolescence • NHL: Immunodeficiency, more common in infants and school-aged children	Hepatomegaly, splenomegaly, swollen lymph node, especially in the neck, armpit or groin, night sweats, pruritus, stridor, breathing difficulties, GI bleeding, back pain	CBC, ESR, Imaging (CT chest, abdomen, pelvis), bone scan, LP, BMA, ferritin, LDH, uric acid

Type of Malignancy (cont.)	Risk Factors/Patient Characteristics	Signs/Symptoms	Initial Workup
Neuroblastoma	Peak incidence 1-5 yrs	Abdominal, head, neck or chest mass; limp, blue subcutaneous nodules, emesis, diarrhea, hypertension, opsoclonus-myoclonus, periorbital ecchymoses, Horner syndrome, stridor, difficulty breathing, persistent cough	Imaging (CT/MRI for staging), BMA, echocardiogram, urine catecholamines (HVA/VMA)
Wilms' tumor	1-5 yrs (peak 2-3 yrs), associated with congenital Aniridia, Beckwith Wiedemann	Abdominal pain, abdominal distention, fever, hypertension, hematuria	Imaging (CT chest/ abdomen/pelvis), abdominal ultrasound with Doppler, echocardiogram
Testicular tumors	• Adolescents • Cryptorchidism	Abdominal pain or tenderness, scrotal swelling or mass, feeling of heaviness in the scrotum	Imaging (CT chest/ abdomen/pelvis), serum β-hCG, AFP, LDH, uric acid
Bone tumors	• Osteosarcoma: Previous treatment with alkylating agents or radiation therapy • Ewing's sarcoma: Caucasian race • Both: Adolescent age	Limp, swelling or tenderness around a bone or joint, back pain, persistent limb pain, weak bones leading to fractures	Imaging (CT chest, primary site), x-ray primary site, bone scan; bilateral BMA (Ewing's sarcoma)

Type of Malignancy (cont.)	Risk Factors/Patient Characteristics	Signs/Symptoms	Initial Workup
Histiocytic disease	Familial disease: Infancy	Hepatomegaly, splenomegaly, polyuria, polydipsia, otorrhea, osteolytic lesions, pulmonary infiltrates, anemia, thrombocytopenia, cutaneous lesions	LDH/ferritin/uric acid, skeletal survey, BMA, chest x-ray
Hepatoblastoma	Peak incidence <3 yrs Beckwith Wiedemann	Abdominal pain and distention, anorexia, loss of appetite, anemia, fatigue, thrombocytosis, vomiting, jaundice	Imaging of abdomen, laboratory studies, β-hCG, AFP
Rhabdomyosarcoma	More common in children >5 yrs and adolescents, NF type 1	Symptoms differ based on location of tumor but bone pain, anemia, thrombocytopenia, neutropenia, and respiratory symptoms are common with metastatic disease	Laboratory studies including LFTs, imaging based on location of suspected disease (CT, MRI, ultrasound), chest x-ray and bone scan to evaluate for metastatic disease
Retinoblastoma	<5 yrs old, genetic associations	Leukocoria, asymmetrical red reflex, orbital inflammation, hyphema, pupil irregularity, problems with eye movements	Ultrasound scan, Brain MRI, lumbar puncture for CSF

Type of Malignancy (cont.)	Risk Factors/Patient Characteristics	Signs/Symptoms	Initial Workup
CNS tumors	• Optic glioma: NF type I, other genetic syndromes • Astrocytoma: Full age range • Ependymoma and medulloblastoma: More common in infants, school-aged children • Craniopharyngioma: Peak 8–10 yrs	Irritability, headache, vomiting, or an enlarging head in infants, seizure, cranial nerve palsies, proptosis, ataxia, visual changes	MRI of brain and spine, lumbar puncture (cytopathology)

12.5 Oncologic Emergencies

Metabolic	Hematologic	Infectious	Inflammatory	Mechanical
• Hypercalcemia • Hyponatremia • Hypoglycemia • Adrenal failure • Lactic acidosis • Tumor lysis syndrome: – Hyperkalemia – Hyperphosphatemia – Elevated uric acid	• Febrile neutropenia • Transfusion reactions • Anemia • Thrombocytopenia • Neutropenia • Hyperleukocytosis • Coagulopathy	• Bacterial • Fungal • Viral	• Pancreatitis • Pneumonitis • Hemorrhagic cystitis • Extravasation of chemotherapy	• Neurologic: – Spinal cord compression – Increased intracranial pressure – Status epilepticus • Respiratory airway obstruction • Cardiac tamponade • Gastrointestinal: – Obstruction – Pseudo-obstruction – Ileus • Urinary obstruction, upper and lower

List of References

81 Nathan D, Oski FA. Hematology of infancy and childhood, 6th ed. Philadelphia, WB Saunders, 2003, p 281-365.

82 Ahsan S, Noether J. Hematology. In Tschudy MM, Arcara KM, eds, The Harriet Lane Handbook, 19th edition, Philadelphia, Mosby, 2012, p 359-386.

83 Albert CM. Oncology. In Tschudy MM, Arcara KM, eds, The Harriet Lane Handbook, 19th edition, Philadelphia, Mosby, 2012, p 603-614.

13 Endocrine Disorders

13.1 Tanner Stages

13.1.1 Tanner scale for males

Stage		Volume	Length
1		3	<2,5 cm
2		4	<2,5-3,2 cm
3		10	<3,6 cm
4		16	4,1-4,5 cm
5		25	>4,5 cm

13.1.2 Tanner scale for females

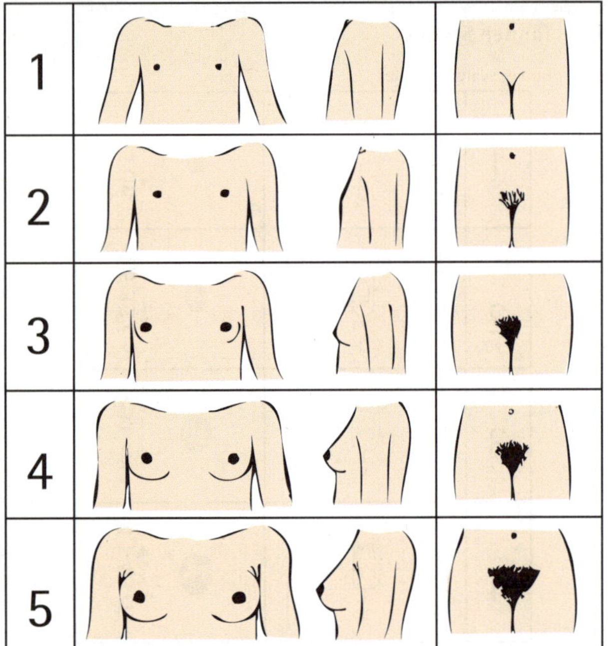

13.2 Suspected Genetic Metabolic Disorders

(see reference [84])

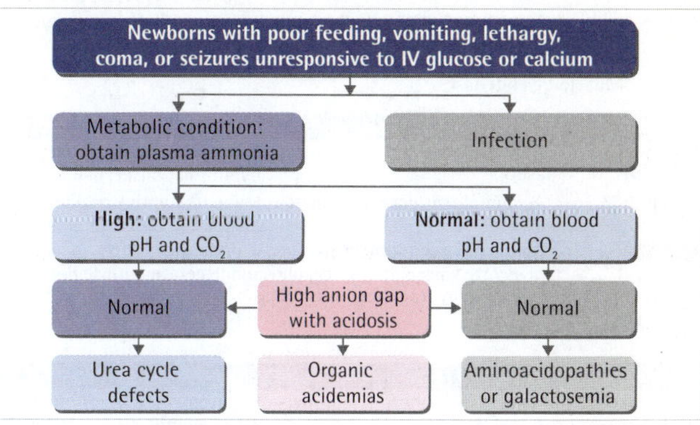

13.3 Disorders of Carbohydrates

13.3.1 Liver glycogenoses

Disorder	Defect	Clinical findings
Ia/von Gierke	Glucose-6-phosphatase	Hepatomegaly, hypoglycemia growth retardation; cholesterol, triglyceride, & uric acid
Ib	Glucose-6-phosphate translo-case	Similar to type Ia; also neutro-penia & impaired neutrophil function
IIIa/Cori or Forbes	Liver & muscle debrancher defi-ciency (amylo-1,6 glucosidase)	Hepatomegaly, muscle weak-ness, hypoglycemia, hyperlipid-emia, growth retardation, transaminase levels; may devel-op liver failure later in life

Disorder (cont.)	Defect	Clinical findings
IIIb	Liver debrancher deficiency; normal muscle enzyme activity	Similar liver symptoms same to type IIIa; no muscle symptoms
Others	IV/Andersen , VI/Hers, phosphorylase kinase deficiency, glycogen synthetase deficiency, Fanconi-Bickel syndrome	

13.3.2 Muscle glycogenoses

Disorder	Defect	Clinical findings
II/Pompe Infantile	Acid α-glucosidase (acid maltase)	Hepatomegaly, cardiomegaly, hypotonia; onset: 0-6 mo
Juvenile	Acid α-glucosidase (acid maltase)	Myopathy with variable cardiomyopathy; onset: childhood
Others	Danon disease, PRKAG2 deficiency, V/McArdle, VII/Tarui, phosphoglycerate kinase deficiency, phosphoglycerate mutase deficiency, lactate dehydrogenase deficiency	

13.3.3 Galactose disorders

Disorder	Defect	Clinical findings
Galactosemia with transferase deficiency	Galactose-1-phosphate uridyltransferase	Hepatomegaly, vomiting, cataracts, aminoaciduria, failure to thrive
Others	Galactokinase deficiency, generalized uridine diphosphate galactose-4-epimerase deficiency	

13.3.4 Disorders of gluconeogenesis

Disorder	Defect	Clinical findings
Fructose-1,6-diphosphatase deficiency	Fructose-1,6-diphosphatase	Apnea, acidosis, episodic hypoglycemia
Others	Phosphoenolpyruvate carboxykinase deficiency, fructose-1,6-diphosphatase deficiency	

13.3.5 Disorders of pyruvate metabolism

Disorder	Defect	Clinical findings
Pyruvate dehydrogenase complex defect	Pyruvate dehydrogenase	Psychomotor retardation, failure to thrive, lactic acidosis; may be severe fatal neonatal to mild later onset
Others	Pyruvate carboxylase, respiratory chain defects (oxidative phosphorylation disease)	

13.3.6 Disorders of fructose metabolism

Disorder	Defect	Clinical Findings
Essential or benign fructosuria	Fructokinase	+Urine reducing substances, otherwise asymptomatic
Others	Aldolase B, hereditary fructose intolerance	

13.3.7 Disorders in pentose metabolism

Disorder	Defect	Clinical Findings
Pentosuria	L-Xylulose reductase	+Urine reducing substances
Others	Transaldolase deficiency, ribose-5-phosphate isomerase deficiency	

13.4 Lysosomal Storage Disorders

(see reference [85])

Algorithm for evaluation:

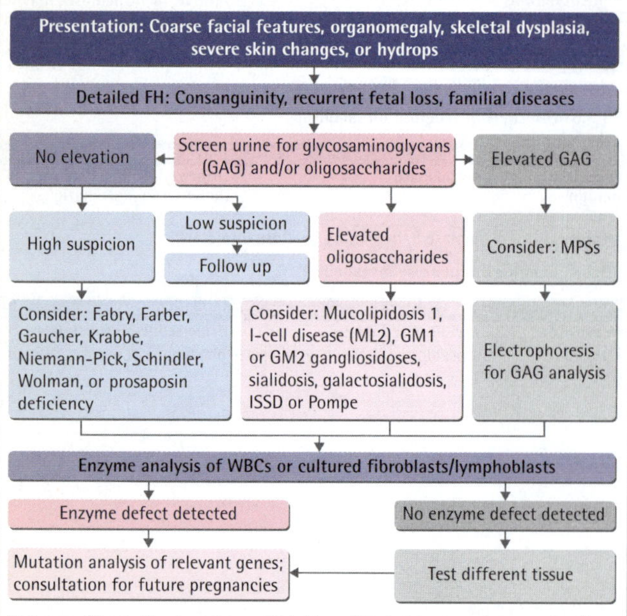

Reference: Staretz-Chacham O, Lang TC, LaMarca ME et al. Lysosomal storage disorders in the newborn. Pediatrics 2009; 123:1191-1207

13.5 Vitamin D Disorders: Rickets

(see reference [86])

Definition	
Rickets results from unmineralized matrix at the growth plates and occurs in children with growing bone.	
Causes	
Vitamin D disorders	• Vitamin D deficiency (congenital, nutritional, secondary) • Vitamin D-dependent rickets type 1 • Vitamin D-dependent rickets type 2 • Chronic renal failure
Calcium deficiency	• Inadequate intake (diet, prematurity) • Malabsorption (celiac disease, abetalipoproteinemia, small bowel resection)
Phosphorus deficiency	Inadequate intake (prematurity, aluminum-containing antacids)
Renal	• X-linked hypophosphatemic rickets • Hypophosphatemic rickets – Autosomal dominant – Autosomal recessive – Hereditary, with hypercalciuria • Overproduction of phosphatonin • Fanconi syndrome • Dent disease • Distal renal tubular acidosis
Clinical features	
General	• Impaired growth • Listlessness • Protruding abdomen • Muscle weakness, secondary to proximal myopathy • Increased fractures
Head	• Frontal bossing (rickets hydrocephalus) • Delayed closure of fontanel • Benign intracranial hypertension • Craniotabes • Dental features: enamel hypoplasia, delayed dentition, caries • Craniosynostosis

Clinical features (cont.)	
Chest	• Pectus carinatum (pigeon chest) • Rachitic rosary • Harrison groove • Respiratory infections, atelectasis
Back	• Kyphosis • Scoliosis
Extremities	• Enlarged wrists and ankles (cartilaginous swelling) • Genu valgum or genu varum deformities • Triradiate or flat pelvis • Anterior bowing of tibia and femur • Coxa vara • Diffuse bone pain
Hypocalcemic symptoms	• Tetany, hypocalcemic seizures, carpopedal spasm, apnea, and stridor

Laboratory findings

Disorder	Ca	Pi	PHT	25-(OH) D	1,25-(OH)$_2$D	Alk Phos	U Ca	U Pi
Vitamin D deficiency	N, ↓	↓	↑	↓	↓, N, ↑	↑	↓	↑
VDDR, type 1	N, ↓	↓	↑	N	↓	↑	↓	↑
VDDR, type 2	N, ↓	↓	↑	N	↑↑	↑	↓	↑
Chronic renal failure	N, ↓	↑	↑	N	↓	↑	N, ↓	↓
Dietary Pi deficiency	N	↓	N, ↓	N	↑	↑	↑	↓
XLH	N	↓	N	N	RD	↑	↓	↑
ADHR	N	↓	N	N	RD	↑	↓	↑
HHRH	N	↓	N, ↓	N	RD	↑	↑	↑
ARHR	N	↓	N	N	RD	↑	↓	↑
Tumor-induced rickets	N	↓	N	N	RD	↑	↓	↑
Fanconi syndrome	N	↓	N	N	RD or ↑	↑	↓ or ↑	↑
Dietary Ca deficiency	N, ↓	↓	↑	N	↑	↑	↓	↑

ADHR: autosomal dominant hypophosphatemic rickets, Alk Phos: alkaline phosphatase, ARHR: autosomal recessive hypophosphatemic rickets, Ca: calcium, HHRH: hereditary hypophosphatemic rickets with hypercalciuria, N: normal, Pi: inorganic phosphorus, PTH: parathyroid hormone, RD: relatively decreased (because should be ↑ given concurrent hypophosphatemia), VDDR: vitamin D-dependent rickets, XLH: X-linked hypophosphatemic rickets, 1,25-(OH)2D: 1,25-dihydroxyvitamin D, 25-OHD: 25-hydroxyvitamin D.

13.6 Diabetes Mellitus

13.6.1 Diagnosis

Criteria for diagnosis

- Symptoms of polyuria, polydipsia or weight loss; and random blood glucose ≥200 mg/dL
- Fasting blood glucose ≥126 mg/dL
- Oral glucose tolerance test (OGTT) with 2 h postload blood glucose of ≥200 mg/dL
- Hemoglobin A1c ≥6.5%

13.6.2 Diabetic ketoacidosis (DKA)[87]

Components

Hyperglycemia, ketonemia, ketosis, and metabolic acidosis (pH <7.30, bicarbonate <15 mEq/L)

Management of DKA

Time	Therapy	Comments
1st h	10-20 mL/kg IV bolus 0.9% NaCl or RL Insulin drip: 0.05-0.10 U/kg/h	Quick volume expansion, may be repeated. NPO. Monitor I/O, neurologic status. Use flow sheet. Have mannitol at bedside; 1g/kg IV push for cerebral edema.
2nd h until DKA resolution	0.45% NaCl: plus continue insulin drip; 20 mEq/L KPhos and 20 mEq/L KAc; 5% glucose if blood sugar >250 mg/dL (14 mmol/L)	IV rate = (85 mL/kg + maintenance - bolus) / 23 h If K <3 mEq/L, give 0.5 to 1.0 mEq/kg as oral K solution OR increase IV K to 80 mEq/L
Variable	Oral intake with subcutaneous insulin	No emesis; CO_2 ≥16 mEq/L; normal electrolytes

Management of DKA (cont.)
• Initial IV bolus is considered part of the total fluid allowed in the 1st 24 h and is subtracted before calculating the IV rate • Maintenance (24 h) = 100 mL/kg (for the 1st 10 kg) + 50 mL/kg (for the 2nd 10 kg) + 25 mL/kg (for all remaining kg)
I/O: Input and output (urine, emesis), KAc: Potassium acetate, KPhos: Potassium phosphate, LR: Lactated Ringer solution, NaCl: Sodium chloride

13.6.3 Type 2 diabetes mellitus

Criteria	• Fasting blood glucose in children >85th percentile BMI + 2 of below: – FH type 2 DM in 1st or 2nd degree relative – Non-Caucasian ethnicity – Signs of insulin resistance (acanthosis nigricans, hypertension, dyslipidemia, polycystic ovaries) • Start screening at 10 yrs or onset of puberty, whichever 1st; repeat every 2 yrs • In adults, HbA1c of 5.7-6.4% indicates increased risk of future DM, 6.0-6.5% requires OGTT and fasting glucose, >6.5% is diagnostic of DM
Treatment	• Primarily diet and exercise • Medications (metformin, insulin) if failure of diet/exercise or symptomatic on presentation

13.6.4 Primary care of all diabetic patients

- Monitor glucose control
  - Daily blood glucose
  - HbA1c every 3 months
- Frequent eye exams
- Screening for hypertension, proteinuria, hyperlipidemia

13.7 Congenital Adrenal Hyperplasia

(see reference [88])

Clinical findings	Lab findings	Therapy
21-Hydroxylase deficiency		
↓ Aldosterone results in salt loss with ↓Na, ↑K Excess of androgens causes dark scrotum, virilization, ambiguous genitalis. There are 2 types: classic & non-classic	↓: Aldosterone, cortisol; ↑: Progesterone, 17-hydroxy-progesterone (very high), sex steroids, urinary pregnanetriol	• Mineralocorticoid (fludrocortisone) replacement; sodium chloride supplementation • Glucocorticoid (hydrocortisone) replacement • Vaginoplasty and clitoral recession • Suppression with glucocorticoids
11β-Hydroxylase deficiency		
↑ Androgen may cause virilization in female fetus, HTN, hypokalemic alkalosis, salt retention	↓Plasma renin; ↑ 11-deoxycortisol & deoxycorticosterone, tetrahydrocompounds-S	• Glucocorticoid (hydrocortisone) replacement • Vaginoplasty & clitoral recession • Suppression with glucocorticoids
17α-Hydroxylase deficiency		
Similar to 11-hydroxylase deficiency except: no virilization & normal genitalia as ↓ androgens	↓ Serum androgens	• Glucocorticoid (hydrocortisone) administration • Orchidopexy or removal of intra-abdominal testes • Sex hormone replacement consonant with sex of rearing • Suppression with glucocorticoids

Clinical findings (cont.)	Lab findings	Therapy
3β-HSD deficiency, classical form		
Rare, causes virilization in female & ambiguous genitalia in newborns	↑ DHEA, ↓ androstenedione, testosterone, & estradiol, ↑ Plasma renin	• Glucocorticoid (hydrocortisone) replacement; Mineralocorticoid (fludrocortisone) replacement; sodium chloride supplementation • Surgical correction of genitals & sex hormone replacement as necessary, consonant with sex of rearing • Suppression with glucocorticoids

13.8 Hypothyroidism

	Primary/congenital	Acquired
Clinical findings	• Hypothermia • Large fontanelles • Lethargy • Constipation • Hoarse cry • Hypotonia • Jaundice	• Decreased growth rate • Other signs include coarse, brittle hair; cool/dry/scaly skin • Delayed dentition • Cold intolerance
Onset	• Symptoms usually by 2-6 wks of life • Some infants may be relatively asymptomatic • Asymptomatic patients still at risk of developmental delay	Can occur as early as 1st 2 yrs of life
Etiology	**Primary**: • Athyrosis • TSH receptor mutation • Thyroid dyshormonogenesis **Central**: • Deficiency of thyrotropin-releasing hormone or TSH	• Hashimoto thyroiditis (diagnosis supported by presence of antithyroglobulin or antimicrosomal antibodies) • Head/neck radiation • Central hypothyroidism (pituitary/hypothalamic insult)

(cont.)	Primary/congenital	Acquired
Management	**Goal:** • T4 in upper half of normal range • TSH <5 (in primary hypothyroidism) • Replacement with L-thyroxine on confirmed diagnosis	Replacement with L-thyroxine
Follow-up	**Weeks 1, 2, & 3-4 weeks after any dose change:** • Monitor T4 & TSH • If levels adequate, follow every 1-3 months during first year	• Same as primary/congenital • After 2 yrs: monitor levels every 6-12 months as dose changes become less frequent

13.9 Hypoglycemia

(see reference [89])

Neonatal transient hypoglycemia
• Inadequate substrate stores or immature enzyme function in otherwise normal newborns (premature, IUGR, normal newborn with inadequate feeding) • Transient neonatal hyperinsulinemic hypoglycemia (TNHI) resolves completely in few days/months (maternal DM, IUGR)
Persistent hypoglycemia (all ages)
Hormone deficiency
• Hypothalamic-pituitary origin • Failure of the adrenal gland (Addison disease) or the thyroid gland • Isolated growth hormone deficiency • Epinephrine deficiency
Hormonal disorders
• Beckwith-Wiedemann syndrome • Syndrome of macroglossia, visceromegaly, and omphalocele • Insulin administration • Hyperinsulinism (usually self limited) • Hyperinsulinism/hyperammonemia syndrome • Focal KATP channel HI • Dominant glucokinase HI, mutation in HNF4A (hepatic nuclear factor 4 alpha) HI with MODY later in life • Dominant mutation in SLC16A1-exercise-induced hypoglycemia • Dominant/recessive KATP channel HI

Hormonal disorders (cont.)
• Recessive HADH (hydroxyl acyl CoA dehydrogenase) mutation HI • Recessive UCP2 (mitochondrial uncoupling protein 2) mutation HI • Acquired islet adenoma • Drugs: oral sulfonylurea • Congenital glycosylation disorders
Fatty acid oxidation disorders
• Acyl CoA dehydrogenase deficiency (SCAD, LCAD, VLACD, MCAD) • Carnitine transporter deficiency (primary carnitine deficiency) • Carnitine palmitoyltransferase deficiency (CPT-1 & CPT-2) • Carnitine translocase deficiency • Secondary carnitine deficiencies
Glycogenolysis and gluconeogenesis disorders & lipolysis disorders
• Glycogen synthetase deficiency (GSD 0, rare) • Fructose-1, 6-diphosphatase deficiency • Glycogen storage disease type Ia and type Ib (G6PD, von Gierke disease) • Glycogen storage disease type III (amylo-1, 6-glucosidase deficiency) • Glycogen storage disease type VI (Hers disease, phosphorylase deficiency • Phosphorylase kinase deficiency (GSD 9) • Galactosemia • Hereditary fructose intolerance • Pyruvate carboxylase deficiency
Other causes
• Liver disease (hepatitis, Reye syndrome, cirrhosis, hepatoma)
• Systemic disorders: – Insulin-dependent diabetes mellitus – Insulin excess – Anti-insulin antibodies – Diarrhea – Burns – Shock – Malnutrition – Sepsis – Postsurgical – Heart failure – Malabsorption – Falciparum malaria – Pseudohypoglycemia – Factitious – Nissen fundoplication (dumping syndrome) – Cancer secreting IGF II – Renal failure
• Substrate-limited: – Poisoning/Drugs (salicylates, pentamidine, Ackee fruit, rat poison, disopyramide, quinine, Trimethoprim-sulfamethoxazole, propranolol) – Oral hypoglycemics, insulin – Ketotic hypoglycemia

- Amino Acid and Organic Acid Disorders:
  - Propionic academia (PROP, propionyl-CoA carboxylase)
  - Methylmalonic academia
  - Maple syrup urine disease
  - Citrullinemia
  - Phenylketonuria (PKU)
  - Tyrosinosis
  - Glutaric acidemia type I (GA-1, glutaryl-CoA dehydrogenase)
  - 3-Hydroxy-3-methylglutaric aciduria (HMG, 3-Hydrox 3-methylglutaryl-CoA lyase)

List of References

84 Rezvani I, Rezvani G. An approach to inborn errors of metabolism. In Kliegman RM et al, eds. Nelson Textbook of Pediatrics, 19th edition, Philadelphia, Elsevier, 2011, 417.

85 Staretz-Chacham O, Lang TC, LaMarca ME et al. Lysosomal storage disorders in the newborn. Pediatrics 2009; 123:1191-1207.

86 Greenbaum LA. Rickets and hypervitaminosis D. In Kliegman RM et al, eds. Nelson Textbook of Pediatrics, 19th edition, Philadelphia, Elsevier, 2011, 202.

87 Alemzadeh R, Ali O. Type 1 diabetes mellitus (immune-mediated). In Kliegman RM et al, eds. Nelson Textbook of Pediatrics, 19th edition, Philadelphia, Elsevier, 2011, p 1979

88 White PC. Congenital adrenal hyperplasia and related disorders. In Kliegman RM et al, eds. Nelson Textbook of Pediatrics, 19th edition, Philadelphia, Elsevier, 2011, p 1932.

89 Sperling M. Hypoglycemia.In Kliegman RM et al, eds. Nelson Textbook of Pediatrics, 19th edition, Philadelphia, Elsevier, 2011, p 517-531.

14 Psychosocial Behavioral Disorders

14.1 Attention Deficit Hyperactivity Disorder (ADHD)

ICD-10 criteria: Attention deficit/ hyperactivity disorder
F90 Hyperkinetic disorders
G1 Inattention
At least six of the following symptoms of attention have persisted for at least 6 months, to a degree that is maladaptive and inconsistent with the developmental level of the child: • Often fails to give close attention to details, or makes careless errors in school work, work, or other activities • Often fails to sustain attention in tasks or play activities • Often appears not to listen to what is being said to him or her • Often fails to follow through on instructions or to finish school work, chores, or duties in the workplace (not because of oppositional behaviour or failure to understand instructions) • Is often impaired in organising tasks and activities • Often avoids or strongly dislikes tasks, such as homework, that require sustained mental effort • Often loses things necessary for certain tasks and activities, such as school assignments, pencils, books, toys, or tools • Is often easily distracted by external stimuli • Is often forgetful in the course of daily activities
G2 Hyperactivity
At least three of the following symptoms of hyperactivity have persisted for at least 6 months, to a degree that is maladaptive and inconsistent with the developmental level of the child: • Often fidgets with hands or feet or squirms on seat • Leaves seat in classroom or in other situations in which remaining seated is expected • Often runs about or climbs excessively in situations in which it is inappropriate (in adolescents or adults, only feelings of restlessness may be present) • Is often unduly noisy in playing or has difficulty in engaging quietly in leisure activities • Exhibits a persistent pattern of excessive motor activity that is not substantially modified by social context or demands

G3 Impulsivity

At least one of the following symptoms of impulsivity has persisted for at least 6 months, to a degree that is maladaptive and inconsistent with the developmental level of the child:

- Often blurts out answers before questions have been completed
- Often fails to wait in lines or await turns in games or group situations
- Often interrupts or intrudes on others (eg, butts into others' conversations or games)
- Often talks excessively without appropriate response to social constraints

G4

Onset of the disorder is no later than the age of 7 yrs.

G5 Pervasiveness

The criteria should be met for more than a single situation, eg, the combination of inattention and hyperactivity should be present both at home and at school, or at both school and another setting where children are observed, such as a clinic. (Evidence for cross-situationality will ordinarily require information from more than one source; parental reports about classroom behaviour, for instance, are unlikely to be sufficient.)

G6

The symptoms in G1 and G3 cause clinically significant distress or impairment in social, academic, or occupational functioning.

G7

The disorder does not meet the criteria for pervasive developmental disorders (F84.-), manic episode (F30.-), depressive episode (F32.-), or anxiety disorders (F41.-)

Evaluation and diagnosis

- Any child between ages 4-18 yrs who presents with academic or behavioral problems & symptoms of inattention, hyperactivity, or impulsivity
- ICD-10 criteria must met to diagnosis ADHD, including documentation of impairment in >1 major setting; required information should be obtained from reports from parents/ guardians, teachers, and mental health clinicians
- Ruled out alternative causes (see DDX below)
- Assessment should be made for other coexisting conditions with ADHD, including:
  - Behavioral or emotional (eg, anxiety, depressive, oppositional defiant, and conduct disorders)
  - Developmental (eg, learning & language disorders or other neurodevelopmental disorders)
  - Physical conditions (eg, tics, sleep apnea)

Differential Diagnoses

- Medical: Sensory impairment, trauma, infection
- Neurological: Brain injury, developmental delays, learning disabilities, mental retardation, seizure disorder, sleep disorders, Tourette syndrome
- Psychiatric: Depression, anxiety disorder, bipolar disorder, psychosis, autism

Treatment and Monitoring

Treatment of 4–5 yrs old children:

- First line of treatment: Evidence-based parent- and/or teacher-administered behavior therapy.
- Prescribe methylphenidate if no significant improvement in behavior interventions and there is moderate to severe continuing disturbance in the child's function.
- In areas in which evidence-based behavioral treatments are not available: Risks of starting medication at an early age should be weighed against the harm of delaying diagnosis and treatment.

Treatment of 6–11 yrs old children:

- FDA-approved medications, and/or evidence-based parent-and/or teacher-administered behavior therapy as treatment for ADHD, preferably both.
- The evidence is particularly strong for stimulant medications and sufficient but less strong for atomoxetine, extended-release guanfacine, and extended-release clonidine (in that order).

Treatment of 12–18 yrs old adolescents:

- FDA-approved medications (assent of the adolescent)
- Behavior therapy

FDA approved medications for ADHD (brands):

- Atomoxetine (Strattera)
- Clonidine (Kapvay)
- Dexmethylphenidate (Focalin, Focalin XR)
- Dextroamphetamine (Dexedrine/Dextrostat, Dexedrine Spansule)
- Guanfacine (Intuniv)
- Lisdexamfetamine (Vyvanse)
- Methylphenidate (Concerta, Daytrana patch, Metadate CD, Methyl ER, Methylin, Ritalin, Ritalin LA, Ritalin SR)
- Mixed amphetamine salts (Adderall, Adderall XR)

Effective behavioral treatments for ADHD:	
Intervention Type	**Description and Typical Outcome(s)**
Behavioral parent training (BPT)	Improving the parents' understanding of the child's behavior and teaching them strategies to improve functioning and communication and discourage unwanted behavior has measurable effect on the children with ADHD. The different educational interventions for the parents are jointly called Parent Management Training. Techniques include operant conditioning: a consistent application of rewards for meeting goals and good behavior (positive reinforcement) and punishments such as time-outs or revocation of privileges for failing to meet goals or poor behavior
Behavioral classroom management	Classroom management is similar to parent management training; educators learn about ADHD and techniques to improve behavior applied to a classroom setting. Strategies utilized include increased structuring of classroom activities, daily feedback, and token economy
Behavioral peer interventions (BPI)	Interventions focused on peer interactions/relationships; these are often group-based interventions provided weekly and include clinic-based social-skills training used either alone or concurrently with behavioral parent training and/or medication. Office-based interventions have produced minimal effects; interventions have been of questionable social validity; some studies of BPI combined with clinic-based BPT found positive effects on parent ratings of ADHD symptoms; no differences on social functioning or parent ratings of social behavior
Clinicians should titrate doses of medication for ADHD to achieve maximum benefit with minimum adverse effects.	
Most frequent stimulant adverse effects are:	
Low appetite, weight loss, headaches, sleep disturbance, irritability	

14.2 Anxiety Disorders

(see reference [90])

Definitions	
Separation anxiety disorder (SAD)	Excessive and developmentally inappropriate fear and distress concerning separation from home or significant attachment figures.
Generalized anxiety disorder (GAD)	Chronic, excessive worry in a number of areas such as schoolwork, social interactions, family, health/safety, world events, and natural disasters with at least one associated somatic symptom.
Social phobia	Feeling scared or uncomfortable in one or more social settings or performance situations.
Specific phobia	Fear of a particular object or situation that is avoided or endured with great distress.
Panic disorder (with and without agoraphobia)	Recurrent episodes of intense fear that occur unexpectedly and include at least 4 of 13 symptoms from ICD-10 such as pounding heart, sweating, shaking, difficulty breathing, chest pressure/pain, feeling of choking, nausea, chills, or dizziness.
Agoraphobia without panic disorder	Fear of having panic-like symptoms in situations from which escape might be difficult.
Posttraumatic stress disorder (PTSD)[91]	For PTSD to be present, the child must report (or there must be other compelling evidence of) a qualifying index traumatic event and specific symptoms in relation to that traumatic experience. Acute PTSD is diagnosed if the symptoms are present after the first month and for less than 3 months after the index trauma; chronic PTSD is diagnosed if the symptoms persist beyond 3 months. **PTSD also requires the presence of:** • Recurrent and intrusive recollections, nightmares, or other senses of reliving the traumatic experience; • Persistent avoidance of trauma reminders and emotional numbing; and • Persistent symptoms of hyperarousal

Definitions (cont.)	
Obsessive compulsive disorder (OCD)[92]	OCD features distressing and intrusive obsessive thoughts, and/or repetitive compulsive physical or mental actions of clinical significance.
Selective mutism	Persistent failure to speak, read aloud, or sing in specific settings despite speaking in other situations.

Diagnosis

- The psychiatric assessment of children and adolescents should routinely include screening questions about anxiety symptoms
- If the screening indicates significant anxiety, then the clinician should conduct a formal evaluation to determine which anxiety disorder may be present, the severity of anxiety symptoms, and functional impairment. Parents or other caregivers should be included in this evaluation, whenever possible
- The psychiatric assessment should consider differential diagnosis of other physical conditions and psychiatric disorders that may mimic anxiety symptoms

Treatment

- Should consider a multimodal treatment approach
- Should consider severity and impairment of the anxiety disorder
- Psychotherapy should be considered as part of the treatment of children and adolescents with anxiety disorders
  - Cognitive behavioral therapy (CBT)
  - Psychodynamic psychotherapy
  - Family interventions
- Trauma-focused psychotherapies should be considered first-line treatments for children and adolescents with PTSD
- CBT is the first-line treatment for mild to moderate cases of OCD in children
- **Medications**:
  - SSRIs may be considered for PTSD. Other medications may be helpful
  - For moderate to severe OCD, medication is indicated in addition to CBT. SSRIs are first-line treatment
  - SSRIs are medications of choice in treating children with other anxiety disorders. Medications other than SSRIs have no controlled trials
- Treatment planning may consider classroom-based accommodations
- Comorbid conditions should be evaluated and treated (depression, substance abuse, ADHD, ODD, learning disabilities, language disorders)

14.3 Depressive Disorders

(see reference [93])

Definitions

Major depressive disorder (MDD)

- At least 2 weeks of persistent change in mood manifested by either depressed or irritable mood and/or loss of interest and pleasure plus:
  - Wishing to be dead, suicidal ideation or attempts;
  - Increased or decreased appetite, weight, or sleep; and
  - Decreased activity, concentration, energy, or self-worth or exaggerated guilt
- These symptoms must represent a change from previous functioning and produce impairment in relationships or in performance of activities.
- Symptoms must not be attributable only to substance abuse, use of medications, other psychiatric illness, bereavement, or medical illness.
- **Subtypes**:
  - Psychotic depression
  - Seasonal affective disorder

Dysthymic disorder (DD)

- Persistent, long-term change in mood that generally is less intense but more chronic than in MDD
- Not as severe as in MDD, but may cause as much or more psychosocial impairment
- Must have depressed mood or irritability on most days for most of the day for a period of 1 yr
- Must have two other symptoms from:
  - Changes in appetite or weight and changes in sleep;
  - Problems with decision-making or concentration; and
  - Low self-esteem, energy, and hope

Comorbidity is frequent

- Anxiety disorders
- Disruptive disorders
- ADHD
- Substance use disorders

Differential diagnosis

Behavioral disorders	Medical disorders
• Anxiety • Dysthymia • ADHD • ODD • PDD • Substance abuse • Bereavement • Adjustment disorder	• Hypothyroidism • Mononucleosis • Anemia • Cancers • Autoimmune diseases • Premenstrual dysphoric disorder • Chronic fatigue syndrome

Diagnosis

- Children and adolescents should routinely be screened for depressive symptoms
- If screening indicates significant depressive symptoms, a complete evaluation should be performed for depressive and comorbid disorders
- The evaluation should include assessment for possible harm to self or others

Treatment

- The treatment of depressive disorders should always include an acute and continuation phase
  - Acute phase goal is response and full remission
  - Continuation phase goal is consolidation of the response during the acute phase and avoidance of relapses
- Some children may also require maintenance treatment to avoid recurrences in more severe, recurrent, and chronic disorders
- Each treatment phase should include psychoeducation, supportive management, and family and school involvement
- Education, support, and case management may be sufficient treatment for depressed children and adolescents with an uncomplicated or brief depression or with mild psychosocial impairment
- Children and adolescents not responsive to supportive psychotherapy or with more complicated depressions should have a trial of specific types of psychotherapy and/or antidepressants
- Treatment should always be continued for 6-12 months to consolidate the response to acute treatment and avoid relapses. Some children and adolescents may require longer treatment
- Depressed children and adolescents with psychosis, seasonal depression, and bipolar disorder may need specific somatic treatments
- Treatment should include management of comorbid conditions
- Frequent follow-up contacts should assure sufficient time to monitor clinical status, environmental conditions, and medication side effects
- Consider factors associated with poor response to pharmacological and/or psychotherapeutic treatments

Treatment (cont.)

- **Medications**: Fluoxetine (Prozac) is the only medication approved by the FDA for use in treating depression in children ages 8 and older
- One large trial indicated that a combination of medication and psychotherapy is the most effective treatment for adolescents with MDD

14.4 Eating Disorders

(see reference [94])

Definitions

F50.0 Anorexia nervosa

Anorexia nervosa is a disorder characterized by deliberate weight loss, induced and/or sustained by the patient.

Diagnostic guidelines

For a definite diagnosis, all the following are required:

- Body weight is maintained at least 15% below that expected (either lost or never achieved), or Quetelet's body-mass index is 17.5 or less. Quetelet's body-mass index = weight (kg) to be used for age 16 or more. Prepubertal patients may show failure to make the expected weight gain during the period of growth
- The weight loss is self-induced by avoidance of "fattening foods". One or more of the following may also be present: self-induced vomiting; self-induced purging; excessive exercise; use of appetite suppressants and/or diuretics
- There is body-image distortion in the form of a specific psychopathology whereby a dread of fatness persists as an intrusive, overvalued idea and the patient imposes a low weight threshold on himself or herself
- A widespread endocrine disorder involving the hypothalamic- pituitary-gonadal axis is manifest in women as amenorrhoea and in men as a loss of sexual interest and potency. (An apparent exception is the persistence of vaginal bleeds in anorexic women who are receiving replacement hormonal therapy, most commonly taken as a contraceptive pill.) There may also be elevated levels of growth hormone, raised levels of cortisol, changes in the peripheral metabolism of the thyroid hormone, and abnormalities of insulin secretion
- If onset is prepubertal, the sequence of pubertal events is delayed or even arrested (growth ceases; in girls the breasts do not develop and there is a primary amenorrhoea; in boys the genitals remain juvenile). With recovery, puberty is often completed normally, but menarche is late

F50.1 Atypical anorexia nervosa

This term should be used for those individuals in whom one or more of the key features of anorexia nervosa (F50.0), such as amenorrhoea or significant weight loss, is absent, but who otherwise present a fairly typical clinical picture. Such people are usually encountered in psychiatric liaison services in general hospitals or in primary care. Patients who have all the key symptoms but to only a mild degree may also be best described by this term. This term should not be used for eating disorders that resemble anorexia nervosa but that are due to known physical illness.

F50.2 Bulimia nervosa

Diagnostic guidelines

For a definite diagnosis, all the following are required:

- There is a persistent preoccupation with eating, and an irresistible craving for food; the patient succumbs to episodes of overeating in which large amounts of food are consumed in short periods of time.
- The patient attempts to counteract the "fattening" effects of food by one or more of the following: self-induced vomiting; purgative abuse, alternating periods of starvation; use of drugs such as appetite suppressants, thyroid preparations or diuretics. When bulimia occurs in diabetic patients they may choose to neglect their insulin treatment.
- The psychopathology consists of a morbid dread of fatness and the patient sets herself or himself a sharply defined weight threshold, well below the premorbid weight that constitutes the optimum or healthy weight in the opinion of the physician. There is often, but not always, a history of an earlier episode of anorexia nervosa, the interval between the two disorders ranging from a few months to several yrs. This earlier episode may have been fully expressed, or may have assumed a minor cryptic form with a moderate loss of weight and/or a transient phase of amenorrhoea.

F50.3 Atypical bulimia nervosa

This term should be used for those individuals in whom one or more of the key features listed for bulimia nervosa (F50.2) is absent, but who otherwise present a fairly typical clinical picture. Most commonly this applies to people with normal or even excessive weight but with typical periods of overeating followed by vomiting or purging. Partial syndromes together with depressive symptoms are also not uncommon, but if the depressive symptoms justify a separate diagnosis of a depressive disorder two separate diagnoses should be made. Includes: normal weight bulimia.

F50.4 Overeating associated with other psychological disturbances

Overeating that has led to obesity as a reaction to distressing events should be coded here. Bereavements, accidents, surgical operations, and emotionally distressing events may be followed by a "reactive obesity", especially in individuals predisposed to weight gain.

F50.5 Vomiting associated with other psychological disturbances

Apart from the self-induced vomiting of bulimia nervosa, repeated vomiting may occur in dissociative disorders (F44.-), in hypochondriacal disorder (F45.2) when vomiting may be one of several bodily symptoms, and in pregnancy when emotional factors may contribute to recurrent nausea and vomiting.

F50.8 Other eating disorders

Includes: pica of nonorganic origin in adults, psychogenic loss of appetite.

F50.9 Eating disorder, unspecified

Presenting signs and symptoms		
General	• Distorted body image: marked weight loss, gain, or fluctuations • Disturbed sleep	• Fatigue or lethargy • Dizziness • Cold intolerance • Weakness
Neurological & psychological	• Insomnia • Poor concentration • Suicidal ideation/attempt • Fear of gaining weight • Irritability	• Depression/Anxiety/Obsessive behavior • Self-harm • Seizures • Lack of emotion
Endocrine	• Menstrual irregularity (eg, amenorrhea)	• Loss of libido • Infertility
Oral and dental	• Dental erosion & caries • Oral trauma/lacerations	• Perimolysis • Parotid enlargement
Cardio-respiratory	• Chest pain • Palpitations	• Arrhythmias
Gastro-intestinal	• Dehydration: dry mouth • Epigastric discomfort • Early satiety	• Hematemesis • Hemorrhoids and prolapse • Constipation
Dermatologic	• Dry skin • Hair loss • Poor healing	• Yellowish discoloration of skin • Russell's sign: Callus or scars on the dorsum of the hand

Assessment	
History	• Rate and amount of weight loss/change • Nutritional status • Methods of weight control • Compensatory behaviors (vomiting, dieting, exercise, insulin misuse, and/or use of diet pills, laxatives, diuretics) • Dietary intake and exercise • Menstrual history in females (hormone replacement therapy, including oral contraceptive pills) • Comprehensive growth and development history, temperament, and personality traits • Family history including symptoms or diagnosis of EDs, obesity, mood and anxiety disorders, alcohol and substance use disorders • Psychiatric history, including symptoms of mood disorders and anxiety disorders
Physical examination	• Supine and standing heart rate and blood pressure • Respiratory rate • Oral temperature • Measurement of height, weight, and determination of body mass index (BMI); record weight, height, and BMI on growth charts for children and adolescents, noting changes from previous height(s) and weight(s) measurements.
Laboratory evaluation	See table below

Lab test	Possible findings
CBC	Leukopenia, anemia, or thrombocytopenia
Calcium	Slightly ↓ (poor nutrition at expense of bone), abnormal levels can cause serious cardiac complications
Sodium	↓ (overhydration or diuretics/ laxatives)
Potassium	↓ (vomiting, use of laxatives/ diuretics, refeeding)
Chloride	↓ (vomiting, diuretics/ laxative use)
Bicarbonate	↑ (vomiting, metabolic alkalosis), ↓ (laxatives, metabolic acidosis)
Glucose	↓ (poor nutrition), ↑ (insulin omission)
BUN	↑ (dehydration)
Creatinine	↑ (dehydration, renal dysfunction), ↓ unusual
Phosphate	↓ (poor nutrition or refeeding, diuretic use, chronic antacid use)
Magnesium	↓ (poor nutrition, diuretics/ laxatives, refeeding)

Lab test (cont.)	Possible findings
Total protein/ albumin	↑ (in early malnutrition at the expense of muscle mass, dehydration), ↓(in later malnutrition)
Total bilirubin	↑ (liver dysfunction), ↓ (poor RBC mass)
AST, ALT	↑ (Elevated liver enzymes, malnutrition)
Amylase	↑ (vomiting, pancreatitis)
Lipase	↑ (pancreatitis)
TFTs	Low to normal thyrotropin (TSH), normal or slightly low thyroxine (T4) (sick euthyroid syndrome)
Gonadotropins and sex steroids	Low luteinizing hormone (LH) and follicle-stimulating hormone (FSH). Low estradiol in females, low testosterone in males.
Pregnancy test	Low weight females can ovulate and are therefore at risk for becoming pregnant if sexually active.
Lipid panel	Not recommended as an initial test since cholesterol may be elevated in early malnutrition or low in advanced malnutrition.
Bone mineral density study	Patients with EDs are at risk of low bone mineral density
ECG	Malnutrition and binge/purge behaviors can lead to bradycardia or other arrhythmias, low-voltage changes, prolonged QTc interval, T-wave inversions, and occasional ST-segment depression

Treatment

Goals of treatment

- Nutritional rehabilitation
- Weight restoration
- Medical stabilization and prevention of morbidity and mortality
- Resumption of menses (where appropriate)
- Cessation of binge eating and/or purging behaviors
- Cessation of eating disordered ideation including body image disturbance
- Restore meal patterns that promote health and social connections
- Re-establish social engagement
- Address comorbidities

Major therapies for eating disorder treatment

- Art Therapy
- Family Therapy
- Medical Nutrition Therapy
- Dialectical Behavioral Therapy
- Dance/Movement Therapy

Complications of treatment

Refeeding syndrome

- Metabolic disturbances (potentially fatal shift of fluid and electrolytes) that can occur as a result of refeeding malnourished patient.
- Refeeding syndrome usually occurs within 4 days of starting to feed
- Can be nonspecific clinical presentation
- Serious consequences include cardiac and/or respiratory failure, gastrointestinal problems, delirium, coma, convulsion and, in some cases, death (cardiac arrhythmias). These require specialized care on an inpatient unit.
- Risk factors for refeeding syndrome: In patients with
  - Anorexia nervosa
  - Rapid or profound weight loss
    Chronically undernourished with little or no energy intake for more than 10 days
  - EDs who are malnourished, especially if significant alcohol intake
  - Obesity and significant weight loss (after bariatric surgery)
  - Prolonged fasting
  - History of diuretic, laxative, or insulin misuse

Underfeeding

- Caused by an improper or insufficient diet either inadequate calories or inadequate specific dietary components for whatever reason
- May lead to further weight loss
- Reported to be fatal in seriously malnourished patients
- Prevention of underfeeding:
  - Avoid overly cautious rates of refeeding.
  - Frequently (12-24 h) reassess and increase calories as soon as it is deemed safe in hospitalized patients.
  - Review electrolytes daily in the initial stages of refeeding.

14.5 Bipolar Disorder

(see reference [95])

Definitions	
Bipolar I disorder	• Requires occurrence of manic (or mixed) episode with duration of at least 7 days, unless hospitalization is required • Episodes represent significant departure from baseline function
Mixed episode	• Requires period of 7 days or more in which symptoms for both a manic and depressive episode are met
Bipolar II disorder	• Requires periods of major depression and hypomania (lasting at least 4 days) but no full manic or mixed manic episodes
Bipolar disorder not otherwise specified (NOS)	• This term is used for cases that do not meet full criteria for other bipolar diagnoses
Rapid cycling	• The occurrence of at least four mood episodes in 1 yr • In adults, episodes still must meet the prerequisite duration criteria above • Durations are reported shorter in children, but ICD criteria for duration should be followed in making diagnosis at all ages

Clinical findings

- Manic mood changes include marked euphoria, grandiosity, and irritability, with associated racing thoughts, increased psychomotor activity, and mood lability
- Paranoia, confusion, and/or psychosis may occur
- Marked sleep disturbance is frequent

Diagnosis

- Psychiatric assessment of children and adolescents should include screening questions for bipolar disorder
- Bipolar disorder NOS should be used to describe children and adolescents with manic symptoms lasting hours to less than 4 days or for those with chronic manic-like symptoms at baseline
- Need careful evaluation of children and adolescents with suspected bipolar disorder for associated problems, including suicidality, comorbid disorders (including substance abuse), psychosocial stressors, and medical problems
- The diagnosis of bipolar disorder in preschool-age children has not been well established

Treatment

- In mania meeting ICD-10 criteria for bipolar I disorder, pharmacotherapy is first- line treatment
- Evidence for specific pharmacotherapy is limited in children. A child psychiatrist should be consulted prior to initiating treatment
- Lithium is approved down to age 12 yrs for acute mania and maintenance therapy
- Aripiprazole, valproate, olanzapine, risperidone, quetiapine, and ziprasidone are approved for acute mania in adults
- Chlorpromazine is also approved for acute mania in adults, but is generally not used as a first-line agent
- Both lamotrigine and olanzapine are approved for maintenance therapy in adults
- The combination of olanzapine and fluoxetine is approved for bipolar depression in adults
- Most children and adolescents will need long-term therapy to prevent relapse, and some will need lifelong treatment
- Baseline and follow-up symptom, side effect (including weight), and laboratory monitoring are required
- In severely impaired adolescents with manic or depressive episodes in bipolar I disorder, electroconvulsive therapy (ECT) may be considered if medications are not helpful or tolerated
- Psychotherapy is an important component of comprehensive treatment

14.6 Autism Spectrum Disorders

Diagnostic criteria

F84.0 Autistic disorder

- Presence of abnormal or impaired development before the age of 3 yrs, in at least one out of the following areas:
  - Receptive or expressive language as used in social communication;
  - The development of selective social attachments or of reciprocal social interaction;
  - Functional or symbolic play.

F84.0 Autistic disorder (cont.)

- Qualitative abnormalities in reciprocal social interaction, manifest in at least one of the following areas:
  - Failure adequately to use eye-to-eye gaze, facial expression, body posture and gesture to regulate social interaction;
  - Failure to develop (in a manner appropriate to mental age, and despite ample opportunities) peer relationships that involve a mutual sharing of interests, activities, and emotions;
  - Lack of socio-emotional reciprocity as shown by an impaired or deviant response to other people's emotions; or lack of modulation of behaviour according to social context, or a weak integration of social, emotional, and communicative behaviours.
- Qualitative abnormalities in communication, manifest in at least two of the following areas:
  - A delay in, or total lack of development of, spoken language that is not accompanied by an attempt to compensate through the use of gesture or mime as alternative modes of communication (often preceded by a lack of communicative babbling);
  - Relative failure to initiate or sustain conversational interchange (at whatever level of language skills are present) in which there is reciprocal to and from responsiveness to the communications of the other person;
  - Stereotyped and repetitive use of language or idiosyncratic use of words or phrases;
  - Abnormalities in pitch, stress, rate, rhythm, and intonation of speech;
- Restricted, repetitive, and stereotyped patterns of behaviour, interests, and activities, manifest in at least two of the following areas:
  - An encompassing preoccupation with one or more stereotyped and restricted patterns of interest that are abnormal in content or focus; or one or more interests that are abnormal in their intensity and circumscribed nature although not abnormal in their content or focus.
  - Apparently compulsive adherence to specific, non-functional routines or rituals;
  - Stereotyped and repetitive motor mannerisms that involve either hand or finger flapping or twisting, or complex whole body movements;
  - Preoccupations with part-objects or non-functional elements of play materials (such as their odour, the feel of their surface, or the noise or vibration that they generate);
  - Distress over changes in small, non-functional details of the environment.
- The clinical picture is not attributable to the other varieties of pervasive developmental disorder; specific developmental disorder of receptive language with secondary socio-emotional problems; reactive attachment disorder or disinhibited attachment disorder; mental retardation with some associated emotional or behavioural disorder; schizophrenia of unusually early onset; and Rett's syndrome

F84.5 Asperger syndrome

A disorder of uncertain nosological validity, characterized by the same kind of qualitative abnormalities of reciprocal social interaction that typify autism, together with a restricted, stereotyped, repetitive repertoire of interests and activities.

Diagnostic guidelines:

Diagnosis is based on the combination of a lack of any clinically significant general delay in language or cognitive development plus, as with autism, the presence of qualitative deficiencies in reciprocal social interaction and restricted, repetitive, stereotyped patterns of behaviour, interests, and activities. There may or may not be problems in communication similar to those associated with autism, but significant language retardation would rule out the diagnosis.

F84.9 Pervasive developmental disorder, not otherwise specified

This is a residual diagnostic category that should be used for disorders which fit the general description for pervasive developmental disorders but in which a lack of adequate information, or contradictory findings, means that the criteria for any of the other F84 codes cannot be met.

Screening

- A standardized screening test for autism spectrum disorders, eg, the M-CHAT, should be performed at 18 and 24 month visits on all children.
- Children with positive screening test should be referred for developmental evaluation and early intervention services.

List of References

90 American Academy of Child and Adolescent Psychiatry. Practice Parameter for the Assessment and Treatment of Children and Adolescents With Anxiety Disorders. J Am Acad Child Adolesc Psychiatry, 2007;46(2):267-283.

91 American Academy of Child and Adolescent Psychiatry. Practice Parameter for the Assessment and Treatment of Children and Adolescents With Posttraumatic Stress Disorder. J Am Acad Child Adolesc Psychiatry, 2010;49(4):414-430.

92 American Academy of Child and Adolescent Psychiatry. Practice Parameter for the Assessment and Treatment of Children and Adolescents with Obsessive Compulsive Disorder. J Am Acad Child Adolesc Psychiatry 2012; 51(1):98-113.

93 American Academy of Child and Adolescent Psychiatry. Practice Parameter for the Assessment and Treatment of Children and Adolescents With Depressive Disorders. J Am Acad Child Adolesc Psychiatry, 2007; 46(11):1503-1526.

94 Academy of Eating Disorders. Eating Disorders: Critical Points for Early Recognition and Medical Risk Management in the Care of Individuals with Eating Disorders. 2nd edition, 2011.

95 American Academy of Child and Adolescent Psychiatry. Practice Parameter for the Assessment and Treatment of Children and Adolescents With Bipolar Disorder. J Am Acad Child Adolesc Psychiatry, 2007;46(1):107-125.

15 Injuries

15.1 Intentional Injuries

(see reference [96])

15.1.1 Reporting

- All health care and child care providers and related professionals are legally required to report suspected child maltreatment to local police and/or child welfare agency or hotline
- Suspicion of child abuse or maltreatment should be supported by objective evidence
- Suspicion should be discussed with the family and the entire medical team
- The professional who makes such a report is protected from civil or criminal liability
- Documentation:
  - Write legibly
  - Reported history and mechanisms of injury
  - History by victim in her/his own words, in quotes
  - Information from other providers
  - Physical exam findings, including drawings and details
  - Photographs when possible

15.1.2 Child physical abuse[97]

Diagnosis
Suspicion if
• Frequent physical injuries that are attributed to the child's being clumsy or accident-prone • Delay in seeking medical care • Evidence of neglect or failure to thrive • Inadequate history of injury • Mechanism of injury not consistent with physical findings – Injury has vague or no explanation – Important detail of explanation changes dramatically – Explanation is not consistent with pattern, age, or severity of injury – Explanation not consistent with child's physical or developmental abilities – Different witnesses provide markedly different explanations • Parental substance abuse; prior history of suspicious events • Often absent or late to school without a credible reason • Child emotional disturbance • Shies away from touch, flinches at sudden movements, or afraid to go home
History clues
• History of abuse to child, sibling, parents • Disciplined family • History of trauma, hospitalizations, chronic illnesses • Violence in home • Child temperament • Substance abuse in home, caregivers • Social stressors • Pregnancy history
Physical examination clues
• Bites: look carefully for shape, size, location • Unusual shapes of bruises, typically in protected areas • Retinal hemorrhages • Duodenal hematoma • Skeletal injuries: – Diaphyseal fracture (nonambulatory infant/child) – Long bone fractures: – Rib fractures (especially posterior) – Skull fractures usually complex, bilateral • Burns: with well-demarcated edges, no splash marks, stocking glove patterns, symmetrically burned areas (palms, soles, buttocks), spared inguinal creases

Physical examination clues (cont.)

- Abusive head trauma/shaken-baby syndrome:
  - Subdural hematomas
  - Retinal hemorrhages
  - CNS dysfunction (seizures, apnea, lethargy)

Management

- Document and report all cases of suspected child abuse or neglect
- Parents will need counseling or an intervention of some type
- Goal is stabilization and prevention of further injuries
- Document with photographs if possible
- Skeletal survey to evaluate suspicious bony trauma
- Bone scan for early fractures
- Noncontrast CT for intracranial hemorrhage
- MRI for posterior fossa and diffuse axonal injury
- Direct/indirect ophthalmoscopy by ophthalmologist for retinal hemorrhages

15.1.3 Child sexual abuse[98]

Definition

Involvement of a child in sexual activities that he or she des not fully comprehend, for which he or she is developmentally unprepared, for which he or she cannot give consent, and/or that violate the law or social taboos of society.

Diagnosis

- Unexplained genital injuries, especially posterior region
- Anal pain, fissure, bleeding
- Vaginal bleeding in prepubertal female
- Bruising, presence of sperm
- Vaginal/penile discharge
- Laceration
- Hemorrhoids
- Scars
- Genital warts
- Circumferential hematoma of anal sphincter
- Pregnancy

Management
• If suspected abuse occurred within 72 h, defer interview, GU exam, and lab collection until expert team is available • Genital exam should be performed by trained specialist • Child should be evaluated by the pediatrician or mental health provider to assess the need for treatment and to measure the level of parental support • Three major modalities for therapy with children and teenagers are – Family therapy – Group therapy – Individual therapy

15.1.4 Munchausen by proxy syndrome[99]

→ (AKA factitious disorder by proxy)

Characteristic features	• Adult caregiver either makes a child appear sick by fabricating symptoms, or actually causes harm to the child • Child is presented persistently for medical assessment, often resulting in multiple procedures • Perpetrator denies cause of child's illness • Acute symptoms and signs of illness stop when the child and perpetrator are separated
Common symptoms	• Dramatic stories about numerous medical problems • Recurrent sepsis from fluid injection • Chronic diarrhea from laxatives • False renal stones from pebbles in urine • Factitious fever • Traumatic rashes • Lab specimens contaminated with foreign substances
Management	• Multidisciplinary child protection team and state social service agencies should be contacted for suspicious cases • Communication with all treating physicians is essential, as abusing parents frequently seek care from multiple providers • Affected children need psychological evaluation and treatment • Therapeutic and medical treatment should center on the underlying psychiatric disorder

15.2 Unintentional Injuries

(see reference [100])

15.2.1 Impact

Mortality:

- 5th leading cause of death <1 yr of age
- 1st leading cause of death 1-21 yrs of age

Morbidity:

Rank	<1	1-4	5-9	10-14	15-24
1	Unintentional fall	Unintentional fall	Unintentional fall	Unintentional fall	Unintentional struck by/ against
2	Unintentional struck by/ against	Unintentional struck by/ against	Unintentional struck by/ against	Unintentional struck by/ against	Unintentional fall
3	Unintentional other bite/ sting	Unintentional other bite/ sting	Unintentional cut/pierce	Unintentional overexertion	Unintentional overexertion
4	Unintentional foreign body	Unintentional foreign body	Unintentional pedal cyclist	Unintentional cut/pierce	Unintentional MV-occupant
5	Unintentional fire/burn	Unintentional overexertion	Unintentional bite/sting	Unintentional pedal cyclist	Unintentional cut/pierce
6	Unintentional other specified	Unintentional cut/pierce	Unintentional overexertion	Unknown/unspecified	Unintentional other specified
7	Unintentional inhalation/ suffocation	Unintentional other specified	Unintentional MV-occupant	Unintentional MV-occupant	Unintentional other bite/ sting
8	Unknown/unspecified	Unintentional fire/burn	Unintentional foreign body	Unintentional other transport	Unknown/unspecified
9	Unintentional overexertion	Unknown/unspecified	Unintentional other transport	Unintentional other bite/ sting	Unintentional other transport
10	Unintentional cut/pierce	Unintentional poisoning	Unknown/unspecified	Unintentional dog bite	Unintentional poisoning

15.2.2 Specific injuries

Motor vehicle injuries	• Leading cause of death 3-14 yrs of age • 6% of pedestrian fatalities are <15 yrs of age • 16% of motor vehicle deaths <15 yrs of age are related to alcohol impairment • Safety seats reduce fatalities by 71% in infants and 54% in toddlers • From 1995-2005, all-terrain vehicles killed at least 1,218 children under 16 yrs of age, accounting for 27% of all ATV-related deaths in this period
Bicycle injuries	• In 2008, 93 children aged 5-15 yrs were killed on bicycles • In 2008, 13,000 children <16 were injured on bicycles
Drowning	• Two peaks: Infant/toddlers and adolescents – Bathtubs are main location <1 year of age – Other infant/toddler locations: toilets, buckets, pools • Boys 3 times at risk • Risk factors: Access, alcohol, lack of supervision, lack of education • Pool isolation fencing more effective than property perimeter fencing
Fires	• 40% of home fire deaths are in homes without smoke alarms • Most victims die from smoke or toxic gases, not burns • Children, elderly, and poor are at highest risk
Choking and suffocation	• 60% choking from food, especially candy and hot dogs • 31% choking from non-food items, especially coins
Playground injuries	• 45% of playground related injuries are severe: fractures, concussions, dislocations, amputations • Of playground deaths, 56% are from strangulation and 20% from falls • In home playgrounds, swings cause most injuries • In public playgrounds, climbing is associated with most injuries
Overexertion and overuse	• Overexertion is 3rd leading cause of nonfatal injuries • Overuse injuries cause half of sports injuries in adolescents • Risk factors: insufficient hydration, inadequate rest breaks in hot weather, insufficient rest after injury

Poisons	• 50% of poisons affect children < 6 yrs of age • Poison Control telephone is 1-800-222-1222 • Top 10 child ingestions: – Cosmetics – Cleaners – Analgesics – Coins, thermometers – Plants – Topical medications – Cough/cold medications – Pesticides – Vitamins/iron – Gastrointestinal medications

List of References

96 American Academy of Pediatrics Section on Radiology. Diagnostic imaging of child abuse. Pediatrics 2009; 123:1430-1435.

97 Kellogg ND and the Committee on Child Abuse and Neglect. Evaluation of suspected child physical abuse. Pediatrics 2007; 119:1232-1241.

98 Kellogg ND and the Committee on Child Abuse and Neglect. The evaluation of sexual abuse in children. Pediatrics 2005; 116:506-512.

99 Brown P, Tierney C. Munchausen syndrome by proxy. Pediatrics in Review 2009;30:414-415.

100 Centers for Disease Control and Preventions: Injury, Violence & Safety. http://cdc.gov/InjuryViolenceSafety (accessed 12/6/2011)

16 Drug Chapter

Note: All below are contraindicated with hypersensitivity to drug, class, or component. Other specific contraindications (CI) are listed below.

16.1 Emergency

MA/EF (albuterol): Selectively stimulates beta-2 adrenergic receptors, relaxing airway smooth muscle
MA/EF (amiodarone): Prolongs action potential phase 3 (class III antiarrhythmic)
MA/EF (methylprednisolone) exact mechanism of anti-inflammatory action unknown; inhibits multiple inflammatory cytokines; produces multiple glucocorticoid and mineralocorticoid effects
MA/EF (propranolol) non-selectively antagonizes beta-1 and beta-2 adrenergic receptors
MA/EF (terbutaline) selectively stimulates beta-2 adrenergic receptors, relaxing airway smooth muscle
MA/EF (verapamil) inhibits calcium ion influx into vascular smooth muscle and myocardium
AE (albuterol) Serious: hypersensitivity reactions, paradoxical bronchospasm, HTN, angina, MI, hypokalemia, arrhythmias, metabolic acidosis; Common: throat irritation, URI sx, cough, bad taste, tremor, dizziness, nervousness, nausea, headache, palpitations, tachycardia
AE (amiodarone) Serious: Bradycardia, severe, AV block, QT prolongation, torsades de pointes, worsened or new ventricular arrhythmias, CHF, hypotension, severe, cardiogenic shock, cardiac arrest, pulmonary toxicity, ARDS, hypersensitivity reaction, skin reactions, severe, rash w/ eosinophilia and systemic sx, hypo- or hyperthyroidism, neonatal gasping syndrome (benzyl alcohol-containing IV forms), rhabdomyolysis, hepatotoxicity, pancreatitis, hallucinations, peripheral neuropathy (long-term use), optic neuritis/neuropathy, blood dyscrasias; Common: corneal deposits (>6 mo use), malaise/fatigue, ataxia, tremor, hyperkinesia, peripheral neuropathy (long-term use), nausea/vomiting, constipation, anorexia, hypotension, pulmonary toxicity, photosensitivity, visual disturbances, dizziness, bradycardia, worsened arrhythmias, elevated LFT, cardiac arrest, CHF, tachycardia, ventricular, ARDS, hypo- or hyperthyroidism
AE (methylprednisolone) Safety: anaphylaxis/anaphylactoid reaction, HPA axis suppression, hyperglycemia, IOP incr., glaucoma, cataracts, growth suppression (long-term use, peds pts), infection, cardiac arrest, arrhythmias, CHF, pulmonary edema, syncope, thromboembolism, vasculitis, osteoporosis, steroid psychosis, GI ulceration/perforation, pancreatitis, pseudotumor cerebri, convulsions, Kaposi sarcoma, tendon rupture, Charcot-like arthropathy, steroid myopathy, angioedema; Common: IOP incr., glucose intolerance, sodium and fluid retention, hypokalemia, HTN, edema, rash, skin disorder, skin atrophy (long-term use), impaired wound healing (long-term use), weight gain, appetite incr., emotional lability, depression, hyperhidrosis, Cushing syndrome (long-term use), hirsutism, menstrual irregularities, nausea, LFTs elevated, hepatomegaly, muscle weakness, muscle atrophy, headache, insomnia, paresthesia, vertigo, neuropathy, psychiatric disorders

AE (propranolo) Serious: CHF, heart block, severe bradycardia, Raynaud phenomenon, bronchospasm, lupus erythematosus, hypersensitivity reaction, Stevens-Johnson syndrome, toxic epidermal necrolysis, exfoliative dermatitis, erythema multiforme, anaphylactic/ anaphylactoid reactions, agranulocytosis; Common: fatigue, dizziness, constipation, bradycardia, hypotension, depression, insomnia, weakness, disorientation, nausea, diarrhea, allergic reaction, purpura, alopecia, impotence
AE (terbutaline) Serious: hypersensitivity reaction, paradoxical bronchospasm, HTN, QT prolongation, arrhythmias, myocardial ischemia, pulmonary edema, hypokalemia, hyperglycemia, seizures, reactive neonatal hypoglycemia, fetal tachycardia; Common: nervousness, tremor, headache, tachycardia, palpitations, drowsiness, nausea, vomiting, sweating, muscle cramps, hypokalemia, hyperglycemia
AE (verapamil): Serious: CHF, severe hypotension, AV block, severe bradycardia, hepatotoxicity, paralytic ileus; Common: constipation, dizziness, nausea, hypotension, headache, edema, CHF, fatigue
CI (albuterol) caution if ischemic heart disease, HTN, arrhythmias, hypokalemia, DM, seizure disorder, hyperthyroidism, pheochromocytoma, pregnancy
CI: (amiodarone) Hypersens to iodine, cardiogenic shock, sinus node dysfunction, severe, 2nd or 3rd degree AV block, syncope, bradycardia-assoc. (w/o pacemaker), neonates or infants (benzyl alcohol-containing INJ forms), pregnancy, breastfeeding; caution if pulmonary disease, thyroid disease, hepatic impairment, QT prolongation, hypokalemia, hypomagnesemia, implantable cardiac device, surgery
CI (methylprednisolone) intrathecal administration, neonates or premature infants (benzyl alcohol-containing INJ forms), thrombocytopenic purpura (IM use), systemic fungal infection, active or recent varicella infection, active or recent measles infection, local infection at injection site, head injury (high dose use), cerebral malaria, avoid abrupt withdrawal, ocular HSV infection, active; caution if ocular HSV infection, inactive, optic neuritis, amebiasis infection, Strongyloides infection, TB infection, recent MI, CHF, HTN, renal impairment, hypo- or hyperthyroidism, GI perforation risk, cirrhosis, osteoporosis, osteoporosis risk, myasthenia gravis, psychiatric disorder, DM
CI (propranolol) cardiogenic shock, sinus bradycardia w/o pacemaker, sick sinus syndrome w/o pacemaker, 2nd or 3rd degree AV block w/o pacemaker, uncompensated heart failure, asthma, avoid abrupt withdrawal; caution if peripheral vascular disease, bronchospastic disease, major surgery, DM, thyroid disorder, WPW syndrome, renal/hepatic impairment, pheochromocytoma, pregnancy 2nd or 3rd trimester, myasthenia gravis, severe anaphylactic reaction hx, caution if musculoskeletal disease
CI (terbutaline): acute or maintenance tocolysis (PO use), prolonged tocolysis >48-72h (SC/ IV use); caution if arrhythmias, cardiovascular disease, HTN, hyperthyroidism, DM, seizure disorder
CI (verapamil) severe LV dysfunction, 2nd or 3rd degree AV block, atrial fibrillation or flutter w/ bypass tract, sick sinus syndrome, severe hypotension, cardiogenic shock, caution if CHF, bradycardia, IHSS, hepatic impairment, renal impairment, muscular dystrophy, myasthenia gravis, GERD, smoking habit changes

Albuterol	PRC C, Lact?
Ventolin HFA, ProAir HFA, Proventil HFA MDI108 µg (90 base)/puff *AccuNeb, Albuterol inhaled neb solution 5 mg/mL, 0.63 mg/3mL, 1.25 mg/3mL, 2.5 mg/3mL*	**Asthma/bronchospasm:** 1-2puffs q4-6h prn; Nebulizer solution: <2y: 0.05-0.15 mg/kg q4-6h, max 1.25 mg/dose; 2-5y: 0.1-0.15 mg/kg q4-6h prn; max 2.5 mg/dose; alt: 1.25-2.5 mg q4-6h prn; >5y: 2.5 mg q4-6h prn, max 10 mg/d
Amiodarone	PRC D, Lact +
Cordarone *Inj 50mg/ml*	**PALS:** VF/pulseless VT, SVT,VT: 5 mg/kg IV/IOx1, max 300 mg/dose, may repeat up to 15 mg/kg
Methylprednisolone	PRC C Lact -
Solu-Medrol *Inj 0.04, 0.125, 0.5g, 1, 2g/vial*	**Status asthmaticus:** 0.5-1 mg/kg IV q6h; 2 mg/kg x1
Propranolol	PRC C, Lact -
Inderal *Inj 1mg/ml; PO 10, 20, 40, 60, 80 mg tabs; 20/5mL, 40/5mL susp*	**HTN:** 1-5 mg/kg/d PO div q6-12h, start 0.5-1 mg/kg/d PO div q6-12h, may incr dose q3-5 d, max 8 mg/kg/d, taper gradually to d/c; Migraine prophylaxis: <35 kg: 10-20 mg PO tid; >35 kg: 20-40 mg PO tid, taper gradually to d/c
Terbutaline	PRC C, Lact -
Bricanyl *Inj 1mg/ml; PO 2.5, 5 mg*	**Asthma:** 6-12yo: 0.05 mg/kg PO tid, q6h while awake, max 0.15 mg/kg/dose or 5 mg/d PO; 0.4 mg/dose SC; alt 0.005-0.01 mg/kg SC q15-30min x2; 12-15yo: 2.5 mg PO tid, q6h while awake, max 7.5 mg/d PO, 0.5 mg/4h SC, alt 0.25 mg SC q15-30 min x2; >15yo: 2.5-5 mg PO tid, q6h while awake, max 15 mg/d PO, 0.5 mg/4h SC, alt 0.25 mg SC q15-30min x2.
Verapamil	PRC C Lact +
Isoptin *Inj 2.5mg/ml; PO 40, 80, 120 mg*	**PSVT conversion:** <1yo: 0.1-0.2 mg/kg IV x1, may repeat x1 in 30min; 1-15yo: 0.1-0.3 mg/kg IV x1, max 5 mg 1st dose, may give 2nd dose up to 10 mg in 30min **HTN:** 4-8 mg/kg/d PO div tid, max 480 mg/d

16.2 Cardiovascular

MA/EF (amiodarone) prolongs action potential phase 3 (class III antiarrhythmic)
MA/EF (guanfacine) stimulates alpha-2 adrenergic receptors (centrally-acting antihypertensive)
MA/EF (mipomersen sodium): reduces LDL-C by preventing the formation of atherogenic lipoproteins; for patients with homozygous familial hypercholesterolemia
MA/EF (procainamide) stabilizes membranes; depresses action potential phase 0 (class IA antiarrhythmic)
AE (amiodarone) Serious: bradycardia, severe, AV block, QT prolongation, torsades de pointes, worsened or new ventricular arrhythmias, CHF, hypotension, severe, cardiogenic shock, cardiac arrest, pulmonary toxicity, ARDS, hypersensitivity reaction, skin reactions, severe, rash w/ eosinophilia and systemic sx, hypo- or hyperthyroidism, neonatal gasping syndrome (benzyl alcohol-containing IV forms), rhabdomyolysis, hepatotoxicity, pancreatitis, hallucinations, peripheral neuropathy (long-term use), optic neuritis/ neuropathy, blood dyscrasias; Common: corneal deposits (>6mo use), malaise/fatigue, ataxia, tremor, hyperkinesia, peripheral neuropathy (long-term use), nausea/vomiting, constipation, anorexia, hypotension, pulmonary toxicity, photosensitivity, visual disturbances, dizziness, bradycardia, worsened arrhythmias, elevated LFT, cardiac arrest, CHF, tachycardia, ventricular, ARDS, hypo- or hyperthyroidism
AE (guanfacine) Serious: syncope, bradycardia, rebound HTN on withdrawal; Common: dry mouth, somnolence, dizziness, constipation, fatigue, asthenia, headache, impotence; Common: dry mouth, somnolence, dizziness, constipation, fatigue, asthenia, headache, impotence
AE (procainamide) Serious: ventricular fibrillation, asystole, seizures, thrombocytopenia, neutropenia, hemolytic anemia, lupus erythematosus, agranulocytosis; Common: hypotension, bradycardia, flushing, urticarial, pruritus, angioedema, rash, fever, nausea, bitter taste, hallucinations, confusion, depression, vomiting, diarrhea, LFTs elevated, dizziness
CI (amiodarone) hypersens. to iodine, cardiogenic shock, sinus node dysfunction, severe, 2nd or 3rd degree AV block, syncope, bradycardia-assoc. (w/o pacemaker), neonates or infants (benzyl alcohol-containing INJ forms), pregnancy, breastfeeding; caution if pulmonary disease, thyroid disease, hepatic impairment, QT prolongation, hypokalemia, hypomagnesemia, implantable cardiac device, surgery
CI (guanfacine) avoid abrupt withdrawal; caution if hepatic/renal impairment, cardiovascular disease, recent MI, CAD
CI (mipomersen sodium): liver disease or abnormal LFT, known hypersensitivity
CI (procainamide) 2nd or 3rd degree AV block, myasthenia gravis, SLE, torsades de pointes; caution if bone marrow depression, renal impairment, CHF

Amiodarone	PRC D, Lact +
Cordarone *Inj 50mg/ml*	**PALS:** VF/pulseless VT, SVT,VT: 5 mg/kg IV/IOx1, max 300 mg/dose, may repeat up to 15 mg/kg

Guanfacine	PRC B, Lact ?
Tenex, Intuniv *1,2*	**ADHD**, 27-40.5 kg: 0.5 mg PO bid-qid; Start: 0.5 mg PO qhs, then may incr. by 0.5 mg/d qwk up to 1.5 mg/d, then may incr. to 2 mg/d after 2wk; Max: 0.5 mg/dose, 2 mg/d; 40.5-45 kg: 0.5 mg PO bid-qid; Start: 0.5 mg PO qhs, then may incr. by 0.5 mg/d qwk up to 1.5 mg/d, then may incr. by 0.5 mg/d q2wk; Max: 1 mg/dose, 3 mg/d; >45 kg: 1 mg PO bid-qid; Start: 1 mg PO qhs, then may incr. by 1 mg/d qwk up to 3 mg/d, then may incr. to 4 mg/d after 2wk; Max: 1 mg/dose, 4 mg/d; Info: taper dose gradually over 4-7 d to D/C
Mipomersen sodium	PRC B, Lact -
Kynamro inj	**Hypercholesterolemia**: SC- The recommended dose is 200 mg/wk
Procainamide	PRC C, Lact -
Procainamide *250,375,500; IM; IV*	**Ventricular & supraventricular arrhythmias:** 20-80 µg/kg/min IV; Start: load 15 mg/kg IV over at least 30min, or 3-6 mg/kg up to 100 mg IV q5-10min; Alt: 15-30 mg/kg/d PO div q3-6h or 20-30 mg/kg/d IM div q4-6h; Max: 15 mg/kg load; 2 g/d IV, 4 g/d PO/IM maintenance **PALS, SVT & VT**: 15mg/kg IV x1; Info: may give additional doses if no response; not 1st-line tx

16.3 Hematology

MA/EF (aminocaproic acid) competitively inhibits plasminogen binding sites, decreasing plasmin formation and fibrinolysis
MA/EF (aspirin) non-selectively and irreversibly inhibits cyclooxygenase, reducing prostaglandin and thromboxane A2 synthesis, producing analgesic, anti-inflammatory, and antipyretic effects and reducing platelet aggregation
MA/EF supplies Factor VIII and von Willebrand factor, promoting coagulation
AE (aminocaproic acid) Serious: anaphylaxis, coagulation disorders, agranulocytosis, leukopenia, thrombocytopenia, thrombosis, rhabdomyolysis, intracranial HTN, stroke, seizures, acute renal failure, bradycardia (IV), arrhythmia (IV), neonatal gasping syndrome (benzyl alcohol-containing injectable forms); Common: nausea, cramps, diarrhea, HTN, headache, rash, dizziness, dyspnea, myopathy, edema

AE (aspirin) Serious: anaphylactic/anaphylactoid reactions, angioedema, bronchospasm, bleeding, GI ulceration/perforation, DIC, pancytopenia, thrombocytopenia, agranulocytosis, aplastic anemia, hypoprothrombinemia, nephrotoxicity, hepatotoxicity (high-dose ASA use), salicylism, Reye syndrome; Common: dyspepsia, nausea, vomiting, abdominal pain, rash, tinnitus, dizziness, hyperuricemia, bleeding, ecchymosis, constipation, diarrhea
AE Serious: anaphylaxis/anaphylactoid reaction, viral transmission risk, thromboembolism; Common: urticarial, dizziness
CI (Aminocaproic acid) active intravascular clotting, neonates or premature infants (benzyl alcohol-containing IV forms); caution if hematuria, subarachnoid hemorrhage, cardiovascular disease, renal or hepatic impairment
CI (aspirin) ASA or NSAID-induced asthma or urticaria, aspirin triad, GI bleed, coagulation disorder, G6PD deficiency, uncontrolled HTN; influenza, varicella, or febrile viral infection (pts <20 yo); caution if thrombocytopenia, surgery or trauma, intracranial lesion, ICP incr., chronic alcohol use, PUD, GI bleed hx, GERD, gout (high-dose ASA use), renal impairment , hepatic impairment sodium restriction (buffered ASA forms)
CI caution if thrombosis risk

Aminocaproic acid	PRC C, Lact?
Aminocaproic acid (generic) *500 mg, 1000 mg; 250/ml sol; IV*	**Bleeding, hyperfibrinolysis:** 100-200 mg/kg IV/PO x1, then 100 mg/kg IV/PO q4-6h; Max 30 g/d
Aspirin	PRC D, Lact +
Aspirin *81,325,500,350; 81 CH; 81,325, 500,650 DR; 60,120,200,300,600 PR*	**Pain/fever:** 10-15 mg/kg PO/PR q4-6h; Max: 60-80 mg/kg/d **JIA**: 60-100 mg/kg/d PO div q6-8h; Start: 60 mg/kg/d; Max: 100 mg/kg/d; Info: incr. 10-20 mg/kg/d q5-7 ds **Kawasaki disease**: 80-100 mg/kg/d PO div q6h; decr. to 3-5 mg/kg PO qd after fever resolves; total duration x8wk
von Willebrand factor complex	PRC C, Lact ?
Alphanate, Humate-P, Wilate *IV*	**von Willebrand disease:** consult pediatric hematologist

16.4 Respiratory

MA/EF (albuterol) stimulates beta-2 adrenergic receptors, relaxing airway smooth muscle
MA/EF (beclomethasone dipropionate): an anti-inflammatory steroid for seasonal and perennial allergic rhinitis
MA/EF (budesonide) inhaled and nasal: exact mechanism of anti-inflammatory action unknown; inhibits multiple inflammatory cytokines; produces multiple glucocorticoid and mineralocorticoid effects
MA/EF (codeine sulfate) binds to various opioid receptors, producing analgesia, sedation and antitussive effects (opioid agonist)

MA/EF (ethambutol) inhibits metabolite synthesis
MA/EF (fluticasone) exact mechanism of anti-inflammatory action unknown; inhibits multiple inflammatory cytokines; produces multiple glucocorticoid and mineralocorticoid effects
MA/EF (fluticasone/salmeterol) see individual drugs
MA/EF (ipratropium) antagonizes acetylcholine receptors, producing bronchodilation
MA/EF (levalbuterol) selectively stimulates beta-2 adrenergic receptors, relaxing airway smooth muscle
MA/EF (lucinactant): non-pyrogenic pulmonary surfactant; compensates for the deficiency of surfactant and restores surface activity to the lungs of these infants
MA/EF (mometasone nasal) exact mechanism of anti-inflammatory action unknown; inhibits multiple inflammatory cytokines; produces multiple glucocorticoid and mineralocorticoid effects
MA/EF (montelukast) selectively binds to cysteinyl leukotriene receptors (leukotriene inhibitor)
MA/EF (omalizumab) inhibits IgE binding to mast cells and basophils, decreasing mediator release
MA/EF (salmeterol inhaled) selectively stimulates beta-2 adrenergic receptors, relaxing airway smooth muscle
MA/EF (theophylline) exact mechanism of action unknown; increases cAMP; antagonizes adenosine receptors (methylxanthine)
MA/EF (triamcinolone nasal) exact mechanism of anti-inflammatory action unknown; inhibits multiple inflammatory cytokines; produces multiple glucocorticoid and mineralocorticoid effects
MA/EF (zileuton) inhibits 5-lipoxygenase, interfering w/ leukotriene formation (leukotriene inhibitor)
AE: (albuterol) Serious: hypersensitivity reactions, paradoxical bronchospasm, HTN, angina, MI, hypokalemia, arrhythmias, metabolic acidosis; Common: throat irritation, URI sx, cough, bad taste, tremor, dizziness, nervousness, nausea, headache, palpitations, tachycardia
AE (beclomethasone dipropionate): nasal discomfort, epistaxis, headache
AE (budesonide) inhaled: Serious: anaphylaxis, bronchospasm, hypersensitivity reaction, angioedema, hypercortisolism, adrenal suppression, Cushing syndrome, growth suppression, eosinophilia, Churg-Strauss syndrome, glaucoma, cataracts, osteoporosis; Common: URI, rhinitis, cough, otitis media, viral infection, oral candidiasis, gastroenteritis, vomiting, diarrhea, abdominal pain, epistaxis, conjunctivitis, rash
AE (budesonide) nasal: Serious: nasal septal perforation, nasal/oral candida, growth suppression, IOP incr., hypercortisolism, adrenal suppression, hypersensitivity reaction, angioedema, bronchospasm, wheezing; Common: epistaxis, pharyngitis, cough, nasal irritation, bronchospasm
AE (codeine sulfate) Serious: respiratory depression, CNS depression, hypotension, bradycardia, syncope, shock, cardiac arrest, ICP incr., seizures, paralytic ileus, dependency/abuse, withdrawal if abrupt D/C, anaphylactoid reactions; Common: lightheadedness,

dizziness, sedation, nausea/vomiting, sweating, dry mouth, anorexia, constipation, urinary hesitancy/retention, weakness, flushing, pruritus, urticarial, headache, rash, visual disturbances, edema, disorientation, euphoria, dysphoria, insomnia, agitation, biliary spasm, palpitations

AE (ethambutol) Serious: anaphylaxis, hypersensitivity syndrome, erythema multiforme, thrombocytopenia, neutropenia, leukopenia, optic neuritis, irreversible blindness, peripheral neuropathy, pulmonary infiltrates, hepatotoxicity; Common: blurred vision, joint pain, anorexia, nausea, vomiting, dyspepsia, abdominal pain, fever, malaise, headache, dizziness, disorientation, hallucinations, rash, hyperuricemia, LFTs elevated, pruritus

AE (fluticasone) propionate nasal: Serious: nasal septal perforation, nasal ulcer, nasal/oral candidiasis, growth suppression, IOP incr., glaucoma, cataracts, hypercortisolism, adrenal suppression, anaphylaxis, angioedema, bronchospasm, wheezing, dyspnea, Common: headache, pharyngitis, epistaxis, nasal burning, nasal irritation, nausea, vomiting, asthma symptoms, cough, dizziness, rhinorrhea, bronchitis, diarrhea, pyrexia, abdominal pain,

AE (fluticasone) inhaled: Serious: bronchospasm, angioedema, anaphylactoid reactions, adrenal suppression, hypercortisolism, growth suppression, eosinophilia, Churg-Strauss syndrome, hyperglycemia, glaucoma, cataracts, osteoporosis, behavioral disturbances; Common: URI, headache, throat irritation, sinusitis, oral candidiasis, pharyngitis, hoarseness, dysphonia, cough, rhinitis, nausea/vomiting, myalgia/arthralgia, rash, pruritus

AE (fluticasone/salmeterol) Serious: paradoxical bronchospasm, asthma exacerbation/death, pneumonia, laryngospasm, angioedema, growth suppression, adrenal suppression, hypercorticalism, ventricular arrhythmias, severe hypokalemia, glaucoma, cataracts, Churg-Strauss syndrome, behavioral disturbances; Common: URI, headache, pharyngitis, cough, sinusitis, nausea/vomiting, dyspepsia, bronchitis, hoarseness, dysphonia, throat irritation, dizziness, palpitations, tremor, taste changes, diarrhea, dermatitis, hypokalemia, oral candidiasis

AE (ipratropium) Serious: hypersensitivity reaction, anaphylaxis, angioedema, laryngospasm, paradoxical bronchospasm, angle-closure glaucoma; Common: cough, nervousness, nausea, dry mouth, GI upset, dizziness, headache, COPD exacerbation, oral irritation, rash/urticaria

AE (levalbuterol) Serious: paradoxical bronchospasm, anaphylaxis, angioedema, MI, cardiac arrest, arrhythmias, hypokalemia; Common: palpitations, dizziness, nervousness, tremor, tachycardia, headache, chest pain, dry mouth, asthenia, rhinitis

AE (lucinactant): ETT reflux, pallor, ETT obstruction, dose interruption

AE (mometasone nasal) Serious: nasal septal perforation, nasal ulcer, nasal/oral candidiasis, growth suppression (peds pts), IOP incr., glaucoma, hypercorticalism, adrenal suppression, anaphylaxis, angioedema; Common: headache, viral infection, pharyngitis, epistaxis, cough, URI, dysmenorrhea, musculoskeletal pain, arthralgia, sinusitis, nausea/vomiting, asthma symptoms, bronchitis, diarrhea, nasal irritation, nasal burning, conjunctivitis, otitis media, wheezing (peds pts), chest pain, dyspepsia, influenza-like sx

AE (montelukast) Serious: angioedema, anaphylaxis, erythema nodosum, Churg-Strauss syndrome, hepatic eosinophilic infiltration, hepatotoxicity, aggressive behavior, hallucinations, depression, suicidality, thrombocytopenia, erythema multiforme; Common:

AE (montelukast) cont.headache, influenza-like sx, abdominal pain, cough, dizziness, fatigue, asthenia, rash, fever, nausea, diarrhea, dyspepsia, gastroenteritis, ALT, AST, bilirubin elevated, pruritus, urticarial, otitis media, URI sx, sleep disorders, anxiety/irritability, restlessness, tremor

AE (omalizumab) Serious: anaphylaxis, malignancy, severe thrombocytopenia, severe injection site reactions; Common: injection site reaction, viral infection, URI, sinusitis, headache, pharyngitis, geohelminth infection, arthralgia, pain, fatigue, dizziness, pruritus, dermatitis, earache, fractures

AE (salmeterol inhaled) Serious: paradoxical bronchospasm, asthma exacerbation, asthma-related death, anaphylaxis, angioedema, laryngospasm, arrhythmias, HTN; Common: headache, throat irritation, nasal congestion, rhinitis, tracheitis/bronchitis, pharyngitis, urticarial, rash, palpitations, tachycardia, tremor, nervousness

AE (theophylline) Serious: seizures, arrhythmias, hypotension, shock, exfoliative dermatitis; Common: nausea,
Vomiting, headache, insomnia, diarrhea, irritability, restlessness, tremor, transient diuresis

AE (triamcinolone nasal) Serious: nasal septal perforation, nasal/oral candidiasis, growth suppression, IOP incr., glaucoma, cataracts, hypercorticalism, adrenal suppression; Common: pharyngitis, epistaxis, cough, headache, vomiting, asthma, infection, otitis media, sinusitis

AE (zileuton) Severe: hepatotoxicity, behavioral disturbances; Common: headache, sinusitis, nausea, pharyngolaryngeal pain, URI, dyspepsia, abdominal pain, myalgia, diarrhea, ALT/AST elevated, leukopenia, sleep disorders

CI (albuterol) caution if ischemic heart disease, HTN, arrhythmias, hypokalemia, DM, seizure disorder, hyperthyroidism, pheochromocytoma, pregnancy

CI (beclomethasone dipropionate): Hypersensitivity

CI (budesonide) inhaled: status asthmaticus, acute asthma or bronchospasm, avoid abrupt withdrawal; caution if untreated local or systemic infection, TB, ocular HSV, measles or varicella exposure, recent long-term systemic corticosteroid tx, glaucoma, incr. IOP, cataracts

CI (budesonide) nasal: unhealed nasal septal ulcer or wound; caution if untreated local or systemic infection, TB, ocular HSV, measles or varicella exposure, recurrent epistaxis, IOP incr., glaucoma, recent long-term systemic corticosteroid tx

CI (codeine sulfate) respiratory depression, paralytic ileus; caution if CNS depression, head injury, ICP incr., seizure disorder, asthma, COPD, acute abdomen, GI/GU obstruction, inflammatory bowel disease, pseudomembranous colitis, biliary disease, urethral stricture, prostatic hypertrophy, severe renal or hepatic impairment, hypothyroidism, Addison disease, alcohol or drug abuse hx, ultra-rapid CYP2D6 metabolizer, pts <2 yo

CI (ethambutol) optic neuritis; caution if gout, eye disorder, renal impairment, concurrent neurotoxic agents, in pts <8 yo, unconscious pts

CI (fluticasone) propionate nasal: unhealed nasal septal ulcer, unhealed nasal surgery or trauma wound; caution if untreated local or systemic infection, TB infection, ocular HSV infection, measles or varicella exposure, recurrent epistaxis, IOP incr., glaucoma, cataracts, recent long-term systemic corticosteroid tx

CI (fluticasone/salmeterol) severe hypersens. to milk protein, status asthmaticus, acute asthma/bronchospasm; caution if HTN, cardiovascular disease, arrhythmias, hypokalemia, DM, seizure disorder, hyperthyroidism, pheochromocytoma, hepatic impairment, untreated local or systemic infection, TB infection, ocular HSV, measles or varicella exposure, recent long-term systemic corticosteroid tx, glaucoma, IOP incr., cataracts, decr. BMD hx, decr. BMD risk
CI (ipratropium) caution if angle-closure glaucoma, prostatic hypertrophy, bladder neck obstruction
CI (levalbuterol) MAO inhibitor use w/in 14 ds; caution if arrhythmias, CAD, HTN, hypokalemia, DM, seizure disorder, hyperthyroidism, pheochromocytoma
CI (mometasone nasal) unhealed nasal septal ulcer, unhealed nasal surgery or trauma wound; caution if untreated local or systemic infection, TB infection, ocular HSV infection, measles or varicella exposure, recurrent epistaxis, glaucoma, cataracts, vision changes, recent long-term systemic corticosteroid tx
CI (montelukast) caution if severe hepatic disease, severe asthma, tapering systemic steroids, PKU (phenylalanine-containing forms)
CI (omalizumab) acute bronchospasm, status asthmaticus
CI (salmeterol inhaled) asthma monotherapy, acute asthma; caution if HTN, cardiovascular disease, arrhythmias, hypokalemia, hyperthyroidism, DM, seizure disorder, pheochromocytoma
CI (theophylline) caution if active PUD, seizure disorder, arrhythmias, CHF, acute pulmonary edema, cor pulmonale, hepatic impairment, hypothyroidism, febrile, sepsis w/ multi-organ failure, shock, smoking habit changes, neonates or infants
CI (triamcinolone nasal) unhealed nasal septal ulcer, unhealed nasal surgery or trauma wound; caution if untreated local or systemic infection, TB infection, ocular HSV infection, measles or varicella exposure, recurrent epistaxis, IOP incr., glaucoma, cataracts, recent long-term systemic corticosteroid tx
CI (zileuton) status asthmaticus, acute asthma, active hepatic disease, AST or ALT >3x ULN; caution if hepatic disease hx, alcohol abuse

Albuterol	PRC C, Lact -
Ventolin HFA, ProAir HFA, Proventil HFA MDI108 μg (90 base)/puff *AccuNeb, Albuterol inhaled neb solution 5 mg/mL, 0.63 mg/3mL, 1.25 mg/3mL, 2.5 mg/3mL*	**Asthma/bronchospasm**: 1-2puffs q4-6h prn; Nebulizer solution: <2y: 0.05-0.15 mg/kg q4-6h, max 1.25 mg/dose; 2-5y: 0.1-0.15 mg/kg q4-6h prn; max 2.5 mg/dose; alt: 1.25-2.5 mg q4-6h prn; >5y: 2.5 mg q4-6h prn, max 10 mg/d
Beclomethasone dipropionate	PRC C, Lact -?
Qnasl *Inh*	**Allergic rhinitis** 320 mcg/d as 2 nasal aerosol sprays in each nostril (80 mcg/aerosol spray od), (maximum total daily dose of four nasal aerosol sprays/d)

Budesonide	PRC B, Lact -
Budesonide inhaled, Pulmicort Flexhaler 90, 180 µg/actuation DPI; Pulmicort Respules *0.25, 0.5, 1 mg/2ml neb*	**Asthma**, maintenance tx, 1-8y; prior bronchodilator alone: 0.25-0.5 mg/d div qd-bid; Start 0.25-0.5 mg/d div qd-bid; Max: 0.5 mg/d; prior inhaled steroid: 0.25-1 mg/d div qd-bid; Start 0.5 mg/d div qd-bid; Max: 1 mg/d; prior oral steroid: 0.25-1 mg/d div qd-bid; Start 1 mg/d div qd-bid; Max: 1 mg/d; taper oral steroids gradually after >1 wk; Info: titrate to lowest effective dose; do not mix w/ other nebulized meds; rinse mouth after use
Budesonide nasal, Rhinocort Aqua *32 µg/spray*	**Allergic rhinitis**, 6-12y: 1-2 sprays/nostril/d; Start 1 spray/nostril/d; Max: 2 sprays/nostril/d; <12y: 1-4 sprays/nostril/d; Start 1 spray/nostril/d; Max: 4 sprays/nostril/d; Info: d/c after 3 wk if no improvement
Codeine sulfate	PRC C, Lact ?
Codeine *15, 30, 60*	Mild-moderate pain, 3-6y: 0.5-1 mg/kg PO q4-6h prn; Max: 60 mg/dose, 360 mg/d; 7-12y: 15-30 mg PO q4-6h prn; Max: 60 mg/dose, 360 mg/d; Alt: 0.5-1 mg/kg PO q4-6h prn; 13-17y: 15-60 mg PO q4-6h prn; Max: 60 mg/dose, 360 mg/d; Alt: 0.5-1 mg/kg PO q4-6h prn **Cough**, 2-5y: 1-1.5 mg/kg/d PO div q4-6h prn; Max: 30 mg/d; 6-11y: 1-1.5 mg/kg/d PO div q4-6h prn; Max: 60 mg/d; >12y: 15-30 mg PO q4-6h prn; Max: 120 mg/d Info for all: give w/ food
Ethambutol	PRC C, Lact -
Myambutol *100,400*	**Active TB**, <5y: 15 mg/kg PO qd; Max: 1000 mg/d; only for isoniazid or rifampin resistance; >5y: 15-20 mg/kg PO qd; Max: 1000 mg/d; Alt: 50 mg/kg PO 2x/wk if directly observed, max 2500 mg/dose; Info for all ages: part of multi-drug regimen

Fluticasone	PRC C, Lact ?
Flonase (nasal) *50 µg/spray* **Flovent HFA** *44,110,220 µg/spray MDI* **Flovent Diskus** *50,100,250 µg/blister DPI*	**Allergic rhinitis**, >4y: 1-2 sprays per nostril qd; Start: 1 spray per nostril qd; Max: 2 sprays per nostril/d **Asthma** maintenance, prior tx, 4-11y: 88 µg inhaled bid; Max: 176 µg/d; prior bronchodilator alone, >12y: 88-440 µg inhaled bid; Start: 88 µg inhaled bid; Max: 880 µg/d; prior inhaled steroid, >12 yo, 88-440 µg inhaled bid; Start: 88-220 µg inhaled bid; Max: 880 µg/d; prior oral steroid, >12 yo, 440-880 µg inhaled bid; Start: 440 µg inhaled bid; Max: 1760 µg/d; Info for all: rinse mouth after use; taper oral steroids gradually after >1wk; titrate to lowest effective dose
Fluticasone/Salmeterol	PRC C, Lact ?
Advair Diskus *100/50, 250/50, 500/50 µg/ blister DPI*	**Asthma** maintenance, 4-11y: 100/50 µg inhaled bid; >12y: 1 puff inhaled bid; Start: varies per disease severity and current asthma tx; Max: 500/50 µg inhaled bid; Info: for pts not controlled on long-term asthma control tx; taper to lowest effective dose; use shortest effective tx duration; not for transferring pts from chronic systemic steroids
Advair HFA *45/21, 115/21, 230/21 µg/spray MDI*	**Asthma** maintenance, >12y: 2 puffs inhaled bid; Start: varies per disease severity and current asthma tx; Max: 460/42 µg inhaled bid; Info: for pts not controlled on long-term asthma control tx; may incr. after 2wk to higher strength; taper to lowest effective dose; use shortest effective tx duration; not for transferring pts from chronic systemic steroids
Ipratropium	PRC B, Lact ?
Atrovent *0.5 mg/2.5 mL neb*	**Acute asthma**, adjunct tx, 5-12y: 0.125-0.25 mg neb q6-8h; >12y: 0.25-0.5 mg neb q6-8h; Info: may mix neb sol w/ albuterol, levalbuterol, or metaproterenol if used w/in 1h

Levalbuterol	PRC C, Lact ?
Xopenex *0.31,0.63,1.25/3 mL neb* **Xopenex HFA** *45 µg/spray MDI*	**Bronchospasm**, 6-11y: 0.31 mg neb tid prn; Max: 0.63 mg neb tid; >11y: 0.63 mg neb tid prn; Max: 1.25 mg neb tid **Bronchospasm**, >4y: 2 puffs inhaled q4-6h prn; Max: 12 puffs/d; Alt: 1 puff inhaled q4h prn
Lucinactant	
Surfaxin *Susp 34 mg/mL*	**RDS** (NICU chart)5.8 mL/kg birth weight. Up to 4 doses of SURFAXIN can be administered in the 1st 48 h. Frequency >6 h
Mometasone nasal	PRC C, Lact ?
Nasonex *50 µg/spray*	**Allergic rhinitis**, 2-12y: 1 spray per nostril qd; Info: not indicated for prophylaxis in this age group; >12y: 2 sprays per nostril qd; Info: start 2-4wk before pollen season for prophylaxis if known seasonal allergen
Montelukast	PRC B, Lact ?
Singulair *10; 4,5 CH; 4 mg granule pkt*	**Asthma** maintenance tx or allergic rhinitis, 1-5y: 4 mg PO qpm; 6-14y: 5 mg PO qpm; >15y: 10 mg PO qpm
Omalizumab	PRC B, Lact ?
Xolair SC	**Asthma** prophylaxis, >12y: 150-375 mg SC q2-4wk; Max: 150 mg/injection site; divide doses >150 mg; Info: actual dose based on pre-tx IgE and wt; avoid abrupt D/C of concurrent asthma meds incl. inhaled, systemic steroids
Salmeterol	PRC C, Lact ?
Serevent Diskus *50 µg/blister DPI*	**Asthma** maintenance, >4y: 50 µg inhaled q12h; Info: for use only in combo w/ asthma controller medication; fixed-dose combination product preferred to incr. compliance; use shortest effective tx duration
Theophylline	PRC C, Lact -
Elixophyllin *100,200,300,400,450,600 ER;80/15 mL; IV*	**Asthma** maintenance or acute bronchospasm: Consult pediatric asthma specialist

Triamcinolone	PRC C, Lact ?
Nasacort AQ *55 µg/spray*	**Allergic rhinitis**, 2-5y: 1 spray per nostril qd; Max: 1 spray in each nostril/d; 6-12y: 1-2 sprays per nostril qd; Start: 1 spray per nostril qd; Max: 2 sprays per nostril/d; <12y: 1-2 sprays per nostril qd; Start: 2 sprays per nostril qd; Max: 2 sprays per nostril/d; Info: D/C after 3wk if no improvement
Zileuton	PRC C, Lact -
Zyflo *600*	**Asthma** maintenance, >12y: 600 mg PO qid; Max: 2400 mg/d

16.5 Gastroenterology

MA/EF (Balsalazide) unknown
MA/EF (Infliximab) binds and inhibits tumor necrosis factor alpha, reducing inflammation and altering immune response
MA/EF (lactulose) increases stool water content; increases stool acidity, trapping NH4 ions (osmotic laxative)
MA/EF (rimantadine) exact mechanism of action unknown; possibly inhibits viral uncoating and replication
MA/EF (Sulfasalazine) unknown
MA/EF (tetracycline) bacteriostatic; inhibits protein synthesis
AE (Balsalazide) Serious: anaphylactic reactions, bronchospasm, hepatotoxicity, ulcerative colitis exacerbation, Reye syndrome; Common: headache, abdominal pain, diarrhea, nausea, vomiting, respiratory infection, arthralgia, insomnia, flatulence, pyrexia, dyspepsia, anorexia, alopecia, skin reactions
AE (Infliximab) Serious: sepsis, pneumonia, opportunistic infection, tuberculosis, malignancy, lymphoma, hepatosplenic T-cell lymphoma, leukemia, HBV reactivation, hepatotoxicity, CHF, anaphylactoid reactions, hypersensitivity reaction, serum sickness, lupus erythematosus, myelosuppression, seizures, optic neuritis, demyelinating CNS disease, skin carcinoma (psoriasis use), severe skin reactions, photosensitivity, severe infusion reaction, pulmonary edema, interstitial lung disease; Common: fever, chills, myalgias, back pain, headache, fatigue, arthralgia, dizziness, nausea, urticarial, pruritus, rash, URI, UTI, ALT/AST elevated, dyspnea, facial or hand edema, hypotension, HTN, chest pain, anemia, leukopenia, neutropenia
AE (lactulose) Serious: severe diarrhea (excessive doses), electrolyte disorders (excessive doses), metabolic acidosis (excessive doses); Common: flatulence, intestinal cramps, abdominal distension, nausea, vomiting
AE (rimantadine) Serious: seizures, ataxia, depression, hallucinations, bronchospasm, HTN, syncope, heart block, cardiac failure; Common: nausea, insomnia, nervousness, impaired concentration, dizziness

AE Serious: anaphylaxis, hypersensitivity reaction, erythema multiforme, Stevens-Johnson syndrome, exfoliative dermatitis, toxic epidermal necrolysis, rash w/ eosinophilia and systemic sx, serum sickness, interstitial lung disease, hypersensitivity pneumonitis, vasculitis, fibrosing alveolitis, pericarditis, allergic myocarditis, polyarteritis nodosa, lupus erythematosus, hepatitis, rhabdomyolysis, photosensitivity, blood dyscrasias, agranulocytosis, aplastic anemia, hemolytic anemia, hepatotoxicity, pancreatitis, infertility, reversible oligospermia, nephrotoxicity, Reye syndrome; Common: anorexia, headache, nausea/vomiting, dyspepsia, reversible oligospermia, skin rash, pruritus, urticarial, fever, hemolytic anemia, cyanosis, crystalluria, hematuria
AE (tetracycline) Serious: tooth discoloration (pts <8 yo), anaphylaxis, angioedema, photosensitivity, lupus erythematosus, serum sickness-like reaction, erythema multiforme, exfoliative dermatitis, Stevens-Johnson syndrome, pancreatitis, thrombocytopenia, neutropenia, hemolytic anemia, pseudotumor cerebri, bulging fontanels (infants), nephrotoxicity, hepatotoxicity, superinfection, Clostridium difficile associated diarrhea, Jarisch-Herxheimer reaction (brucellosis or spirochetal infection use); Common: nausea, vomiting, diarrhea, anorexia, flatulence, abdominal discomfort, epigastric discomfort, rash, urticarial, oral or vulvovaginal candidiasis, headache, dizziness, tinnitus, photosensitivity
CI (Balsalazide) hypersens. to salicylates; influenza, varicella, or febrile viral infection (pts <20 yo); caution if pyloric stenosis, renal impairment
CI (Infliximab) hypersens. to murine proteins, concurrent live vaccination, active infection, NYHA Class III-IV CHF; caution if NYHA Class I-II CHF, chronic or recurrent infections, opportunistic infection hx, infection risk, co-morbid conditions, uncontrolled DM, latent tuberculosis, tuberculosis risk, concurrent immunosuppressants, HBV carrier, CNS demyelinating disease, seizure disorder, myelosuppression, mod-severe COPD, malignancy hx, malignancy risk, resides/travels in area w/ endemic TB or mycoses, adolescent or young adult males, restarting after tx interruption
CI (lactulose) galactosemia; caution if DM, colorectal electrocautery procedures
CI (rimantadine) caution if seizure disorder, renal/hepatic impairment
CI (Sulfasalazine) hypersens. to sulfonamides, hypersens. to salicylates, porphyria, GI/GU obstruction; influenza, varicella, or febrile viral infection (pts <20 yo); caution if renal/hepatic impairment, G6PD deficiency, severe allergies, asthma, blood dyscrasia, dehydration, pregnancy near-term, breastfeeding
CI (tetracycline) pregnancy, pts <8 yo; caution if renal/hepatic impairment, SLE, recent abx-assoc. colitis hx

Aminosalicylates	
(see sulfasalazine, balsalazide)	
Balsalazide	PRC B, Lact ?
Colazal *750*	**Ulcerative colitis**, active mild-moderate, 5-17 yo: 2.25 g PO tid x8wk; Alt: 750 mg PO tid x8wk; Max: 6.75 g/ x8wk; Info: 6.75 g/d balsalazide = 2.4 g/d mesalamine

Infliximab	PRC B, Lact ?
Remicade *IV*	**Crohn disease or active ulcerative colitis,** mod-severe: 5 mg/kg IV q8wk; Start: 5 mg/kg IV x1 on wk 0,2,6; Info: In Crohn disease, D/C if no response by 14wk; weigh risk/benefit of reinduction tx if maintenance tx interrupted
Lactulose	PRC B, Lact ?
Kristalose *10 g/15 mL sol*	**Constipation**: 1 mL/kg PO qd-bid; Max: 60 mL/d; Info: response may require 24-48h
Rimantadine	PRC C, Lact +
Flumadine *100*	**Influenza** A prophylaxis (high resistance), 1-10y: 5 mg/kg/d PO div qd-bid; Start: prior to or immed. upon exposure; Max: 150 mg/d; >10y: 100 mg PO bid; Start: prior to or immed. upon exposure; Max: 200 mg/d; Alt: 5 mg/kg/d PO div bid
Sulfasalazine	PRC B, Lact ?
Azulfidine *500; 500 DR*	**Ulcerative colitis**: 30 mg/kg/d PO div q6h; Start: 40-60 mg/kg/d PO div q6-8h; Max: 6 g/d initial dose; 2 g/d maint. dose; Info: give w/ food; JIA, >6y: 30-50 mg/kg/d PO div q6-12h; Start: 10 mg/kg/d PO div q6-12h, incr. over 4wk; Max: 2 g/d; Info: give w/ food
Tetracycline	PRC D, Lact +
Tetracycline *250,500; 125/5 mL*	**Bacterial & chlamydial infections**, >8y: 25-50 mg/kg/d PO div q6h; Max: 3 g/d **Acne vulgaris,** adolescents: 250-500 mg PO q6-12h x1-2wk, then 250-500 mg PO qd Info for all uses: give at least 1h before or 2h after meals

16.6 Metabolic, Endocrine

MA/EF (Fluoride) stabilizes apatite crystals in bones and teeth, promotes tooth enamel remineralization, interferes w/dental plaque bacteria, and increases tooth enamel acid-resistance, preventing dental caries
MA/EF (glycerol phenylbutyrate): nitrogen-binding agent, prescribed for the treatment of Urea Cycle Disorders (UCD) in pediatric patients >2 y & adults
MA/EF (Insulin regular) stimulates peripheral glucose uptake, inhibits hepatic glucose production, inhibits lipolysis and proteolysis, regulating glucose metabolism
MA/EF (Isoniazid): bactericidal; inhibits lipid and nucleic acid synthesis

MA/EF (Levothyroxine) produces various physiologic effects, including increasing metabolism (synthetic T4)
MA/EF (metformin): decreases hepatic glucose production and intestinal glucose absorption; increases insulin sensitivity
MA/EF (prednisolone/prednisone): exact mechanism of anti-inflammatory action unknown; inhibits multiple inflammatory cytokines; produces multiple glucocorticoid and mineralocorticoid effects
AE (Fluoride) Serious: allergic reactions, dental fluorosis (excessive doses), skeletal fluorosis (large doses), fractures (large doses), rheumatic effects (large doses), GI bleed (large doses); Common: nausea, vomiting, abdominal pain, rash, mucositis/stomatitis
AE (glycerol phenylbutyrate): upper abdominal pain, rash, nausea, vomiting, diarrhea, decreased appetite, hyperammonemia, headache, dizziness
AE (Insulin regular) Serious: severe hypoglycemia, hypokalemia, generalized hypersensitivity reaction, anaphylaxis; Common: hypoglycemia, injection site reaction, lipoatrophy at injection site, pruritus, rash, weight gain
AE (Isoniazid): Serious: agranulocytosis, aplastic anemia, thrombocytopenia, hepatotoxicity, optic neuritis, peripheral neuropathy, toxic psychosis, seizures, hypersensitivity reaction; Common: paresthesia, nausea, vomiting, epigastric discomfort, ALT/AST elevated, hypersensitivity reaction, pyridoxine deficiency
AE (Levothyroxine) Serious: arrhythmias, CHF, HTN, angina, pseudotumor cerebri, craniosynostosis (infants), premature epiphyseal closure, seizures; Common: palpitations, appetite incr., tachycardia, nervousness, tremor, weight loss, diaphoresis, diarrhea, abdominal cramps, insomnia, fever, headache, alopecia, heat intolerance, menstrual irregularities, nausea, anxiety
AE (metformin): Serious: lactic acidosis, megaloblastic anemia; Common: diarrhea, nausea/vomiting, flatulence, asthenia, indigestion, abdominal discomfort, anorexia, headache, metallic taste, rash, ovulation induction
AE (prednisolone): Serious: adrenal insufficiency, Cushing syndrome, immunosuppression, infection, HTN, CHF, DM, steroid psychosis, GI ulceration/perforation, osteopenia/osteoporosis, hypokalemic alkalosis, steroid myopathy, tendon rupture, pseudotumor cerebri, ICP incr., seizures, glaucoma, cataract formation (long-term use), pancreatitis, growth suppression (long-term use, peds pts), exophthalmos, anaphylaxis; Common: sodium and fluid retention, sweating incr., headache, vertigo, insomnia, nervousness, mood swings, edema, muscle weakness, BP elevated, glucose intolerance, petechiae/ecchymosis, facial erythema, menstrual irregularities, hypokalemia, IOP incr., impaired wound healing (long-term use), Cushing syndrome, skin pigmentation abnormality, hirsutism, urticarial
AE (prednisone): Serious: adrenal insufficiency, Cushing syndrome, immunosuppression, infection, HTN, CHF, DM, steroid psychosis, GI ulceration/perforation, osteopenia/osteoporosis, hypokalemic alkalosis, steroid myopathy, tendon rupture, pseudotumor cerebri, ICP incr., seizures, glaucoma, cataract formation (long-term use), pancreatitis, growth suppression (long-term use), exophthalmos, anaphylaxis; Common: sodium and fluid retention, sweating incr., headache, vertigo, insomnia, nervousness, mood swings, edema, muscle weakness, BP elevated, glucose intolerance, petechiae/ecchymosis,

AE (prednisone) cont: facial erythema, menstrual irregularities, hypokalemia, IOP incr., impaired wound healing (long-term use), Cushing syndrome, skin pigmentation abnormality, hirsutism, urticarial
CI (Fluoride) drinking water fluoride >0.7 ppm; caution if active GI ulcer, severe renal impairment, arthralgia, rheumatoid arthritis
CI (glycerol phenylbutyrate): Children I<2 mo of age, allergic to phenylbutyrate
CI (Insulin regular) hypoglycemia; caution if infection, illness, stress, hypokalemia, hepatic/renal impairment
CI (Isoniazid): prior isoniazid-assoc. hepatic injury, acute hepatic disease, avoid tyramine- or histamine-containing foods; caution if hepatic impairment, caution if severe renal impairment, peripheral neuropathy, pregnancy, HIV infection, alcohol abuse, IV drug abuse
CI (Levothyroxine): thyrotoxicosis, acute MI, adrenal insufficiency, pre-existing TSH suppression; caution if cardiovascular disease, DM
CI (metformin): dysfunction or disease, metabolic acidosis, diabetic ketoacidosis, lactic acidosis, iodinated contrast, hypoxemia, dehydration, sepsis, surgery, hepatic disease; caution if CHF, alcohol abuse, hypoglycemia risk
CI (prednisolone): systemic fungal infection, active or recent varicella infection, active or recent measles infection, avoid abrupt withdrawal (long-term use); caution if active infection, TB infection, ocular HSV, immunosuppressed, HTN, CHF, DM, seizure disorder, PUD, ulcerative colitis, diverticulitis, recent intestinal anastomosis, psychiatric disorder, hypothyroidism, osteoporosis, myasthenia gravis, severe renal/hepatic impairment; caution if thromboembolic disorder, coagulation disorder
CI (prednisone): systemic fungal infection, active or recent varicella infection, active or recent measles infection, avoid abrupt withdrawal (long-term use); caution if active infection, TB infection, ocular HSV, immunosuppressed, HTN, CHF, DM, seizure disorder, PUD, ulcerative colitis, diverticulitis, recent intestinal anastomosis, psychiatric disorder, hypothyroidism, osteoporosis, myasthenia gravis, severe renal/hepatic impairment; caution if thromboembolic disorder, coagulation disorder

Fluoride	PRC C, Lact -
Fluoride *0.5,1 CH; 1; 0.5/mL*	**Dental caries** prophylaxis: Info: dose stratified by fluoride ion levels in drinking water; ADA rec. cont. until 13 yo, AAP rec. cont. until 16 yo in areas w/o fluoridated water (<0.7 ppm)
Glycerol phenylbutyrate	PRC C, Lact?
Ravicti *oral liq 1.1 g/mL*	**UCD**: 3 equally divided dosages, each rounded up to the nearest 0.5 mL to max total dosage is 17.5 mL/d (19 g) (must use with dietary protein restriction, in some cases, dietary supplements) **Switching From Sodium Phenylbutyrate to RAVICTI:** total daily dosage of sodium phenylbutyrate (g) x 0.8

Insulin regular	PRC B, Lact ?
Humulin R, Novolin SC, *IV Inj 100 U/ml*	**Diabetic ketoacidosis**: 0.1 U/kg IV bolus, then 0.1 U/kg/h; decrease when blood glucose falls to < 250mg/dl
Isoniazid	PRC C, Lact +
Isoniazid *100,300; 50/5 mL; IM*	**Active TB,** 1mo-15y: 10-15 mg/kg PO/IM qd x6-18mo; Max: 300 mg/d; Alt: 20-30 mg/kg PO/IM 2x/wk x6-18mo if directly observed tx, max 900 mg/dose; >15y: 5 mg/kg PO/IM qd x6-9mo; Max: 300 mg/d; Alt: 15 mg/kg PO/IM 1-3x/wk x6-18mo if directly observed tx, max 900 mg/dose; Info: admin. as part of multi-drug regimen; give on empty stomach **Latent TB,** mono tx, >1mo: 10-20 mg/kg PO/IM qd x9mo; Max: 300 mg/d; Alt: 20-40 mg/kg PO/IM 2x/wk x9mo if directly observed tx, max 900 mg/dose; combo tx, >2y: 15 mg/kg PO qwk x12wk; Max: 900 mg/dose; Info: for directly observed tx; give w/ rifapentine; give on empty stomach TB, 1o prevention, <5y: 10 mg/kg PO/IM qd x3mo; Info: for PPD-negative pts exposed to TB; repeat PPD in 3mo; give on empty stomach
Levothyroxine	PRC A, Lact -
Synthroid *25, 50, 75, 88, 100, 112, 125, 137, 150, 175, 200, 300 µg*	**Hypothyroidism**: consult with pediatric endocrinologist
Metformin	PRC B, Lact -
Metformin *500,850,1000*	**DM, type 2**, 10-16y: 500 mg PO bid, incr. 500 mg qwk; Max: 2000 mg/d; Info: give w/ meals; hold for iodinated contrast study
Prednisolone	PRC C, Lact -
Orapred, Pediapred, Prelone *5; 5,15/5 mL*	**Acute asthma**: 1-2 mg/kg/d PO div qd-bid x3-10 d; Max: 60 mg/d **Corticosteroid-responsive conditions**: 0.14-2 mg/kg/d PO div qd-qid; Alt: 4-60 mg/m2/d PO div qd-qid; Info: dose, frequency varies by condition; taper dose gradually after long-term use

Prednisone	PRC C, Lact -
Prednisone *1,2.5,5, 10,20,50; 5/5 mL*	**Acute asthma**: 1-2 mg/kg/d PO div qd-bid x3-10 d; Max: 60 mg/d **Corticosteroid-responsive conditions**: 0.05-2 mg/kg/d PO div qd-qid; Info: dose, frequency varies by condition; taper dose gradually after long-term use

16.7 Antimicrobials

MA/EF (amantadine) blocks viral particle uncoating and nucleic acid release into host cell, inhibiting viral replication
MA/EF (amoxicillin) bactericidal; inhibits cell wall mucopeptide synthesis
MA/EF (amoxicillin-clavulanic acid) bactericidal; inhibits cell wall mucopeptide synthesis / inhibits beta-lactamases
MA/EF (ampicillin) bactericidal; inhibits cell wall mucopeptide synthesis
MA/EF (azithromycin) bacteriostatic; binds to P site of 50S ribosomal subunit, interfering w/ protein synthesis
MA/EF (cefixime) 3rd generation ceph.; bacteriocidal; inhibits cell wall mucopeptide synthesis
MA/EF (cefotaxime) 3rd generation ceph.; bactericidal; inhibits cell wall mucopeptide synthesis
MA/EF (cefprozil) 2nd generation ceph.; bactericidal; inhibits cell wall mucopeptide synthesis
MA/EF (ceftriaxone) 3rd generation ceph.; bactericidal; inhibits cell wall mucopeptide synthesis
MA/EF (cephalexin)1st generation ceph; bactericidal; inhibits cell wall mucopeptide synthesis
MA/EF (clarithromycin) binds to P site of 50S ribosomal subunit, interfering w/ protein synthesis
MA/EF (erythromycin) binds to P site of 50S ribosomal subunit, interfering w/ protein synthesis
MA/EF (fexofenadine) selectively antagonizes peripheral histamine H1 receptors
MA/EF (gentamycin) bactericidal; binds to bacterial 30S ribosomal subunit, inhibiting protein synthesis
MA/EF (isoniazid): bactericidal; inhibits lipid and nucleic acid synthesis
MA/EF (metronidazole): exact mechanism of action unknown; disrupts DNA and inhibits nucleic acid synthesis
MA/EF (midazolam): binds to benzodiazepine receptors; enhances GABA effects
MA/EF (oseltamivir): inhibits influenza neuraminidase
MA/EF (palivizumab) binds to A antigenic site of RSV F protein (monoclonal antibody)
MA/EF (pyrazinamide): unknown
MA/EF (rifampin): inhibits DNA-dependent RNA polymerase (rifamycin)

MA/EF (sulfamethoxazole): bacteriostatic; competitively inhibits bacterial or fungal dihydropteroate synthetase, preventing PABA conversion to folic acid and inhibiting growth
MA/EF (trimethoprim): selectively inhibits bacterial dihydrofolate reductase (folate antagonist)
MA/EF (vancomycin) bactericidal; inhibits cell wall synthesis; inhibits RNA synthesis
MA/EF (zanamivir) inhibits influenza neuraminidase
MA/EF (zidovudine) inhibits reverse transcriptase; incorporates into viral DNA (nucleoside reverse transcriptase inhibitor)
AE (amantadine) Serious: CHF, arrhythmias, cardiac arrest, psychosis, coma, neuroleptic malignant syndrome, visual impairment, respiratory failure, pulmonary edema, anaphylactoid reactions, suicidal ideation, agranulocytosis, neutropenia, leukopenia, seizures, oculogyric crisis, heat stroke; Common: nausea, dizziness, insomnia, depression, anxiety, irritability, hallucinations, confusion, anorexia, dry mouth, constipation, ataxia, livedo reticularis, peripheral edema, orthostatic hypotension, headache, somnolence, abnormal dreams, diarrhea, compulsive behaviors
AE (amoxicillin) Serious: anaphylaxis, immediate or delayed hypersensitivity reaction, serum sickness-like reaction, erythema multiforme, exfoliative dermatitis, Stevens-Johnson syndrome, toxic epidermal necrolysis, acute generalized exanthematous pustulosis, hypersensitivity vasculitis, superinfection, Clostridium difficile associated diarrhea, hemolytic anemia, leukopenia, thrombocytopenia, thrombocytopenic purpura, agranulocytosis, hepatitis, cholestatic jaundice, seizures; Common: nausea, vomiting, diarrhea, urticaria, rash, eosinophilia, black hairy tongue, oral or vulvovaginal candidiasis, LFT elevated
AE (amoxicillin-clavulanic acid) Serious: anaphylaxis, immediate or delayed hypersensitivity reaction, serum sickness-like reaction, erythema multiforme, exfoliative dermatitis, Stevens-Johnson syndrome, toxic epidermal necrolysis, acute generalized exanthematous pustulosis, hypersensitivity vasculitis, superinfection, Clostridium difficile associated diarrhea, hemolytic anemia, leukopenia, thrombocytopenia, thrombocytopenic purpura, agranulocytosis, hepatitis, cholestatic jaundice, seizures; Common: nausea, vomiting, diarrhea, urticaria, rash, eosinophilia, black hairy tongue, oral or vulvovaginal candidiasis, LFT elevated
AE (ampicillin) Serious: anaphylaxis, immediate or delayed hypersensitivity reaction, serum sickness-like reaction, erythema multiforme, exfoliative dermatitis, Stevens-Johnson syndrome, superinfection, Clostridium difficile associated diarrhea, hemolytic anemia, leukopenia, thrombocytopenia, thrombocytopenic purpura, agranulocytosis, seizures; Common: nausea, vomiting, diarrhea, urticaria, rash, eosinophilia, black hairy tongue, oral or vulvovaginal candidiasis
AE (azithromycin) Serious: angioedema, anaphylaxis, cholestatic jaundice, hepatotoxicity, pancreatitis, Stevens-Johnson syndrome, toxic epidermal necrolysis, Clostridium difficile associated diarrhea, QT prolongation, torsades de pointes, myasthenia gravis exacerbation; Common: diarrhea, nausea, abdominal pain, vaginitis, dyspepsia, dizziness, rash, vomiting, anorexia pruritus

AE (cefixime) Serious: anaphylaxis, erythema multiforme, Stevens-Johnson syndrome, toxic epidermal necrolysis, acute renal failure, hemolytic anemia, blood dyscrasia, superinfection, C. difficile associated diarrhea, seizures; Common: diarrhea, abdominal pain, nausea, dyspepsia, flatulence, rash, headache, dizziness, urticaria, pruritus, elevated LFTs, elevated BUN/Cr, eosinophilia

AE (cefotaxime) Serious: anaphylaxis, toxic epidermal necrolysis, Stevens-Johnson syndrome, erythema multiforme, interstitial nephritis, agranulocytosis, hemolytic anemia, neutropenia, thrombocytopenia, seizures, C. difficile associated diarrhea; Common: injection site reaction, rash, pruritus, fever, eosinophilia

AE (cefprozil) Serious: anaphylaxis, seizures, nephrotoxicity, leukopenia, thrombocytopenia, hemolytic anemia, erythema multiforme, Stevens-Johnson syndrome, toxic epidermal necrolysis, superinfection, C. difficile associated diarrhea; Common: nausea, diarrhea, dyspepsia, vomiting, abdominal pain, LFTs elevated, vulvovaginal candidiasis, dizziness, rash, pruritus, eosinophilia

AE: (ceftriaxone) Serious: anaphylaxis, bronchospasm, Stevens-Johnson syndrome, toxic epidermal necrolysis, erythema multiforme, serum sickness, allergic pneumonitis, neutropenia, leukopenia, hemolytic anemia, thrombocytopenia, hypoprothrombinemia, agranulocytosis, superinfection, C. difficile associated diarrhea, colitis, biliary/gallbladder sludge, jaundice, pancreatitis, seizures, nephrolithiasis, lung/kidney Ca-ceftriaxone precipitate, incl. fatal (neonates); Common: local injection site reactions, eosinophilia, thrombocytosis, LFTs elevated, diarrhea, leukopenia

AE (cephalexin) Serious: anaphylaxis, angioedema, erythema multiforme, Stevens-Johnson syndrome, toxic epidermal necrolysis, C. difficile associate diarrhea, neutropenia, thrombocytopenia, hemolytic anemia, aplastic anemia, hemorrhage, hepatitis, cholestatic jaundice, seizures; Common: diarrhea, nausea, vomiting, rash, headache, dizziness, LFTs elevated, eosinophilia

AE (clarithromycin) Serious: superinfection, C. difficile associated diarrhea, hepatic impairment, hepatitis,
interstitial nephritis, pancreatitis, QT prolongation, ventricular arrhythmias, torsades de pointes, thrombocytopenia, leukopenia, neutropenia, reversible hearing loss, seizures, behavioral disturbances, psychosis, hallucinations, psychiatric disturbances, anaphylaxis, erythema multiforme, Stevens-Johnson syndrome, toxic epidermal necrolysis, hypoglycemia, myasthenia gravis exacerbation; Common: diarrhea, nausea/vomiting, taste changes, abdominal pain, dyspepsia, headache, rash

AE (erythromycin) oral: Serious: Clostridium difficile associated diarrhea, superinfection, hepatic impairment, hepatitis, QT prolongation, ventricular arrhythmias, torsades de pointes, anaphylaxis, erythema multiforme, Stevens-Johnson syndrome, toxic epidermal necrolysis, reversible hearing loss, infantile hypertrophic pyloric stenosis, pancreatitis, convulsions, myasthenia gravis exacerbation, interstitial nephritis; Common: nausea/vomiting, abdominal pain, diarrhea, anorexia, rash, urticarial, ALT/AST elevated, jaundice

AE (fexofenadine) Serious: hypersensitivity reaction; Common: headache, dyspepsia, fever, cough, URI, myalgia, pain, diarrhea, otitis media, rhinorrhea, dizziness, somnolence

AE (gentamycin): Serious: nephrotoxicity, Fanconi syndrome, vestibular ototoxicity, auditory ototoxicity, neurotoxicity, neuromuscular blockade, seizures, pseudotumor cerebri, hypersensitivity reaction, endotoxin-like reaction (peds doses >5.5 mg/kg), anaphylactoid reactions, exfoliative dermatitis, toxic epidermal necrolysis, erythema multiforme, Stevens-Johnson syndrome, superinfection, agranulocytosis; Common: BUN/Cr elevated, dizziness, vertigo, tinnitus, hearing loss, injection site reaction
AE (isoniazid): Serious: agranulocytosis, aplastic anemia, thrombocytopenia, hepatotoxicity, optic neuritis, peripheral neuropathy, toxic psychosis, seizures, hypersensitivity reaction; Common: paresthesia, nausea, vomiting, epigastric discomfort, ALT/AST elevated, hypersensitivity reaction, pyridoxine deficiency
AE (metronidazole): Serious: seizures, aseptic meningitis, peripheral neuropathy, optic neuropathy, encephalopathy, hypersensitivity reaction, Stevens-Johnson syndrome, toxic epidermal necrolysis, leukopenia; Common: nausea, vomiting, dyspepsia, diarrhea, metallic taste, dry mouth, rash, pruritus, headache, dizziness, syncope, ataxia, confusion, thrombophlebitis (IV use), fever, vertigo, paresthesia, furry tongue, dark, red-brown urine, candidiasis, dysarthria
AE (midazolam): Serious: respiratory depression, apnea, respiratory failure, cardiac arrest, hypotension, bradycardia, tachycardia, syncope, seizures, paradoxical CNS stimulation, dependency/abuse, withdrawal if abrupt D/C, bronchospasm, anaphylactic/anaphylactoid reactions; Common: sedation, nausea, vomiting, injection site pain, hiccups, hypotension, agitation, dystonia, amnesia, diplopia, disinhibition, confusion, ataxia, weakness, dysarthria, euphoria, rash
AE (oseltamivir): Serious: delirium, behavioral disturbances, self-injury, anaphylaxis, Stevens-Johnson syndrome, toxic epidermal necrolysis, erythema multiforme; Common: nausea, vomiting, diarrhea, abdominal pain, headache, epistaxis, ear disorder
AE (palivizumab): Serious: anaphylaxis, hypersensitivity reactions, severe thrombocytopenia; Common: URI sx, otitis media, rhinitis, rash, pain, injection site reaction, hernia, ALT/AST elevated, pharyngitis
AE (pyrazinamide): Serious: hepatotoxicity, thrombocytopenia, anemia, interstitial nephritis, porphyria; Common: anorexia, rash, urticarial, nausea, vomiting, malaise, arthralgia, photosensitivity, hyperuricemia, gout, LFTs elevated
AE (rifampin): Serious: hepatitis, thrombocytopenia, leukopenia, hemolytic anemia, agranulocytosis, hemorrhage, DIC, interstitial nephritis, renal failure, anaphylaxis, shock, psychosis, porphyria exacerbation, erythema multiforme, Stevens-Johnson syndrome, toxic epidermal necrolysis, Clostridium difficile associated diarrhea; Common: reddish-orange body fluids, anorexia, nausea/vomiting, headache, ALT/AST elevated, fatigue, drowsiness, dizziness, abdominal pain, diarrhea, hypersensitivity reaction, influenza-like sx, dyspnea, ataxia, visual changes, contact lens staining

AE Serious: Stevens-Johnson syndrome, toxic epidermal necrolysis, photosensitivity, fulminant hepatic necrosis, agranulocytosis, aplastic anemia, blood dyscrasias, anaphylactoid reactions, hepatitis, hepatotoxicity, interstitial nephritis, nephrotoxicity, pulmonary infiltrates, kernicterus (neonates), aseptic meningitis, myelosuppression, methemoglobinemia, hyperkalemia, goiter, lupus erythematosus, Clostridium difficile-associated diarrhea; Common: nausea/vomiting, anorexia, allergic rash, urticarial, hypersensitivity reaction, photosensitivity, diarrhea, dizziness, GI upset, headache, lethargy
AE (vancomycin): Serious: anaphylactic/anaphylactoid reactions, severe hypotension (rapid IV use), thrombophlebitis, tissue necrosis (if extravasated), vasculitis, exfoliative dermatitis, Stevens-Johnson syndrome, toxic epidermal necrolysis, rash w/ eosinophilia and systemic sx, interstitial nephritis, nephrotoxicity, ototoxicity, neutropenia, thrombocytopenia, superinfection, Clostridium difficile associated diarrhea; Common: red-man syndrome (rapid IV use), hypotension (rapid IV use), fever, nausea, chills, eosinophilia, rash, urticarial, phlebitis, tinnitus, dizziness/vertigo, BUN/Cr elevated, vomiting (PO use), flatulence (PO use)
AE (zanamivir): Serious: bronchospasm, anaphylaxis, angioedema, severe skin reactions, erythema multiforme, Stevens-Johnson syndrome, toxic epidermal necrolysis, delirium, hallucinations, behavioral disturbances, self-injury, arrhythmias, syncope, seizures; Common: nausea, dizziness, headache, bronchitis, cough, nasal sx, ear/nose/throat infection, fever/chills, malaise, myalgia, appetite changes
AE (zidovudine): Serious: lactic acidosis, hepatomegaly w/ steatosis, hepatotoxicity, severe anemia, neutropenia, pancytopenia, aplastic anemia, myopathy, myositis, rhabdomyolysis, pancreatitis, seizures, anaphylactoid reactions, Stevens-Johnson syndrome, toxic epidermal necrolysis, immune reconstitution syndrome, autoimmune disorders; Common: headache, malaise, nausea, anorexia, vomiting, asthenia, constipation, abdominal cramps/pain, arthralgia, chills, dyspepsia, fatigue, insomnia, musculoskeletal pain, myalgia, neuropathy, ALT/AST elevated, anemia, fever, cough, hepatomegaly, rash, URI sx, diarrhea, stomatitis, lipodystrophy
CI (amantadine) caution in depression, psychiatric disorder, CHF, cardiovascular disease, peripheral edema, angle-closure glaucoma, seizure disorder, renal or hepatic impairment, high environmental temperature
CI (amoxicillin) anaphylactic reaction to beta-lactams, mononucleosis; caution if non-anaphylactic hypersens. to beta-lactams, hypersens. to multiple allergens, asthma or hx, ALL, if HIV infection, recent abx-assoc. colitis hx, seizure disorder, renal impairment, PKU (phenylalanine-containing forms)
CI (amoxicillin-clavulanic acid) anaphylactic reaction to beta-lactams, mononucleosis; caution if non-anaphylactic hypersens. to beta-lactams, hypersens. to multiple allergens, asthma or hx, ALL, HIV infection, recent hx abx-assoc. colitis, seizure disorder, renal impairment, PKU (phenylalanine-containing forms)
CI (ampicillin) anaphylactic reaction to beta-lactams, mononucleosis; caution if non-anaphylactic hypersens. to beta-lactams, hypersens. to multiple allergens, asthma or hx, ALL, HIV infection, recent hx abx-assoc. colitis, seizure disorder, renal impairment

CI (azithromycin) azithromycin-assoc. cholestatic jaundice hx, azithromycin-assoc. hepatic impairment hx; caution if hepatic impairment, renal impairment, QT prolongation, QT prolongation risk, myasthenia gravis, recent abx-assoc. colitis hx
CI (cefixime) caution if renal impairment, concurrent nephrotoxic agents, seizure disorder, recent hx abx-assoc. colitis
CI (cefotaxime) caution if hypersens. to PCN, renal impairment, concurrent nephrotoxic agents, seizure disorder, hx recent abx-assoc. colitis
CI (cefprozil) PKU (phenylalanine-containing forms); caution if hypersens. to PCN, renal impairment, concurrent nephrotoxic agents, seizure disorder, hx recent abx-assoc. colitis
CI (ceftriaxone) hyperbilirubinemia (neonates <28 ds old), IV Ca-containing product use (neonates <28 d old); caution if hypersens. to PCN, seizure disorder, hyperbilirubinemia, concurrent nephrotoxic agents, concomitant hepatic and renal impairment, vitamin K deficiency, hx GI disorder, recent hx abx-assoc. colitis
CI (cephalexin) caution if hypersens. to PCN, renal impairment, recent hx abx-assoc. colitis, hx GI disorder
CI (clarithromycin) hx clarithromycin-assoc. hepatic impairment; caution if pregnancy, severe renal impairment, QT prolongation or risk, hypokalemia, hypomagnesemia, bradycardia, myocardial ischemia or MI, cardiomyopathy, myasthenia gravis, recent abx-assoc. colitis hx
CI (erythromycin) caution if hepatic impairment, myasthenia gravis, QT prolongation, QT prolongation risk, hypokalemia, hypomagnesemia, bradycardia, myocardial ischemia or MI, cardiomyopathy, recent abx-assoc. colitis hx
CI (fexofenadine) caution if renal impairment, PKU (phenylalanine-containing forms)
CI (gentamycin): caution if hypersens. to sulfites, renal impairment, dehydration, concurrent nephrotoxic agents, impaired vestibular fxn, impaired auditory fxn, concurrent ototoxic agents, concurrent neurotoxic agents, neuromuscular disease, electrolyte abnormalities, prolonged use, high dose tx, in neonates or infants
CI (isoniazid): prior isoniazid-assoc. hepatic injury, acute hepatic disease, avoid tyramine- or histamine-containing foods; caution if hepatic impairment, caution if severe renal impairment, peripheral neuropathy, pregnancy, HIV infection, alcohol abuse, IV drug abuse
CI (metronidazole): pregnancy (single dose bacterial vaginosis use), pregnancy 1st trimester (trichomoniasis use), alcohol use during and x72h after tx; caution if severe hepatic impairment, blood dyscrasia, CNS disorder
CI (midazolam): neonates or premature infants (benzyl alcohol-containing INJ forms); caution if pulmonary/renal/hepatic impairment, sleep apnea, CHF, CNS depression, alcohol use, alcohol or drug abuse hx, abrupt withdrawal, seizure hx, debilitated pts
CI (oseltamivir): pts <1 yo; caution if renal/hepatic impairment, hereditary fructose intolerance (PO susp form)
CI (palivizumab): none
CI (pyrazinamide): severe hepatic damage, acute gout; caution if hepatic impairment, DM, alcohol abuse
CI (rifampin): IM or SC administration; caution if DM, hepatic impairment, porphyria, recent abx-assoc. colitis hx

CI hypersens. to sulfonamides, megaloblastic anemia, folate deficiency, G6PD deficiency, pts <2 mo, pregnancy near-term, breastfeeding, significant hepatic impairment; caution if hepatic/renal impairment, chronic alcohol use, anticonvulsant use, bone marrow suppressants, malabsorption, malnutrition, asthma, severe allergies, hyperkalemia, recent abx-assoc. colitis hx
CI (vancomycin): caution if renal impairment, concurrent nephrotoxic agents, hearing impairment, concurrent ototoxic agents, intestinal inflammation (PO use), recent abx-assoc. colitis hx
CI (zanamivir): hypersens. to milk proteins, unable to learn administration technique, caution if asthma or COPD
CI (zidovudine): breastfeeding not recommended; caution if myelosuppression, advanced HIV disease, severe renal impairment, hepatic impairment, hepatic disease risk, obesity, female pts, long-term nucleoside tx

Amantadine	PRC C, Lact ?
Symmetrel *100 mg tab/cap, 50 mg/5ml syrup*	**Influenza A** tx, 1-10y: 5 mg/kg/d PO div bid x3-5 d; Start: w/in 48h of sx onset; Max: 150 mg/d; D/C w/in 24-48h of sx resolution; >10y: 100 mg PO bid x3-5 d; Start: w/in 48h of sx onset; Max: 200 mg/d; Alt: 5 mg/kg/d PO div bid x3-5 d; D/C w/in 24-48h of sx resolution **Influenza A** prophylaxis, 1-10y: 5 mg/kg/d PO div bid; Start: prior to or immed. upon exposure; Max: 150 mg/d; >10y: 100 mg PO bid; Start: prior to or immed. upon exposure; Max: 200 mg/d; Alt: 5 mg/kg/d PO div bid
Amoxicillin	PRC B, Lact -
Amoxil *250,500,875; 125,200,250,400 CH; 125,200,250,400/5 mL*	**Acute otitis media:** <2 mo: 30 mg/kg/d PO div q12h x10 d; >3 mo: 80-90 mg/kg/d PO div q12h x5-7 d; Max: 1000 mg/dose **Acute sinusitis:** >3 mo: 80-90 mg/kg/d PO div q12h x5-7 d; Max: 1000 mg/dose **Streptococcal pharyngitis:** 50 mg/kg PO qd x10 d; Max: 1000 mg/dose **Community-acquired pneumonia:** 4mo-5y: 90 mg/kg/d PO div q8h x10 ds; Max: 500 mg/dose; >5y: 90 mg/kg/d PO div q8-12h x10 d; Max: 875 mg/dose bid; 500 mg/dose tid **Endocarditis prophylaxis**: 50 mg/kg PO x1; Max: 2000 mg/dose; give 1h before procedure

	Lyme disease, early: 50 mg/kg/d div q8h x 14-21 d; Max: 500 mg/dose
Amoxicillin-clavulanic acid	PRC B, Lact -
Augmentin *250/125, 500/125, 875/125; 125/31.25/5 mL, 250/62.5/5 mL*	**Bacterial infections:** <3mo: 30 mg/kg/d PO div q12h; Info: use 125 mg/31.25 mg/5 mL susp; >3 mo, <40 kg: 25-45 mg/kg/d PO div q12h, use 200 mg/28.5 mg or 400 mg/57 mg forms; Alt: 20-40 mg/kg/d PO div q8h, use 125 mg/31.25 mg or 250 mg/62.5 mg forms; dose based on amoxicillin component; >3 mo, >40 kg: 500/125 mg - 875/125 mg PO q8h; give w/ food or milk
Ampicillin	PRC B, Lact -
Ampicillin *250,500; 125,250/5 mL; IM; IV*	**Bacterial infections:** <7 d old, <2000 g: 50-100 mg/kg/d IM/IV div q12h; <7 d old, >2000 g: 75-150 mg/kg/d IM/IV div q8h; >7 d old, <1200 g: 50-100 mg/kg/d IM/IV div q12h; >7 d old, 1200-2000 g: 75-150 mg/kg/d IM/IV div q8h; >7 d old, >2000 g: 100-200 mg/kg/d IM/IV div q6h; infants/children: 100-400 mg/kg/d IM/IV div q4-6h; Max: 2-3 g/d PO; 12 g/d IM/IV; Alt: 50-100 mg/kg/d PO div q6h; give 1-2h before food on empty stomach **Bacterial meningitis:** <7 d old, <2000 g: 100 mg/kg/d IM/IV div q12h; <7 d old, >2000 g: 150 mg/kg/d IM/IV div q8h; >7 d old, <1200 g: 100 mg/kg/d IM/IV div q12h; >7 d old, 1200-2000 g: 150 mg/kg/d IM/IV div q8h; >7 d old, >2000 g: 200 mg/kg/d IM/IV div q6h; infants/children: 200-400 mg/kg/d IM/IV div q4-6h; Max: 12 g/d **Endocarditis prophylaxis:** 50 mg/kg PO x1; Max: 2000 mg/dose; give 1h before procedure
Azithromycin	PRC B, Lact ?
Zithromax, Zmax *250,500,600; 100,200/5 mL; 1 g pwdr pkt*	**Otitis media, acute**, >6 mo: 10 mg/kg PO x1 on d 1, then 5 mg/kg PO q24h x4 d; Alt: 30 mg/kg PO x1 dose, or 10 mg/kg PO q24h x3 d **Pharyngitis/tonsillitis, streptococcal,** >2 yo: 12 mg/kg PO q24h x5 d; Max: 500 mg/d

	Pneumonia, community-acquired, >6 mo: 10 mg/kg PO x1 on d 1, then 5 mg/kg PO q24h x4 d **Sinusitis, acute bacterial,** >6 mo: 10 mg/kg PO q24h x3 d **Infection tx, chlamydial**, <8 yo & <45 kg: 20 mg/kg PO x1; >8 yo or >45 kg: 1 g PO x1
Cefixime	PRC B, Lact ?
Suprax *400; 100/5mL, 200/5mL*	**Bacterial infections**; 6mo-11y, <50 kg: 8 mg/kg/d PO div qd-bid; 6mo-11y, >50 kg; or >12y: 400 mg PO qd or 200 mg PO bid; Info: use susp for otitis media
Cefotaxime	PRC B, Lact -
Claforan *IM*	**Bacterial infections**, neonates <7 ds old, <2000 g: 50 mg/kg IM/IV q12h; neonates <7 ds old, >2000 g: 50 mg/kg IM/IV q8-12h; neonates >7 ds old, <1200 g: 50 mg/kg IM/IV q12h; neonates >7 ds old, 1200-2000 g: 50 mg/kg IM/IV q8h; neonates >7 ds old, >2000 g: 50 mg/kg IM/IV q6-8h; infants/children, <50 kg: 50 mg/kg IM/IV q6-8h; Max: 12 g/d; Alt: 50-75 mg/kg IM/IV q6-8h for PCN-resistant pneumococci; Children >50 kg: 1-2 g IM/IV q8-12h; Max: 12 g/d; Info: duration varies w/ infection type, severity
Cefprozil	PRC B, Lact -
Cefzil *250, 500; 125/5mL, 250/5mL susp*	**otitis media**, 6 mo-12 yo: 30 mg/kg/d PO div q12h x10 d; Max: 1000 mg/d **sinusitis**, 6 mo-12 yo: 15-30 mg/kg/d PO div q12h x10 d: Max: 1000 mg/d **pharyngitis/tonsillitis, streptococcal,** 2-12 yo: 15 mg/kg/d PO div q12h x10 d: Max: 1000 mg/d **skin/skin structure infections, uncomplicated bacterial,** 2-12 yo: 20 mg/kg PO q24h x10 d: Max: 1000 mg/d

Ceftriaxone	PRC B, Lact -
Rocephin *IM, IV*	**Bacterial infections,** neonates, <7 d old: 50 mg/kg IM/IV q24h; Info: duration varies w/ infection type, severity; neonates, >7 d old, <2000 g: 50 mg/kg IM/IV q24h; Info: duration varies w/ infection type, severity; neonates, >7 d old, >2000 g: 75 mg/kg IM/IV q24h; Info: duration varies w/ infection type, severity; infants/children: 50-75 mg/kg/d IM/IV div q12-24h for mild/moderate infections, 80-100 mg/kg/d IM/IV div q12-24h for severe infections; Max: 2 g/24h; Info: dose, duration varies w/ infection type, severity **Meningitis**: infants/children: 80-100 mg/kg/d IV div q12-24h x7-21 d; Start: 100 mg/kg IV x1; Max: 4 g/24h **Acute otitis media,** infants/children: 50 mg/kg IM/IV q24h x1-3 d; Max: 1 g/dose; Info: give x1 d if initial tx in penicillin allergic pts, give x3 d if previous tx failure **GC prophylaxis,** neonates: 25-50 mg/kg IM/IV x1; Max: 125 mg/dose; Info: for neonates born to mothers w/ gonococcal infection; children/ adolescents: 125 mg IM x1; Info: for sexual assault victims GC tx, neonates: 25-50 mg/kg IM/IV q24h x7 d; Info: give x10-14 d if meningitis; children, <45 kg: 125 mg IM x1; Info: for **uncomplicated infections of pharynx, cervix, urethra, rectum; dual tx for chlamydial co-infection recommended**; children, >45 kg: 250 mg IM x1; Info: for uncomplicated infections of pharynx, cervix, urethra, rectum; dual tx for chlamydial co-infection recommended; adolescents: 250 mg IM x1; Info: for uncomplicated infections of pharynx, cervix, urethra, rectum; dual tx for chlamydial co-infection recommended **Ophthalmia neonatorum:** 25-50 mg/kg IM/IV x1; Max: 125 mg/dose PID, mild-mod, adolescents: 250 mg IM x1; Info: use w/ doxycycline or clindamycin

Cephalexin	PRC B, Lact -
Keflex *250, 500; 125/5mL, 250/5mL*	**Bacterial infections**: 25-50 mg/kg/d PO div q6-12h; Max: 4000 mg/24h; Alt: 25-50 mg/kg/d PO div q12h for strep pharyngitis or skin infections in pts>1 yo or uncomplicated cystitis in pts >15 yo; Info: dose, duration vary by infection type, severity; may give 50-100 mg/kg/d PO div q6h for severe infection
Clarithromycin	PRC C, Lact ?
Biaxin *250,500; 125,250/5 mL*	**Bacterial infections,** >6mo: 15 mg/kg/d PO div q12h; Max: 1 g/d
Erythromycin	PRC B, Lact -
Erythromycin base *250,500; 250 DR* **Erythromycin ethylsuccinate** *400, 2*	**Bacterial infections**: 30-50 mg/kg PO qd div q6-8h; Max: 4 g/d; Info: give IR on empty stomach **Pertussis:** 40-50 mg/kg/d PO div Q6h x 14 d
Erythromycin ophthalmic *0.5% oint*	Bacterial ocular infections: Apply 1 cm ribbon to lower conjunctival sac or affected structure
Fexofenadine	PRC C, Lact -
Allegra *30,60,180, oral susp*	**Allergic rhinitis or chronic idiopathic urticaria**, 2-11y: 30 mg PO bid; >12y: 180 mg PO qd; Alt: 60 mg PO bid **Chronic idiopathic urticarial**, 6mo-2y: 15 mg PO bid; Info: some pts may benefit from higher doses, weigh risk/benefit
Gentamycin	PRC D, Lact -
Gentamycin *IV, IM*	**Bacterial infections**, <8 ds old: <28 wk gest: 2.5 mg/kg IV/IM q24h; Alt: 5 mg/kg IV/IM q48h 28-29 wk gest: 2.5 mg/kg IV/IM q18h; Alt: 5 mg/kg IV/IM q48h 30-33 wk gest: 2.5 mg/kg IV/IM q18h; Alt: 4.5 mg/kg IV/IM q36-48h; 3.5 mg/kg IV/IM q24h 34 wk gest: 2.5 mg/kg IV/IM q18h; Alt: 4 mg/kg IV/IM q24-36h; 3.5 mg/kg IV/IM q24h 35-36 wk gest: 2.5 mg/kg IV/IM q12h; Alt: 4 mg/kg IV/IM q24-36h; 3.5 mg/kg IV/IM q24h Full term: 2.5 mg/kg IV/IM q12h;

	Alt: 4 mg/kg IV/IM q24h 8 d-1 mo old: <30 wk gest: 2.5 mg/kg IV/IM q18h; Alt: 4 mg/kg IV/IM q24-36h 30-33 wk gest: 2.5 mg/kg IV/IM q12h; Alt: 4 mg/kg IV/IM q24h 34 wk gest: 2.5 mg/kg IV/IM q12h; Alt: 4 mg/kg IV/IM q18h 35-36 wk gest: 2.5 mg/kg IV/IM q8h; Alt: 4 mg/kg IV/IM q12h Full term: 2.5 mg/kg IV/IM q8h; Alt: 5 mg/kg IV/IM q24h 1-6 mo: 2.5 mg/kg IV/IM q8h; Alt: 6.5 mg/kg IV/IM q24h >6 mo: 2.5 mg/kg IV/IM q8h; Alt: 6.5-7.5 mg/kg IV/IM q24h; Info: use IBW if >2 yo Info: adjust dose based on levels
Isoniazid	PRC C, Lact +
Isoniazid *100,300; 50/5 mL; IM*	**Active TB**, 1mo-15y: 10-15 mg/kg PO/IM qd x6-18mo; Max: 300 mg/d; Alt: 20-30 mg/kg PO/IM 2x/wk x6-18mo if directly observed tx, max 900 mg/dose; >15y: 5 mg/kg PO/IM qd x6-9mo; Max: 300 mg/d; Alt: 15 mg/kg PO/IM 1-3x/wk x6-18mo if directly observed tx, max 900 mg/dose; Info: admin. as part of multi-drug regimen; give on empty stomach **Latent TB,** mono tx, >1mo: 10-20 mg/kg PO/IM qd x9mo; Max: 300 mg/d; Alt: 20-40 mg/kg PO/IM 2x/wk x9mo if directly observed tx, max 900 mg/dose; combo tx, >2y: 15 mg/kg PO qwk x12wk; Max: 900 mg/dose; Info: for directly observed tx; give w/ rifapentine; give on empty stomach TB, 1o prevention, <5y: 10 mg/kg PO/IM qd x3mo; Info: for PPD-negative pts exposed to TB; repeat PPD in 3mo; give on empty stomach

Metronidazole	PRC B, Lact ?
Flagyl *250,375,500; IV*	**Bacterial infections**, neonates <1200g: 7.5 mg/kg PO/IV q48h; neonates <7d, >1200g: 7.5-15 mg/kg/d PO/IV div q12-24h; neonates >7d, >1200g: 15-30 mg/kg/d PO/IV div q12h; infants/children: 30 mg/kg PO/IV/d div q6h; Max: 4 g/d **PID**, adolescents: 500 mg PO q12h x14 d; Info: use w/ doxycycline and w/cefoxitin plus probenecid or ceftriaxone **Bacterial vaginosis**, adolescents: 500 mg PO bid x7 ds; Info: may also consider 250 mg PO tid x7 ds in pregnant pts C. difficile-associated diarrhea: 30 mg/kg/d PO div q6h x7-10 d
Midazolam	PRC D, Lact +
Versed *2/mL syrup; IM; IV*	Procedural sedation, IV, 6mo-5y: 0.05-0.1 mg/kg IV x1, repeat q2-3min prn; Max: 0.6 mg/kg total; Info: cumulative dose >6 mg rarely needed; give 5min before procedure; IV, 6-12y: 0.025-0.05 mg/kg IV x1, repeat q2-3min prn; Max: 0.4 mg/kg total; Info: cumulative dose >10 mg rarely needed; give 5min before procedure; IV, >12y: 0.5-2 mg IV x1, repeat q2-3min prn; Info: cumulative dose >10 mg rarely needed; give 5min before procedure; PO, >6mo: 0.25-0.5 mg/kg PO x1; Max: 20 mg; Info: give 20-30min before procedure; children <6 yo may require up to 1 mg/kg/dose; Info: use IBW in obese pts; dose, response vary w/ concomitant medications/clinical status
Oseltamivir	PRC C, Lact ?
Tamiflu *30,45,75; 6/mL*	**Influenza A & B** tx, uncomplicated, <1y: 3 mg/kg PO bid x5 d; Start: ASAP after sx onset; Alt: 0.5 mL/kg (6 mg/mL) PO bid x5 d; Info: use in full-term infants only; >1y, <15 kg: 30 mg PO bid x5 d; Start: w/in 48h of sx onset; Alt: 5 mL (6 mg/mL) PO bid x5 d; >1y, 15-23 Kg: 45 mg PO bid x5 d; Start: w/in 48h of sx onset; Alt: 7.5 mL (6 mg/mL) PO bid x5

	d; 23-40 kg: 60 mg PO bid x5 d; Start: w/in 48h of sx onset; Alt: 10 mL (6 mg/mL) PO bid x5 d; >40 kg: 75 mg PO bid x5 d; Start: w/in 48h of sx onset; Alt: 12.5 mL (6 mg/mL) PO bid x5 d **Influenza A & B** prophylaxis: Same doses as above but qd x 10 ds
Palivizumab	PRC C, Lact ?
Synagis *IM*	**RSV prophylaxis,** high-risk patients: 15 mg/kg IM qmo; Max: 3-5 doses; varies based on gestational age, chronologic age at start of RSV season, & major risk factors; refer to AAP guidelines
Pyrazinamide	PRC C, Lact ?
Pyrazinamide *500*	**Active TB**, 2-15y: 15-30 mg/kg PO qd x2mo; Max: 2 g/d; Alt: 50 mg/kg PO 2x/wk x2mo if directly observed tx, max 2 g/dose; Info: as part of multi-drug regimen; >15y: 20-25 mg/kg PO qd x2mo; Max: 2 g/d; Alt: 40-50 mg/kg PO 2x/wk x2mo if directly observed tx, max 4 g/dose; 30-40 mg/kg PO 3x/wk x2mo if directly observed tx, max 3 g/dose; Info: as part of multi-drug regimen; monitor LFTs
Rifampin	PRC C, Lact -
Rifampin *150,300; IV*	**Active TB**, <15y: 10-20 mg/kg PO/IV qd x4-6mo; Max: 600 mg/d; Alt: 10-20 mg/kg PO/IV 2x/wk x4-6mo if directly observed, max 600 mg/dose; >15y: 10 mg/kg PO/IV qd x4-6mo; Max: 600 mg/d; Alt: 10 mg/kg PO/IV 2-3x/wk x4-6mo if directly observed, max 600 mg/dose; Info: admin. as part of multi-drug regimen; give on empty stomach **Latent TB**, <15y: 10-20 mg/kg PO/IV qd x4mo; Max: 600 mg/d; >15y: 10 mg/kg PO/IV qd x4mo; Max: 600 mg/d; Info: to prevent progression in PPD-positive pts; not first line regimen; give on empty stomach **H influenza** prophylaxis, <1mo: 10 mg/kg PO/IV q24h x4 d; Max: 600 mg/d; >1mo: 20 mg/kg PO/IV q24h x4 d: Max: 600 mg/d

	Meningococcal prophylaxis, <1mo: 5 mg/kg PO/IV q12h x2 d; Max: 600 mg/d; >1mo: 10 mg/kg PO/IV q12h x2 d; Max: 600 mg/d; Info: for asymptomatic meningococcal carriers; not for meningococcal infection tx
Trimethoprim-sulfamethozasole	PRC C, Lact +
Bactrim, Septra *80/400, 160/800; 40/200/ 5 mL; IV*	**Infections, bacterial**, >2 mo: 8-10 mg/kg/d TMP PO/IV div q12h; Info: dose, duration varies w/ infection type, severity infections, severe bacterial, >2 mo: 15-20 mg/kg/d TMP PO/IV div q6-8h; Info: dose, duration varies w/ infection type, severity PCP prophylaxis, >2 mo: 150 mg/m2/d TMP PO div q12h 3x/wk; Max: 320 mg/d TMP; Alt: 5-10 mg/kg/d TMP PO div q12h 3x/wk PCP tx, >2 mo: 15-20 mg/kg/d TMP PO div q6h x14-21 d; Alt: 15-20 mg/kg/d TMP IV div q6-8h x14 d
Vancomycin	PRC C, Lact -
Vancocin *125,250; IV*	**Severe bacterial infections**, severe bacterial, neonates <7 ds old, <1200 g: 15 mg/kg IV q24h; neonates <7 ds old, 1200-2000 g: 10-15 mg/kg IV q12-18h; neonates <7 ds old, >2000 g: 10-15 mg/kg IV q8-12h; neonates >7 ds old, <1200 g: 15 mg/kg IV q24h; neonates >7 ds old, 1200-2000 g: 10-15 mg/kg IV q8-12h; neonates >7 ds old, >2000 g: 15-20 mg/kg IV q8h; 1mo-12 yo: 10-15 mg/kg IV q6-8h; Max: 1 g/dose; Info: dose, duration varies by infection site/ severity; 12-16 yo: 1000 mg IV q12h; Alt: 10-15 mg/ kg IV q12h; Info: pts w/ high clearance may require 1200-1500 mg IV q12h or 10 mg/kg IV q8h
Zanamivir	PRC C, Lact
Relenza *5 mg/blister DPI*	**Influenza A & B** tx, >7y: 10 mg inhaled q12h x5 d; Info: give two 10 mg doses on d 1 at least 2h apart; 10 mg inhaled = 2 blisters; start w/in 48h of sx onset Influenza A & B prophylaxis, household

	setting, >5y: 10 mg inhaled q24h x10 da; Info: 10 mg inhaled = 2 blisters; start w/in 36h of sx onset in index case; CDC recommends duration 10 ds after a household exposure or 7 ds after other known exposure; community outbreak, adolescents: 10 mg inhaled q24h x28 d; Info: 10 mg inhaled = 2 blisters; start preexposure prophylaxis w/in 5 d of identified community outbreak, continue for duration of influenza activity; institutional setting, >5y: 10 mg inhaled q24h; Info: 10 mg inhaled = 2 blisters; CDC recommends duration 14 d minimum and up to 7 ds after last known case
Zidovudine	PRC C, Lact +
Retrovir, AZT *100,300; 50/5 mL*	**HIV infection**, >4wk old, 4-8 kg: 24 mg/kg/d PO div bid-tid; Max: 600 mg/d; Alt: 480 mg/m2/d PO div bid-tid; 9-29 kg: 18 mg/kg/d PO div bid-tid; Max: 600 mg/d; Alt: 480 mg/m2/d PO div bid-tid; >30 kg: 600 mg/d PO div bid-tid; Max: 600 mg/d; Alt: 480 mg/m2/d PO div bid-tid HIV prevention, premature neonates, <30wk gest: 4 mg/kg/d PO div q12h x4wk, then 6 mg/kg/d PO div q8h; Info: initiate tx w/in 12h after birth; premature neonates, >30wk gest: 4 mg/kg/d PO div q12h x2wk, then 6 mg/kg/d PO div q8h; Info: initiate tx w/in 12h after birth; term neonates: 8 mg/kg/d PO div q6h x6wk; Info: initiate tx w/in 12h after birth

16.8 Immunology

MA/EF (azathioprine): inhibits T-lymphocytes
MA/EF (cyclosporine) exact mechanism of action unknown; inhibits T-lymphocytes
MA/EF (6-mercaptopurine): inhibits DNA synthesis
MA/EF (methotrexate) immunosuppressant: inhibits dihydrofolate reductase; inhibits lymphocyte proliferation (folate antagonist)
AE (azathioprine): Serious: leukopenia, thrombocytopenia, anemia, myelosuppression, immunosuppression, infection, GI hypersensitivity reaction, pancreatitis, hepatotoxicity, hepatic veno-occlusive disease, lymphoma, malignancy, acute febrile neutrophilic

dermatosis; Common: leukopenia, thrombocytopenia, anemia, infection, nausea ,vomiting, anorexia, diarrhea, ALT/AST elevated, malaise, myalgia, fever, rash, malignancy
AE (cyclosporine): Serious: severe HTN, immunosuppression, severe or fatal infection, opportunistic infection, BK virus-assoc. nephropathy, severe hyperkalemia, nephrotoxicity, hepatotoxicity, glomerular capillary thrombosis, DM, leukopenia, thrombocytopenia, hemolytic anemia, malignancy, seizures, encephalopathy, neurotoxicity, intracranial HTN, optic disc edema, allergic reaction, MI, depression, pancreatitis, GI bleed; Common: BUN/Cr elevated, HTN, hirsutism, infection, tremor, gingival hyperplasia, headache, hypertriglyceridemia (psoriasis use), nausea/vomiting, diarrhea, leg cramps, paresthesia, influenza-like sx, edema, dizziness, rash, acne, chest pain, stomatitis, hypomagnesemia, arthralgia, flushing, bronchospasm, hyperkalemia, hyperglycemia, hyperuricemia
AE (6-mercaptopurine): Serious: myelosuppression, immunosuppression, hepatotoxicity, hepatosplenic T-cell lymphoma, hepatic encephalopathy, ascites, pancreatitis (IBD uses), GI ulceration, tumor lysis syndrome; Common: anemia, leukopenia, thrombocytopenia, jaundice, diarrhea, nausea, vomiting, anorexia, abdominal pain, hyperuricemia, hyperuricosuria, hepatotoxicity, rash, hyperpigmentation, alopecia, oligospermia
AE (methotrexate): Serious: severe ulcerative stomatitis, severe diarrhea, thrombocytopenia, leukopenia, severe anemia, aplastic anemia, agranulocytosis, lymphoproliferative disorders, hepatotoxicity, cirrhosis, hepatic fibrosis, nephrotoxicity, pulmonary fibrosis, pneumonitis, immunosuppression, opportunistic infection, leukoencephalopathy, acute transient stroke-like encephalopathy, seizures, neurotoxicity, arachnoiditis (IT use), subacute myelopathy (IT use), Stevens-Johnson syndrome, exfoliative dermatitis, erythema multiforme, toxic epidermal necrolysis, radiation recall reaction, anaphylactoid reactions; Common: LFTs elevated, nausea/vomiting, stomatitis, malaise, fatigue, abdominal discomfort, chills, fever, dizziness, diarrhea, anemia, thrombocytopenia, leukopenia, rash, pruritus, alopecia, photosensitivity
CI (azathioprine): pregnancy (RA use), avoid pregnancy, caution if renal impairment , prior alkylating agents
CI modified (cyclosporine) : uncontrolled HTN (RA or psoriasis use), renal impairment (RA or psoriasis use), malignancy (RA or psoriasis use), PUVA/UVB tx (psoriasis use), concurrent immunosuppressants (psoriasis use), coal tar tx (psoriasis use), concomitant XRT (psoriasis use); caution if hepatic or renal impairment, concurrent nephrotoxic agents, concurrent immunosuppressants
CI unmodified (cyclosporine): hypersens. to castor oil derivatives (IV form); caution if hepatic or renal impairment, concurrent nephrotoxic agents, concurrent immunosuppressants, malabsorption
CI (6-mercaptopurine): mercaptopurine or thioguanine resistance; caution if renal impairment, thiopurine methyltransferase (TPMT) deficiency, concurrent hepatotoxic agents
CI (methotrexate): pregnancy (RA or psoriasis use), breastfeeding, immunodeficiency syndromes, alcohol abuse hx (RA or psoriasis use), hepatic disease or impairment (RA or psoriasis use), blood dyscrasias (RA or psoriasis use), myelosuppression (RA or psoriasis use); caution if myelosuppression, active infection, hepatic impairment, renal impairment,

ulcerative colitis, PUD, pleural effusion, ascites, concomitant XRT, debilitated pts, avoid conception (female or male pts)	
Azathioprine	PRC D, Lact +
Imuran, Azasan *50; IV*	**JIA**, severe: 1-2.5 mg/kg/d PO div qd-bid]; Start: 1 mg/kg/d PO div qd-bid; Max: 2.5 mg/kg/d; Info: after 6-8wks may incr. 0.5 mg/kg/d q4wk
Cyclosporine	PRC C, Lact ?
Cyclosporine modified, Gengraf, Neoral *25,100; 100/mL* **Cyclosporine unmodified, Sandimmune** *25,100; 100/mL; IV*	**Organ transplant rejection prophylaxis, modified:** 7-9 mg/kg/d PO div bid, give 1st dose 4-12h pre-transplant or postop; Info: for heart, kidney, or liver transplant; adjust dose based on target levels, rejection status, adverse effects; unmodified PO: dosing protocols vary; Start: 15 mg/kg PO x1 given 4-12h pre-transplant or postop, then 10-15 mg/kg/d PO x1-2wk, then decr. 5%/wk to 5-10 mg/kg/d PO div bid; Info: for heart, kidney, or liver transplant; adjust dose based on target levels, rejection status, adverse effects; unmodified IV: dosing protocols vary; Start: 5-6 mg/kg/d IV, give 1st dose 4-12h pre-transplant or postop; Info: for heart, kidney, or liver transplant; adjust dose based on target levels, rejection status, adverse effects; IV dose = 1/3 PO dose, switch to PO form ASAP Info: modified and non-modified cyclosporine products not bioequivalent; caution advised if switching between products
6-mercaptopurine	PRC D, Lact ?
Purinethol *50*	**Acute lymphoblastic leukemia:** consult with pediatric oncologist
Methotrexate	PRC X, Lact +
Methotrexate *2.5; IM; IV; IT; intra-arterial*	**JIA**, 2-16y: 5-15 mg/m2 PO/IM qwk; Start: 10 mg/m2 PO/IM qwk; Max: 30 mg/m2/wk; Alt: may give div doses PO q12h x3 doses qwk; Info: use lowest effective dose; give w/ folic acid 1 mg qd or leucovorin 5 mg qwk; injectable product may be given PO

	Cancer chemotherapy: Consult pediatric oncologist

16.9 Antirheumatics/Analgesics

MA/EF (acetaminophen): analgesic mechanism unknown; antipyretic effect via direct action on hypothalamus
MA/EF (adalimumab): binds & inhibits tumor necrosis factor, reducing inflammation & altering immune response
MA/EF (anakinra): recombinant human IL 1 antagonist, reduce the pain and swelling in moderate to severe RA. Inhibits the binding of the IL 1 to its receptor
MA/EF (aspirin) non-selectively and irreversibly inhibits cyclooxygenase, reducing prostaglandin and thromboxane A2 synthesis, producing analgesic, anti-inflammatory, and antipyretic effects and reducing platelet aggregation
MA/EF (Beclomethasone): exact mechanism of anti-inflammatory action unknown; inhibits multiple inflammatory cytokines; produces multiple glucocorticoid and mineralocorticoid effects
MA/EF (codeine sulfate) binds to various opioid receptors, producing analgesia, sedation and antitussive effects (opioid agonist)
MA/EF (fentanyl) binds to various opioid receptors, producing analgesia and sedation (opioid agonist)
MA/EF (flunisolide nasal) exact mechanism of anti-inflammatory action unknown; inhibits multiple inflammatory cytokines; produces multiple glucocorticoid and mineralocorticoid effects
MA/EF (hydromorphone) binds to various opioid receptors, producing analgesia and sedation (opioid agonist)
MA/EF (ibuprofen) exact mechanism of action unknown; inhibits cyclooxygenase, reducing prostaglandin and thromboxane synthesis
MA/EF (indomethacin) exact mechanism of action unknown; inhibits cyclooxygenase, reducing prostaglandin and thromboxane synthesis
MA/EF (ketorolac) exact mechanism of action unknown; inhibits cyclooxygenase, reducing prostaglandin and thromboxane synthesis
MA/EF (meperidine) binds to various opioid receptors, producing analgesia and sedation (opioid agonist)
MA/EF (morphine) binds to various opioid receptors, producing analgesia and sedation (opioid agonist)
MA/EF (naproxen) exact mechanism of action unknown; inhibits cyclooxygenase, reducing prostaglandin and thromboxane synthesis
MA/EF (oxycodone) binds to various opioid receptors, producing analgesia and sedation (opioid agonist)
AE (acetaminophen): Serious: anaphylaxis, hepatoxicity, acute RTA, chronic nephropathy, anemia, thrombocytopenia; Common: nausea, rash, headache
AE (adalimumab): Serious: sepsis, TB, RA flare, malignancy, HBV reactivation, CHF, anaphylaxis, angioneurotic edema, SLE, myelosuppression, aplastic anemia, demyelinating disease, skin reactions, photosensitivity; Common: injection site reaction, URI, headache,

rash, sinusitis, nausea, UTI, hyperlipidemia, flu syndrome, abdominal pain, back pain, HTN, hematuria, allergic reactions; alk phos, ALT, AST, CK
AE (anakinra):redness, bruising, swelling & pain at injection site, chest infection, UTI, headache, nausea, diarrhea, sinusitis, joint pain, flu like-symptoms, and abdominal pain
AE (aspirin): Serious: anaphylactic/anaphylactoid reactions, angioedema, bronchospasm, bleeding, GI ulceration/perforation, DIC, pancytopenia, thrombocytopenia, agranulocytosis, aplastic anemia, hypoprothrombinemia, nephrotoxicity, hepatotoxicity (high-dose ASA use), salicylism, Reye syndrome; Common: dyspepsia, nausea, vomiting, abdominal pain, rash, tinnitus, dizziness, hyperuricemia, bleeding, ecchymosis, constipation, diarrhea
AE (Beclomethasone) inhaled: Serious: bronchospasm, hypersensitivity reaction, adrenal suppression, hypercortisolism, growth suppression, eosinophilia, Churg-Strauss syndrome, glaucoma, cataracts, osteoporosis; Common: headache, pharyngitis, URI, rhinitis, sinusitis, pain, back pain, nausea, dysphonia, dysmenorrheal, cough, oral candidiasis
AE (Beclamethasone) nasal: Serious: nasal septal perforation, nasal ulcer, nasal/oral candidiasis, growth suppression, IOP incr., glaucoma, cataracts, hypercortisolism, adrenal suppression, anaphylaxis, angioedema, bronchospasm, wheezing; Common: nasal irritation, headache, nausea, lightheadedness, epistaxis, rhinorrhea, watery eyes, sneezing, dry nose, dry throat, dysgeusia
AE (codeine sulfate): Serious: respiratory depression, CNS depression, hypotension, bradycardia, syncope, shock, cardiac arrest, ICP incr., seizures, paralytic ileus, dependency/abuse, withdrawal if abrupt D/C, anaphylactoid reactions; Common: lightheadedness, dizziness, sedation, nausea/vomiting, sweating, dry mouth, anorexia, constipation, urinary hesitancy/retention, weakness, flushing, pruritus, urticarial, headache, rash, visual disturbances, edema, disorientation, euphoria, dysphoria, insomnia, agitation, biliary spasm, palpitations
AE (fentanyl): Serious: respiratory depression, respiratory arrest, dependency/abuse, severe bradycardia, severe hypotension, anaphylaxis, laryngospasm, bronchoconstriction, severe muscle rigidity, cardiac arrest, circulatory collapse, arrhythmias, ICP incr., delirium, seizures, paralytic ileus; Common: somnolence, nausea, vomiting, confusion, asthenia, constipation, dry mouth, sweating, dizziness, urinary retention, nervousness, euphoria, hallucinations, dyspnea, pruritus, hypotension, bradycardia, muscle rigidity, biliary spasm, incoordination
AE (flunisolide nasal): Serious: nasal septal perforation, nasal ulcer, nasal/oral candidiasis, growth suppression, hypercortisolism, adrenal suppression; Common: dysgeusia, nasal burning/stinging, nasal irritation, epistaxis, nasal dryness, pharyngitis, cough, nausea, headache, watery eyes, sneezing, nasal congestion, nausea/vomiting
AE (hydromorphone): Serious: respiratory depression, circulatory depression, severe hypotension, ICP incr., seizures, dependency/abuse, withdrawal if abrupt D/C, neonatal withdrawal (long-term maternal use), paralytic ileus, biliary spasm, hypersensitivity reaction; Common: dizziness, somnolence, nausea/vomiting, hyperhidrosis, flushing, dysphoria/euphoria, xerostomia, pruritus, headache, constipation, anorexia, rash, insomnia, anxiety/agitation, muscle spasms, depression, abdominal cramps, injection site reaction (IV)
AE (ibuprofen): Serious: GI bleed, GI ulceration/perforation, MI, stroke, thromboembolism, HTN, CHF, renal papillary necrosis, nephrotoxicity, hepatotoxicity, anaphylactic/anaphylactoid reactions, bronchospasm, exfoliative dermatitis, Stevens-Johnson syndrome,

toxic epidermal necrolysis, thrombocytopenia, agranulocytosis, aplastic anemia, hemolytic anemia, neutropenia, pancytopenia; Common: dyspepsia, nausea, abdominal pain, constipation, headache, dizziness, drowsiness, rash, ALT/AST elevated, fluid retention, tinnitus, ecchymosis, photosensitivity

AE (indomethacin): Serious: pulmonary hemorrhage (neonates), GI bleed, GI ulceration/perforation, MI, stroke, thromboembolism, HTN, CHF, renal papillary necrosis, nephrotoxicity, acute renal failure (neonates), hepatotoxicity, anaphylactoid reactions, bronchospasm, exfoliative dermatitis, Stevens-Johnson syndrome, toxic epidermal necrolysis, anemia, blood dyscrasias, prolonged bleeding time, DIC (neonates), platelet aggregation decr. (neonates), thrombocytopenia (neonates), hyponatremia (neonates), hyperkalemia (neonates), psychiatric disturbances; Common: dyspepsia, nausea, abdominal pain, constipation, headache, dizziness, somnolence, rash, ALT/AST elevated, peripheral edema, fluid retention, tinnitus, ecchymosis, corneal deposits, photosensitivity

AE (ketorolac): Serious: GI bleed, GI ulceration/perforation, ulcerative stomatitis, severe bleeding, MI, stroke, thromboembolism, HTN, CHF, renal papillary necrosis, nephrotoxicity, hepatotoxicity, bronchospasm, anaphylactoid reactions, exfoliative dermatitis, Stevens-Johnson syndrome, toxic epidermal necrolysis, anemia, blood dyscrasias, inflammatory bowel disease exacerbation; Common: headache, nausea, abdominal pain, dyspepsia, dizziness, somnolence, constipation, diarrhea, edema, rash, ALT/AST elevated, fluid retention, tinnitus, injection site pain, HTN, pruritus, flatulence, sweating, ecchymosis, photosensitivity

AE (meperidine): Serious: respiratory depression, apnea, respiratory arrest, severe hypotension, circulatory depression, shock, cardiac arrest, syncope, bradycardia, urinary retention, hallucinations, seizures, biliary spasm, hypersensitivity reactions, anaphylaxis, withdrawal if abrupt D/C, dependency/abuse; Common: lightheadedness, dizziness, sedation, nausea/vomiting, sweating, dry mouth, constipation, dysphoria/euphoria, flushing, orthostatic hypotension, weakness, palpitations/tachycardia, headache, anxiety/agitation, pruritus/rash/urticaria, visual disturbances, tremor, involuntary movements, urinary retention, bradycardia

AE (morphine): Serious: respiratory depression, apnea, severe hypotension, cardiac arrest, shock, bradycardia, paralytic ileus, toxic megacolon, seizures, ICP incr., dependency/abuse, withdrawal if abrupt D/C, neonatal withdrawal (long-term maternal use), anaphylaxis, anemia, thrombocytopenia; Common: somnolence, constipation, nausea/vomiting, dizziness, hypotension, histamine release, dysphoria, euphoria, sweating, edema, abdominal pain, pruritus, flushing, dry mouth, asthenia, paresthesia, urinary retention, biliary spasm, libido decr., miosis

AE (naproxen): Serious: GI bleed, GI ulceration/perforation, MI, stroke, thromboembolism, HTN, CHF, renal papillary necrosis, nephrotoxicity, hepatotoxicity, anaphylactic/anaphylactoid reactions, bronchospasm, exfoliative dermatitis, Stevens-Johnson syndrome, toxic epidermal necrolysis, thrombocytopenia, agranulocytosis, aplastic anemia, hemolytic anemia, neutropenia, leukopenia, angioedema; Common: dyspepsia, nausea, abdominal pain, constipation, headache, dizziness, drowsiness, rash, ALT/AST elevated, fluid retention, tinnitus, ecchymosis, dyspnea, photosensitivity

AE (oxycodone): Serious: respiratory depression, circulatory depression, severe hypotension, ICP incr., seizures, dependency/abuse, withdrawal if abrupt D/C (long-term use), neonatal withdrawal (long-term maternal use), paralytic ileus, biliary spasm, hypersensitivity reaction, exfoliative dermatitis; Common: constipation, nausea/vomiting, headache, pruritus, insomnia, dizziness, asthenia, somnolence, dry mouth, sweating, anorexia, nervousness, fever/chills, confusion, diarrhea, abdominal pain, dyspepsia, rash, anxiety, dysphoria/euphoria, orthostatic hypotension
CI (acetaminophen): caution if hepatic impairment, renal impairment, severe hypovolemia, PKU, malnutrition, chronic alcohol use
CI (adalimumab): concurrent live vaccine, active infection; caution if chronic/recurrent infection, infection risk, opportunistic infection hx, co-morbid conditions, uncontrolled DM, TB latent or risk, concurrent immunosuppressants, HBV carrier, demyelinating disease, myelosuppression, CHF, malignancy hx, TB/mycoses exposure, latex hypersensitivity
CI (anakinra): Hypersensitivity to E. coli -derived proteins, anakinra, or its any component
CI (aspirin): ASA or NSAID-induced asthma or urticaria, aspirin triad, GI bleed, coagulation disorder, G6PD deficiency, uncontrolled HTN; influenza, varicella, or febrile viral infection (pts <20 yo); caution if thrombocytopenia, surgery or trauma, intracranial lesion, ICP incr., chronic alcohol use, PUD, GI bleed hx, GERD, gout (high-dose ASA use), renal impairment , hepatic impairment, sodium restriction (buffered ASA forms)
CI (Beclomethasone) inhaled: status asthmaticus, acute asthma, acute bronchospasm, avoid abrupt withdrawal; caution if untreated local or systemic infection, TB infection, ocular HSV, measles or varicella exposure, recent long-term systemic corticosteroid tx, glaucoma, IOP incr., cataracts, decr. BMD hx, decr. BMD risk
CI (Beclomethasone) nasal unhealed nasal septal ulcer, unhealed nasal surgery or trauma wound; caution if untreated local or systemic infection, TB infection, ocular HSV infection, measles or varicella exposure, recurrent epistaxis, IOP incr., glaucoma, cataracts, recent long-term systemic corticosteroid tx
CI (codeine sulfate): respiratory depression, paralytic ileus; caution if CNS depression, head injury, ICP incr., seizure disorder, asthma, COPD, acute abdomen, GI/GU obstruction, inflammatory bowel disease, pseudomembranous colitis, biliary disease, urethral stricture, prostatic hypertrophy, severe renal or hepatic impairment, hypothyroidism, Addison disease, alcohol or drug abuse hx, ultra-rapid CYP2D6 metabolizer, pts <2 yo
CI (fentanyl): caution if renal/hepatic impairment, head injury, ICP incr., pulmonary impairment, impaired cardiovascular fxn, GI obstruction, prostatic hypertrophy, CNS depressant use, resp. depressant use, hypotension, biliary disease, seizure disorder, inflammatory bowel disease
CI (flunisolide nasal): unhealed nasal septal ulcer, unhealed nasal surgery or trauma wound; caution if untreated local or systemic infection, TB infection, ocular HSV infection, measles or varicella exposure, recurrent epistaxis, glaucoma, recent long-term systemic corticosteroid tx
CI (hydromorphone): hypersens. to sulfites, opioid non-tolerant pts (high potency dosage form), severe respiratory depression, acute or severe asthma, hypercarbia, GI obstruction, paralytic ileus, labor and delivery, avoid abrupt withdrawal; caution if hypersens. to latex (branded vial form), pregnancy 3rd trimester, hepatic/renal/pulmonary impairment, CNS

depression, CNS depressant use, alcohol use, delirium tremens, hypothyroidism, adrenal insufficiency, ICP incr., seizure disorder, toxic psychosis, cardiovascular disease, volume depletion, circulatory shock, GI motility disorder, acute abdomen, biliary surgery or disease, prostatic hypertrophy, urethral stricture, substance abuse hx

CI (ibuprofen): ASA or NSAID-induced asthma or urticarial, aspirin triad, pregnancy 3rd trimester, CABG surgery period use; caution if cardiovascular disease, cardiac disease risk, HTN, CHF, fluid retention, dehydration, PUD, GI bleed hx, coagulation disorder, chronic alcohol use, smoker, debilitated pts, renal/hepatic impairment, asthma, prolonged use

CI (indomethacin): ASA or NSAID-induced asthma or urticarial, aspirin triad, pregnancy 3rd trimester, untreated infection (neonates), active bleeding (neonates), thrombocytopenia (neonates), coagulation disorder (neonates), necrotizing enterocolitis (neonates), , renal impairment, significant (neonates), pulmonary atresia (neonates), tetralogy of Fallot, severe (neonates), aortic coarctation, severe (neonates), CABG surgery period use, proctitis hx (supp form), recent rectal bleeding (supp form); caution if cardiovascular disease, cardiac disease risk, HTN, CHF, fluid retention, GI bleed or ulcer hx, coagulation disorder, debilitated pts, alcohol use, smoker, renal/hepatic impairment, concurrent nephrotoxic agents, dehydration, sepsis, asthma, psychiatric disorder, neurologic disease, prolonged use

CI (ketorolac): ASA or NSAID-induced asthma or urticarial, aspirin triad, GI bleed or PUD hx, cerebrovascular hemorrhage, coagulation disorder, active bleeding, CABG surgery periop use, major surgery preop use, epidural or intrathecal use, pregnancy 3rd trimester, labor and delivery, breastfeeding if infant <1 mo, severe renal impairment, volume depletion; caution if inflammatory bowel disease, coagulation disorder, alcohol use, smoker, asthma, hepatic impairment, mild-moderate renal impairment, CHF, HTN, cardiovascular disease, cardiac disease risk

CI (meperidine): MAO inhibitor use w/in 14 ds, severe respiratory depression, avoid abrupt withdrawal; caution in labor and delivery, neonates or infants, debilitated pts, hepatic/renal/pulmonary impairment, cor pulmonale, asthma or COPD, respiratory depression, head injury or intracranial lesion, ICP incr., CNS depression, seizure disorder, SVT, hypotension, acute abdomen, prostatic hypertrophy or urethral stricture, adrenal insufficiency, hypothyroidism, substance abuse, acute alcoholism, sickle cell anemia, pheochromocytoma, delirium tremens, toxic psychosis, prolonged use

CI (morphine): respiratory depression, acute or severe asthma, hypercarbia, paralytic ileus, <24h postop (opioid-naive pts, ER form), labor and delivery, avoid abrupt withdrawal; caution if renal impairment, hepatic impairment, pulmonary impairment, CNS depression, head injury or intracranial lesion, ICP incr., seizure disorder, substance abuse, acute alcoholism, delirium tremens, toxic psychosis, kyphoscoliosis, circulatory shock, adrenal insufficiency, hypothyroidism, prostatic hypertrophy or urethral stricture, acute abdomen, acute pancreatitis or biliary disease, pregnancy 3rd trimester, debilitated pts

CI (naproxen): ASA or NSAID-induced asthma or urticarial, aspirin triad, pregnancy 3rd trimester; caution if cardiovascular disease or risk, HTN, CHF, fluid retention, dehydration, PUD, GI bleed hx, coagulation disorder, renal/hepatic impairment, asthma, sodium restriction, prolonged use, chronic alcohol use, smoking habit changes, debilitated pts

CI (oxycodone): severe respiratory depression, asthma, hypercarbia, paralytic ileus, labor and delivery, avoid abrupt withdrawal (long-term use); caution in debilitated pts, 3rd trimester, hepatic/pulmonary/renal impairment, CNS depression, alcohol use, delirium tremens, hypothyroidism, adrenal insufficiency, ICP incr., seizure, volume depletion, CVS disease, circulatory shock, GI motility disorder, GI obstruction or stricture, acute abdomen, biliary surgery or disease, prostatic hypertrophy, urethral stricture, substance abuse hx	
Acetaminophen	PRC B, Lact -
Tylenol *325, 500 mg tab; 80, 160 mg chewable; 160 mg/5ml susp* *FeverAll rectal supp 80, 120, 325 mg*	**Fever, pain**: 10-15 mg/kg q4h, max 75 mg/kg/d
Adalimumab	PRC B, Lact ?
Brand1 Humira, SC	**JIA**, moderate-severe, >4y: 15-30 kg: 20 mg SC q2wk; >30 kg: 40 mg SC q2wk
Anakinra	PRC B, Lact ?
Kineret, SC	**NOMID**:1-2 mg/kgto8 mg/kg/d
Aspirin	PRC D, Lact +
Aspirin *81,325,500,350; 81 CH; 81,325, 500,650 DR; 60,120,200,300,600 PR*	**Pain/fever**: 10-15 mg/kg PO/PR q4-6h; Max: 60-80 mg/kg/d **JIA**: 60-100 mg/kg/d PO div q6-8h; Start: 60 mg/kg/d; Max: 100 mg/kg/d; Info: incr. 10-20 mg/kg/d q5-7 ds **Kawasaki disease:** 80-100 mg/kg/d PO div q6h; decr. to 3-5 mg/kg PO qd after fever resolves; total duration x8wk
Beclomethasone	PRC C, Lact ?
Beclomethasone inhaled, Qvar *40,80 µg/ spray MDI*	**Asthma**, maintenance tx: Prior bronchodilator alone, 5-11 yo: 40-80 µg inhaled bid; Start: 40 µg inhaled bid; Max: 160 µg/d; Prior bronchodilator alone, >12 yo: 40-320 µg inhaled bid; Start: 40-80 µg inhaled bid; Max: 640 µg/d; Prior inhaled steroid, 5-11 yo: 40-80 µg inhaled bid; Start: 40 µg inhaled bid; Max: 160 µg/d; Prior inhaled steroid, >12 yo: 40-320 µg inhaled bid; Start: 40-160 µg inhaled bid; Max: 640 µg/d; Prior oral steroid, 5-11 yo: 40-80 µg inhaled bid; Start: varies based on oral steroid maintenance dose; Max: 160 µg/d; Info: titrate to lowest effective dose; rinse mouth after use; taper oral steroids gradually after >1wk; Prior oral steroid, >12 yo:

	40-320 µg inhaled bid; Start: varies based on oral steroid maintenance dose; Max: 640 µg/d; Info: titrate to lowest effective dose; rinse mouth after use; taper oral steroids gradually after >1wk; Info for all above: titrate to lowest effective dose
Beclomethasone nasal, Beconase AQ, Qnasl *42 µg/spray*	**Allergic rhinitis,** 6-12 yo: 1-2 sprays in each nostril bid; Start: 1 spray in each nostril bid; Max: 4 sprays in each nostril/d; Info: D/C after 3wk if no improvement; >12 yo: 1-2 sprays in each nostril bid; Max: 4 sprays in each nostril/d; Info: D/C after 3wk if no improvement
Codeine sulfate	PRC C, Lact ?
Codeine *15, 30, 60*	**Mild-moderate pain,** 3-6y: 0.5-1 mg/kg PO q4-6h prn; Max: 60 mg/dose, 360 mg/d; 7-12y: 15-30 mg PO q4-6h prn; Max: 60 mg/dose, 360 mg/d; Alt: 0.5-1 mg/kg PO q4-6h prn; 13-17y: 15-60 mg PO q4-6h prn; Max: 60 mg/dose, 360 mg/d; Alt: 0.5-1 mg/kg PO q4-6h prn **Cough**, 2-5y: 1-1.5 mg/kg/d PO div q4-6h prn; Max: 30 mg/d; 6-11y: 1-1.5 mg/kg/d PO div q4-6h prn; Max: 60 mg/d; >12y: 15-30 mg PO q4-6h prn; Max: 120 mg/d Info for all: give w/ food
Fentanyl	PRC C, Lact -
Sublimaze *IM, IV*	**Sedation/analgesia**, 1-3y: 2-3 µg/kg IV q1-4h prn; Alt: 1-2 µg/kg IV x1 then 0.5-1 µg/kg/h infusion; 3-12y: 1-2 µg/kg IV q1-4h prn; Alt: 1-2 µg/kg IV x1 then 0.5-1 µg/kg/h infusion; >12y: 0.5-1 µg/kg IV q1-4h prn; Alt: 1-2 µg/kg IV x1 then 0.5-1 µg/kg/h infusion; Info all ages: titrate upward
Flunisolide nasal	PRC C, Lact ?
Nasarel *25,29 µg spray*	**Allergic rhinitis**, 6-14y: 2 sprays per nostril bid; Alt: 1 spray per nostril tid; Max: 4 sprays per nostril/d; >14y: 2 sprays per nostril bid-tid; Start: 2 sprays per nostril bid; Max: 8 sprays per nostril/d

Hydromorphone	PRC C, Lact -
Dilaudid *2,4,8; SC; IV*	**Moderate-severe pain,** <6mo: 0.005 mg/kg SC/IV q2-6h; Start: 0.005 mg/kg SC/IV q4-6h; Alt: 0.0015 mg/kg/h IV; >6mo, <50 kg: 0.03-0.08 mg/kg PO q3-6h; 0.015-0.02 mg/kg SC/IV q2-6h; Start: 0.03-0.08 mg/kg PO q4-6h; 0.015-0.02 mg/kg SC/IV q4-6h; Alt: 0.006 mg/kg/h IV; >6mo, >50 kg: 2-4 mg PO q3-6h; 1-2 mg SC/IV q3-6h; Start: 1-2 mg PO q4-6h; 1 mg SC q4-6h; 0.2-0.6 mg IV q2-4h; Alt: 0.3 mg/h IV
Ibuprofen	PRC B, Lact -
Advil, Motrin *100,200,400, 600,800; 50,100 CH; 20,40/mL susp*	**Fever, mild-moderate pain**, 6mo-12y: 5-10 mg/kg PO q6-8h prn; Max: 40 mg/kg/d; Info: use lower dose for fever <102.5 F, higher dose for fever >102.5 F; >12y: 200-400 mg PO q4-6h; Info: use shortest effective tx duration; give w/ food
Indomethacin	PRC B, Lact +
Indocin *25,50; 75 ER; 50 PR; IV*	**Patent ductus arteriosus,** <48h: start 0.2 mg/kg IV x1, then 0.1 mg/kg q12-24h x2; 2-7 d: start 0.2 mg/kg IV x1, then 0.2 mg/kg q12-24h x2; >7d: start 0.2 mg/kg IV x1, then 0.25 mg/kg q12-24h x2
Ketorolac	PRC C, Lact ?
Toradol *10; IM; IV*	**Pain, mod-severe**, >6mo: 0.5 mg/kg IM/IV q6h up to 72h; Alt: 1 mg/kg IM/IV q6h up to 24-48h; Max: 30 mg/dose IM, 15 mg/dose IV; Info: single dose tx FDA-approved for >2 yo; limited data on multiple dose tx; use lowest effective dose, shortest effective tx duration
Meperidine	PRC C, Lact -
Demerol *50,100; 10/mL; SC; IM; IV*	**Pain, mod-severe**: 1-1.75 mg/kg PO/SC/IM q3-4h; Max: 100 mg/dose; Info: PO route least effective; IM preferred over SC for repeat doses; decr. dose if given IV, dilute prior to use, admin. slowly or via PCA; incr. risk of excitatory neurotoxicity, seizure if dose >600 mg/24h IM/SC/IV or duration >48h

	Preoperative sedation: 1-2.2 mg/kg SC/IM x1; Max: 100 mg/dose; Info: give 30-90min before anesthesia
Morphine	PRC C, Lact -
Morphine sulfate *Inj 0.5, 1, 2, 3, 4, 5, 8, 10, 15, 20, 25, 50mg/ml*	**Pain**: <6mo: 0.05-0.2 mg/kg SC/IM/IV q4h prn (avoid IM if possible); 6mo-12yo: 0.1-0.2 mg/kg SC/IM/IV q2-4h, max 15 mg/dose; alt 0.01-0.04 mg/kg/h IV for postop pain; 0.04-0.07 mg/kg/h IV for sickle cell or cancer pain; >12yo: 2.5-10 mg SC/IM/IV q2-6h prn, alt 0.05-0.1 mg/kg IV load, then 0.8-1.0 mg/h IV; **Neonatal opioid withdrawal**: 0.08-0.2 mg IV q3-4h prn
Naproxen	PRC C, Lact +
Naprosyn, Aleve *250,375,500; 375,500 DR; 125/5 mL*	**Pain, fever, JIA:** 10-20 mg/kg/d PO div q8-12h; Max: 1000 mg/d; Info: use lowest effective dose, shortest effective tx duration
Oxycodone	PRC B, Lact -
Roxycodone *5,10,15,20,30*	**Mod-severe pain:** 0.05-0.15 mg/kg PO q4-6h prn; Max: 5 mg/dose; Info: give w/ food; taper dose gradually to D/C if physical dependence risk

16.10 Anesthetics

MA/EF inhibits Na ion channels, stabilizing neuronal cell membranes and inhibiting nerve impulse initiation and conduction (amide local anesthetic); depresses action potential phase 0 (class IB antiarrhythmic)
AE Serious: seizures, respiratory arrest, worsened arrhythmias, status asthmaticus, heart block, bradycardia, coma, anaphylaxis, methemoglobinemia; Common: injection site pain, lightheadedness, tremor, confusion, hypotension, blurred vision, tinnitus, anxiety, dizziness, euphoria, drowsiness, lethargy, nausea, vomiting, agitation, hallucinations
CI Adams-Stokes syndrome, WPW syndrome, heart block w/o pacemaker, intra-articular continuous infusion; caution if impaired cardiac fxn, heart block, CHF, bradycardia, marked hypoxia, severe respiratory depression, hypovolemia, shock, hepatic impairment, renal impairment

Lidocaine	PRC B, Lact -
Xylocaine *Inj 0.5% (5mg/ ml), 1% (10mg/ml), 2% (20mg/ml), 4% (40mg/ml)* **Zingo (lidocaine intradermal system)** **LidoSite (lidocaine/epinephrine iontophoretic topical)** **EMLA (lidocaine/prilocaine topical)**	**Ventricular arrhythmias:** 20-50 µg/kg/min IV; start 1 mg/kg slow IV, may repeat q10-15min x2, up to 3-5 mg/kg in 1st h; max 20 µg/kg/min if in shock or CHF; PALS, VF/ pulseless VT: 1 mg/kg IV/IO prn, max 100 mg/ dose; Topical/intradermal/ **oronasopharyngeal**: apply/inject prior to procedure (various pre-procedure times according to product

16.11 Neurology

MA/EF (almotriptan) activates vascular serotonin 5-HT1 receptors, producing vasoconstriction (selective serotonin agonist)
MA/EF (amantadine) blocks viral particle uncoating and nucleic acid release into host cell, inhibiting viral replication
MA/EF (divalproex sodium) exact mechanism of action unknown; increases GABA effects, may inhibit glutamate/NMDA receptor-mediated neuronal excitation
MA/EF (eletriptan) activates vascular serotonin 5-HT1 receptors, producing vasoconstriction (selective serotonin agonist)
MA/EF (fosphenytoin) modulates neuronal voltage-dependent sodium and calcium channels
MA/EF (gabapentin)(lamotrigine)(levetiracetam)(topiramate)(zonisamide) unknown
MA/EF (oxcarbazepine ER): produces blockade of voltage-sensitive sodium channels, partial seizures in adults and in children 6 years to 17 years of age
MA/EF (perampanel): selective AMPA-type glutamate receptor antagonist. Indicated as adjunctive therapy for the treatment of partial-onset seizures with or without secondarily generalized seizures in patients with epilepsy .12 y
MA/EF (rizatriptan) (sumatriptan)activates vascular serotonin 5-HT1 receptors, producing vasoconstriction (selective serotonin agonist)
MA/EF (valproic acid) exact mechanism of action unknown; increases GABA effects, may inhibit glutamate/NMDA receptor-mediated neuronal excitation
AE (almotriptan): Serious: coronary vasospasm, myocardial ischemia, MI, ventricular tachycardia, ventricular fibrillation, arrhythmias, severe HTN, stroke, cerebral hemorrhage, subarachnoid hemorrhage, peripheral vascular ischemia, intestinal ischemia, vision loss, serotonin syndrome, headache exacerbation; Common: nausea, somnolence, dizziness, vomiting, headache, paresthesia, dry mouth; chest, jaw or neck pain/pressure/tightness, jaw pain/pressure/tightness
AE (amantadine): Serious: CHF, arrhythmias, cardiac arrest, psychosis, coma, neuroleptic malignant syndrome, visual impairment, respiratory failure, pulmonary edema, anaphylactoid reactions, suicidal ideation, agranulocytosis, neutropenia, leukopenia, seizures, oculogyric crisis, heat stroke; Common: nausea, dizziness, insomnia, depression, anxiety, irritability, hallucinations, confusion, anorexia, dry mouth, constipation, ataxia, livedo reticularis, peripheral edema, orthostatic hypotension, headache, somnolence, abnormal dreams, diarrhea, compulsive behaviors

AE (divalproex sodium): Serious: hepatotoxicity, pancreatitis, SIADH, hyponatremia, pancytopenia, thrombocytopenia, multi-organ hypersensitivity reaction, hyperammonemia, hypothermia, myelosuppression, aplastic anemia, bleeding, erythema multiforme, Stevens-Johnson syndrome, toxic epidermal necrolysis, anaphylaxis, hallucinations, psychosis, suicidality, congenital anomalies, congenital neural tube defects, encephalopathy, coma, polycystic ovary syndrome; Common: headache, nausea/vomiting, asthenia, somnolence, thrombocytopenia, dyspepsia, dizziness, diarrhea, abdominal pain, tremor, alopecia, weight changes, appetite changes, constipation, nervousness, emotional lability, insomnia, peripheral edema, petechiae/ecchymosis, rash, depression, dyspnea, tinnitus, ALT/AST elevated, amnesia, abnormal gait, visual changes, blurred vision, nystagmus, myalgia, photosensitivity
AE (eletriptan): Serious: coronary vasospasm, myocardial ischemia, MI, ventricular tachycardia, ventricular fibrillation, life-threatening arrhythmias, severe HTN, hypertensive crisis, stroke, cerebral hemorrhage, subarachnoid hemorrhage, peripheral vascular ischemia, intestinal ischemia, serotonin syndrome, seizure, headache exacerbation (use >10 ds/mo); Common: dizziness, somnolence, asthenia, nausea, headache, paresthesia, dry mouth, chest pain/pressure/ tightness, jaw pain/pressure/tightness, neck pain/pressure/tightness, dysphagia, dyspepsia, abdominal cramps/pain
AE (fosphenytoin): Serious: cardiovascular collapse, toxic delirium, severe hypotension, bradycardia, arrhythmias, exfoliative dermatitis, Stevens-Johnson syndrome, toxic epidermal necrolysis, rash w/ eosinophilia and systemic sx, hepatotoxicity, thrombocytopenia, leukopenia, agranulocytosis, pancytopenia, anemia, purple glove syndrome (IV use); Common: nystagmus, dizziness, pruritus, paresthesia, headache, somnolence, ataxia, nausea, rash, tremor, hypotension, dry mouth, confusion, blurred vision, taste changes, fever, injection site reaction, constipation, hypokalemia
AE (gabapentin): Serious: leukopenia, thrombocytopenia, withdrawal seizures, withdrawal if abrupt D/C, dyskinesia, depression, suicidality, hostility, erythema multiforme, Stevens-Johnson syndrome, rash w/ eosinophilia and systemic sx, acute renal failure; Common: dizziness, somnolence, ataxia, fatigue, peripheral edema, nystagmus, nausea/vomiting, viral infection, fever, hostility, tremor, emotional lability, blurred vision, asthenia, diarrhea, infection, dry mouth, hyperkinesia, headache, constipation, URI, abnormal thinking, dysarthria, dyspepsia, weight gain
AE (lamotrigine): Serious: severe rash, Stevens-Johnson syndrome, toxic epidermal necrolysis, angioedema hypersensitivity reaction, multiple organ failure, rash w/ eosinophilia and systemic sx, DIC, neutropenia, leukopenia, thrombocytopenia, pancytopenia, anemia, aplastic anemia, hemolytic anemia, pure red cell aplasia, withdrawal seizures, status epilepticus, aseptic meningitis, sudden death, hepatic failure, pancreatitis, rhabdomyolysis, suicidality, worsening depression, neonatal cleft lip/palate (1st trimester use); Common: nausea/vomiting, dizziness/vertigo, visual disturbances, somnolence, ataxia, pruritus/rash, headache, pharyngitis, rhinitis, diarrhea, fever, asthenia, insomnia, tremor, abdominal pain, cough, accidental injury, constipation, dysmenorrhea, incoordination, anxiety, seizures, back pain, dyspepsia, irritability, anorexia, xerostomia, photosensitivity

AE (levetiracetam): Serious: depression, hostility, aggressive behavior, psychosis, suicidality, leukopenia, neutropenia, withdrawal seizures, Stevens-Johnson syndrome, toxic epidermal necrolysis; Common: somnolence, asthenia, vomiting, headache, URI sx, anorexia, infection, hostility, fatigue, nervousness, dizziness, diarrhea, behavior changes, irritability, pain, agitation, emotional lability, depression, nausea, vertigo, ataxia, leukopenia, neutropenia, anxiety, confusion, amnesia, alopecia
AE (oxcarbazepine ER): dizziness, headache, tremor, vomiting, diplopia, asthenia, fatigue
AE (perampanel): dizziness, drowsiness, fatigue, irritability, falls, upper respiratory tract infection, weight increase, vertigo, ataxia, gait disturbance, balance disorder, anxiety, blurred vision, dysarthria, asthenia, aggression, hypersomnia
AE (rizatriptan): Serious: anaphylaxis, hypersensitivity reaction, toxic epidermal necrolysis, coronary vasospasm, myocardial ischemia, MI, ventricular tachycardia, ventricular fibrillation, life-threatening arrhythmias, severe HTN, hypertensive crisis, stroke, cerebral hemorrhage, subarachnoid hemorrhage, peripheral vascular ischemia, intestinal ischemia, splenic infarction, Raynaud phenomenon, serotonin syndrome, headache exacerbation (use >10 ds/mo); Common: dizziness, somnolence, asthenia, fatigue, nausea, paresthesia, chest pain/pressure/tightness, jaw pain/pressure/tightness, neck pain/pressure/tightness, dry mouth
AE (sumatriptan): Serious: coronary vasospasm, myocardial ischemia, MI, ventricular tachycardia, ventricular fibrillation, life-threatening arrhythmias, severe HTN, hypertensive crisis, stroke, cerebral hemorrhage, subarachnoid hemorrhage, peripheral vascular ischemia, intestinal ischemia, partial vision loss, transient/permanent blindness, anaphylaxis, seizures, corneal defects (animal studies), serotonin syndrome, headache exacerbation (use >10 ds/mo); Common: injection site reactions (SC use), paresthesia, hot or cold sensation, malaise/fatigue, chest pain/pressure/tightness, neck pain/pressure/tightness, jaw pain/pressure/tightness, dizziness/vertigo, flushing (SC use), weakness (SC use), drowsiness/sedation (SC use)
AE (topiramate): Serious: severe metabolic acidosis, nephrolithiasis, osteomalacia, osteoporosis, growth suppression, acute myopia, maculopathy, 2o angle-closure glaucoma, oligohidrosis, hyperthermia, DM, leukopenia, anemia, psychosis, suicidality, erythema multiforme, Stevens-Johnson syndrome, toxic epidermal necrolysis, pemphigus, hepatotoxicity, Pancreatitis, DVT, pulmonary embolism, syncope, neonatal cleft lip/palate (1st trimester use); Common: metabolic acidosis, paresthesia, somnolence, dizziness, weight loss, fatigue, nervousness, anorexia, cognitive dysfunction, UTI, ataxia, abnormal vision, diarrhea, mood disturbances, nystagmus, nausea, diplopia, insomnia, depression, infection, fever, tremor, rhinitis/sinusitis, dyspepsia, asthenia, anxiety, abdominal pain, hypoesthesia, taste changes, alopecia
AE (valproic acid): Serious: hepatotoxicity, pancreatitis, SIADH, hyponatremia, pancytopenia, thrombocytopenia, multi-organ hypersensitivity reaction, hyperammonemia, hypothermia, myelosuppression, aplastic anemia, bleeding, erythema multiforme, Stevens-Johnson syndrome, toxic epidermal necrolysis, anaphylaxis, hallucinations, psychosis, suicidality, congenital anomalies, congenital neural tube defects, encephalopathy, coma, polycystic ovary syndrome; Common: headache, nausea/vomiting, asthenia, somnolence, thrombocytopenia, dyspepsia, dizziness, diarrhea, abdominal pain, tremor, alopecia, weight changes, appetite changes, constipation, nervousness, emotional lability, insomnia, peripheral edema, petechiae/ecchymosis, rash, depression, dyspnea, tinnitus, ALT/AST elevated, amnesia, abnormal gait, visual changes, blurred vision, nystagmus, myalgia,

AE (zonisamide): Serious: Stevens-Johnson syndrome, toxic epidermal necrolysis, aplastic anemia, agranulocytosis, oligohidrosis (peds pts), hyperthermia (peds pts), heat stroke, nephrolithiasis, metabolic acidosis, pancreatitis, depression, psychosis, suicidality, withdrawal seizures, status epilepticus, rhabdomyolysis; Common: somnolence, dizziness, anorexia, nausea, headache, irritability, agitation, fatigue, impaired concentration, impaired memory, confusion, depression, insomnia, diplopia, ataxia, abdominal pain, speech disturbance, diarrhea, nystagmus, mental slowing, paresthesia, flu syndrome, rash, anxiety, dyspepsia, weight loss, BUN/Cr elevated, taste changes, dry mouth, constipation
CI (almotriptan): ischemic heart disease, coronary vasospasm, uncontrolled HTN, cerebrovascular disease, peripheral vascular disease, ischemic bowel disease, basilar or hemiplegic migraine; caution if hypersensitivity to sulfonamides, cardiac disease risk, hepatic or renal impairment
CI (amantadine) : caution in depression, psychiatric disorder, CHF, cardiovascular disease, peripheral edema, angle closure glaucoma, seizure disorder, renal or hepatic impairment, high environmental temperature
CI (divalproex sodium): hepatic disease, hepatic impairment, urea cycle disorders; caution in infants or young children, if renal impairment, organic brain disease, head injury, mental retardation w/ seizure disorder, congenital metabolic disorders, multiple anticonvulsant tx, myelosuppression, bleeding risk, depression or hx
CI (eletriptan): uncontrolled HTN, ischemic heart disease, coronary vasospasm, cerebrovascular disease, basilar migraine, hemiplegic migraine, PVD, ischemic bowel disease, severe hepatic impairment, caution if cardiac disease risk
CI (fosphenytoin): sinus bradycardia, SA block, 2nd or 3rd degree AV block, Adams-Stokes syndrome; caution if hypotension, cardiovascular disease, hepatic impairment, renal impairment, phosphate restriction, DM, alcohol use, pregnancy, HLA-B*1502-positive
CI (gabapentin): avoid abrupt withdrawal; caution if renal impairment, depression or hx, CNS depressant use, alcohol use, drug abuse hx
CI (lamotrigine): avoid abrupt withdrawal; caution if hypersens. to antiepileptic drugs, hepatic/renal impairment, pregnancy, suicide risk
CI (levetiracetam): abrupt withdrawal; pregnancy, renal impairment, psychiatric disorder
CI (rizatriptan): uncontrolled HTN, ischemic heart disease, coronary vasospasm, basilar or hemiplegic migraine; caution if cerebrovascular disease, peripheral vascular disease, ischemic bowel disease, cardiac disease risk, dialysis, hepatic impairment, PKU (phenylalanine-containing forms)
CI (sumatriptan): uncontrolled HTN, ischemic heart disease, coronary vasospasm, cerebrovascular disease, basilar or hemiplegic migraine, PVD, ischemic bowel disease, severe hepatic impairment, avoid breastfeeding x12h after dose; caution if cardiac disease risk, mild-mod hepatic impairment (PO use), seizure disorder, HTN
CI (valproic acid): hepatic disease, hepatic impairment, urea cycle disorders; caution in infants or young children, renal impairment, organic brain disease, head injury, mental retardation w/ seizure disorder, congenital metabolic disorders, multiple anticonvulsant tx, myelosuppression, bleeding risk, depression

CI (topiramate): avoid abrupt withdrawal; caution if renal/hepatic impairment, nephrolithiasis hx, dehydration, diarrhea, severe respiratory disease, surgery, ketogenic diet, congenital metabolic disorders, valproic acid use, status epilepticus, depression or hx
CI (valproic acid): Serious: hepatotoxicity, pancreatitis, SIADH, hyponatremia, pancytopenia, thrombocytopenia, multi-organ hypersensitivity reaction, hyperammonemia, hypothermia, myelosuppression, aplastic anemia, bleeding, erythema multiforme, Stevens-Johnson syndrome, toxic epidermal necrolysis, anaphylaxis, hallucinations, psychosis, suicidality, congenital anomalies, congenital neural tube defects, encephalopathy, coma, polycystic ovary syndrome; Common: headache, nausea/vomiting, asthenia, somnolence, thrombocytopenia, dyspepsia, dizziness, diarrhea, abdominal pain, tremor, alopecia, weight changes, appetite changes, constipation, nervousness, emotional lability, insomnia, peripheral edema, petechiae/ecchymosis, rash, depression, dyspnea, tinnitus, ALT/AST elevated, amnesia, abnormal gait, visual changes, blurred vision, nystagmus, myalgia
CI (zonisamide): hypersens. to sulfonamides, renal failure (GFR <50 mL/min), avoid pregnancy, avoid abrupt withdrawal; caution if renal/hepatic impairment, nephrolithiasis, metabolic acidosis, ketogenic diet, diarrhea, severe respiratory disease, surgery, high environmental temperature, depression or hx

Almotriptan	PRC C, Lact ?
Axert *6.25, 12.5 mg tab*	**Migraine headache**, 12-17y: 6.25-12.5 mg PO x1; Max: 25 mg/24h; may repeat dose x1 after 2h if HA recurs
Amantadine	PRC C, Lact ?
Symmetrel *100 mg tab/cap, 50 mg/5ml syrup*	**Influenza A** tx, 1-10y: 5 mg/kg/d PO div bid x3-5 d; Start: w/in 48h of sx onset; Max: 150 mg/d; D/C w/in 24-48h of sx resolution; >10y: 100 mg PO bid x3-5 d; Start: w/in 48h of sx onset; Max: 200 mg/d; Alt: 5 mg/kg/d PO div bid x3-5 d; D/C w/in 24-48h of sx resolution Influenza A prophylaxis, 1-10y: 5 mg/kg/d PO div bid; Start: prior to or immed. upon exposure; Max: 150 mg/d; >10y: 100 mg PO bid; Start: prior to or immed. upon exposure; Max: 200 mg/d; Alt: 5 mg/kg/d PO div bid
Divalproex sodium	PRC D, Lact -
Depakote *125 DR cap; 125,250,500 DR tab; 250,500 ER tab* *divalproex sodium ER and DR tabs not bioequivalent; incr. total daily dose by 8-20% if switching from DR tab to ER tab*	**Partial complex seizures,** >10y, DR: 30-60 mg/kg/d PO div bid-tid; Start: 10-15 mg/kg/d PO div qd-tid, incr. 5-10 mg/kg/d q7 d; Max: 60 mg/kg/d; Info: divide doses >250 mg/d; give w/ food; may open caps, sprinkle on soft food, and swallow w/o chewing

	Partial complex seizures, >10y, ER: 30-60 mg/kg PO qd; Start: 10-15 mg/kg PO qd, incr. 5-10 mg/kg/d q7 d; Max: 60 mg/kg/d; Info: incr. total daily dose 8-20% when converting from delayed-release forms; give w/ food; do not cut/crush/chew Absence seizures, >10y, DR: 30-60 mg/kg/d PO div bid-tid; Start: 15 mg/kg/d PO div qd-tid, incr. 5-10 mg/kg/d q7 d; Max: 60 mg/kg/d; Info: divide doses >250 mg/d; give w/ food; may open caps, sprinkle on soft food, and swallow w/o chewing Absence seizures, >10y, ER: 30-60 mg/kg PO qd; Start: 15 mg/kg PO qd, incr. 5-10 mg/kg/d q7 d; Max: 60 mg/kg/d; Info: incr. total daily dose 8-20% when converting from delayed-release forms; give w/ food; do not cut/crush/chew
Eletriptan	PRC C, Lact ?
Relpax *20, 40*	**Acute migraine headache (adult dosing):** 80 mg/24h; Info: may repeat q2h x1 if HA recurs
Fosphenytoin	PRC D, Lact ?
Cerebyx *IM, IV*	Info: fosphenytoin doses expressed as phenytoin equivalents (PE) to avoid need for dose conversions between products; fosphenytoin should be prescribed and dispensed in PE units; each vial contains 75 mg/mL fosphenytoin equivalent to 50 mg/mL phenytoin **Status epilepticus**: 4-8 mg PE/kg/d IM/IV div qd-tid; Start: 15-20 mg PE/kg IV x1; Max: 3 mg PE/kg/min up to 150 mg PE/min IV; Info: begin maint. dose 12h after loading dose Seizure disorder, short-term tx: 4-6 mg PE/kg/d IM/IV div qd-tid; Start: 10-20 mg PE/kg IM/IV x1; Max: 3 mg PE/kg/min up to 150 mg PE/min IV; Info: begin maint. dose 12h after loading dose; switch to PO phenytoin as soon as possible

Gabapentin	PRC C, Lact -
Neurontin *100,300, 400,600,800; 50/mL*	**Partial seizures**, 3-4y: 40 mg/kg/d PO div tid; Start: 10-15 mg/kg/d PO div tid, titrate up over 3 d; Max: 50 mg/kg/d; 5-12y: 25-35 mg/kg/d PO div tid; Start: 10-15 mg/kg/d PO div tid, titrate up over 3 d; Max: 50 mg/kg/d; >12y: 300-800 mg PO tid; Start: 300 mg PO tid; Max: 3600 mg/d; Info: taper dose over >7 d to D/C
Lamotrigine	PRC C, Lact +
Lamictal *25,100,150,200; 5,25 CH*	**Seizures**: consult with pediatric neurologist
Levetiracetam	
Keppra *250,500,750,1000; 500,750 ER; 100/mL; IV* **Keppra XR** *500,750 ER*	**Seizures:** consult pediatric neurologist
Oxcarbazepine ER	PRC C, Lact +
Oxtellar XR Tb	8-10 mg/kg od, not to exceed 600 mg/d in the 1st wk.
Perampanel	PRC C, Lact -
Fycompa *Tb*	**Seizures**: 2 mg/od hs to 4-8 mg/od hs
Rizatriptan	PRC C, Lact ?
Maxalt *5,10*	**Acute migraine headache,** 6-17y, <40 kg: 5 mg PO x1; 6-17y, >40 kg: 10 mg PO x 1
Sumatriptan	PRC C, Lact -
Imitrex *25,50,100; SC*	**Acute migraine headache (adult dosing),** PO: 25-100 mg PO x1, may repeat x1 after 2h if HA recurs; Max: 200 mg/24h; Info: may follow initial 4-6 mg SC dose after 1h w/ 25-100 mg PO q2h x1-2 doses, up to 100 mg/24h PO; SC route: 4-6 mg SC x1, may repeat x1 after 1h if HA recurs; Max: 2 doses/24h; 12 mg/24h
Topiramate	PRC D, Lact ?
Topamax *25,50,100,200 tabs; 15,25 caps*	**Seizures**: consult pediatric neurologist
Valproic acid	PRC D, Lact -
Depakene *250; 250/5 mL*	**Complex partial seizures,** >10y: 30-60 mg/kg/d PO div bid-tid; Start: 10-15 mg/kg/d PO div qd-tid, incr. 5-10 mg/kg/d q7 ds; Max:

	60 mg/kg/d; Info: divide doses >250 mg/d; give w/ food; do not cut/crush/ chew/open capsules **Simple and complex absence seizures**, >10y: 30-60 mg/kg/d PO div bid-tid; Start: 15 mg/kg/d PO div qd-tid, incr. 5-10 mg/kg/d q7 ds; Max: 60 mg/kg/d; Info: divide doses >250 mg/d; give w/ food; do not cut/crush/ chew/open capsules
Zonisamide	PRC C, Lact ?
Zonegran *25,50,100*	**Partial seizures**, >16y: 100-600 mg/d PO div qd-bid; Start: 100 mg PO qd, titrate up q2wk at minimum; Max: 600 mg/d

16.12 Psychiatry

MA/EF (amitriptyline) exact mechanism of action unknown; inhibits norepinephrine and serotonin reuptake
MA/EF (aripiprazole) exact mechanism of action unknown; partially agonizes dopamine D2 and serotonin 5-HT1A receptors, antagonizes serotonin 5-HT2A receptors
MA/EF (atomoxetine) exact mechanism of action unknown; selectively inhibits norepinephrine reuptake
MA/EF (chlorpromazine) exact mechanism of action unknown; selectively antagonizes dopamine D2 receptors
MA/EF (dexmethylphenidate) exact mechanism of action unknown; stimulates CNS activity; blocks reuptake and increases release of norepinephrine and dopamine in extraneuronal space (sympathomimetic)
MA/EF (dextroamphetamine) exact mechanism of action unknown; stimulates CNS activity; blocks reuptake and increases release of norepinephrine and dopamine in extraneuronal space (sympathomimetic)
MA/EF (dextroamphetamine/amphetamine) exact mechanism of action unknown; stimulates CNS activity; blocks reuptake and increases release of norepinephrine and dopamine in extraneuronal space (sympathomimetic)
MA/EF (epinephrine) stimulates alpha and beta adrenergic receptors (sympathomimetic)
MA/EF (fluoxetine) selectively inhibits serotonin reuptake
MA/EF (lisdexamfetamine) exact mechanism of action unknown; stimulates CNS activity (sympathomimetic)
MA/EF (lithium) exact mechanism of action unknown; alters neuronal sodium transport
MA/EF (methylphenidate) exact mechanism of action unknown; stimulates CNS activity; blocks reuptake and increases release of norepinephrine and dopamine in extraneuronal space (sympathomimetic)
MA/EF (pentobarbital) alters sensory cortex, cerebellar, and motor activities; produces sedation, hypnosis, and anesthesia (barbiturate)

MA/EF (quetiapine) exact mechanism of action unknown; antagonizes dopamine D2 receptors, serotonin 5-HT2 receptors, others
MA/EF (risperidone) exact mechanism of action unknown; antagonizes dopamine D2 receptors, serotonin 5-HT2 receptors, others
MA/EF (ziprasidone) exact mechanism of action unknown; antagonizes dopamine D2 receptors, serotonin 5-HT2A receptors, others
AE (amitriptyline): Serious: orthostatic hypotension, HTN, syncope, ventricular arrhythmias, QT prolongation, torsades de pointes, AV block, MI, stroke, seizures, extrapyramidal symptoms, ataxia, tardive dyskinesia, paralytic ileus, IOP incr., agranulocytosis, leukopenia, thrombocytopenia, hallucinations, psychosis exacerbation, hypomania/mania, worsening depression, suicidality, SIADH, hepatitis, angioedema, anticholinergic psychosis, hyperthermia, heat stroke; Common: drowsiness, dry mouth, dizziness, constipation, blurred vision, palpitations, tachycardia, incoordination, appetite incr., nausea/vomiting, sweating, weakness, disorientation, confusion, restlessness, insomnia, anxiety/agitation, urinary retention, urinary frequency, rash/urticaria, pruritus, weight gain, libido changes, impotence, gynecomastia, galactorrhea, tremor, hypo/hyperglycemia, paresthesia, photosensitivity
AE (aripiprazole): Serious: neuroleptic malignant syndrome, extrapyramidal symptoms, tardive dyskinesia, dystonia, stroke, TIA, syncope, orthostatic hypotension, seizures, severe hyperglycemia, DM, severe dysphagia, aspiration, hyperthermia, HTN, tachycardia/bradycardia, hemorrhage, intestinal obstruction, cholecystitis, pancreatitis, blood dyscrasias, leukopenia, neutropenia, agranulocytosis, hypokalemia, hyperkalemia, rhabdomyolysis, suicidality, worsening depression, neonatal extrapyramidal sx or withdrawal (3rd trimester use); Common: headache, weight gain, anxiety, insomnia, nausea/vomiting, lightheadedness, dizziness, somnolence, sedation, akathisia, injection site reactions (IM use), constipation, incontinence, blurred vision, extrapyramidal symptoms, tremor, dry mouth, cough, restlessness, fatigue, arthralgia/myalgia, sialorrhea, diarrhea, pyrexia, appetite incr., dystonia, dyslipidemia
AE (atomoxetine): Serious: angioedema, anaphylactic reaction, psychosis, mania, aggressive behavior, suicidal ideation, Raynaud phenomenon, orthostatic hypotension, syncope, HTN, tachycardia, QT prolongation, MI, stroke, sudden death, seizures, hepatotoxicity, priapism; Common: dry mouth, abdominal pain, dyspepsia, nausea/vomiting, insomnia, sleep disorders, abnormal dreams, appetite decr., somnolence, constipation, urinary hesitancy/retention, erectile dysfunction, ejaculatory dysfunction, hot flashes, libido decr., dysmenorrheal, dysuria, fatigue, dizziness, sweating incr., palpitations, paresthesia; BP, HR incr.
AE (chlorpromazine): Serious: seizures, leukopenia, neutropenia, agranulocytosis, aplastic anemia, thrombocytopenia, neuroleptic malignant syndrome, tardive dyskinesia, heat stroke, neonatal extrapyramidal sx (3rd trimester use),neonatal withdrawal (3rd trimester use); Common: drowsiness, jaundice, hypotension, agitation, insomnia, photosensitivity

AE (dexmethylphenidate): Serious: dependency/abuse, psychosis, mania, aggressive behavior, Tourette syndrome, arrhythmias, MI, stroke, sudden death, seizures, growth suppression (long-term use), hypersensitivity reaction, exfoliative dermatitis, erythema multiforme, thrombocytopenic purpura; Common: anorexia, headache, anxiety, dyspepsia, dry mouth (ER form), throat pain (ER form), dizziness, insomnia, weight loss, BP changes, visual disturbances

AE (dextroamphetamine): Serious: dependency/abuse, withdrawal if abrupt d/c, psychosis, mania, aggressive behavior, Tourette syndrome, severe HTN, MI, stroke, sudden death, cardiomyopathy (long-term use), seizures, growth suppression (long-term use); Common: palpitations, tachycardia, restlessness, dizziness, tremor, euphoria, anorexia, headache, dyskinesia, dysphoria, tic exacerbation, unpleasant taste, dry mouth, throat pain (ER form), insomnia, weight loss, BP elevated, visual disturbances, constipation, libido changes, urticaria

AE (dextroamphetamine/amphetamine): Serious: dependency/abuse, withdrawal if abrupt D/C (long-term use), depression, psychosis, mania, aggressive behavior, Tourette syndrome, severe HTN, MI. stroke. sudden death, cardiomyopathy (long-term use), seizures, growth suppression (long-term use), hypersensitivity reaction, anaphylaxis, angioedema, Stevens-Johnson syndrome, toxic epidermal necrolysis, dermatillomania; Common: anorexia, insomnia, abdominal pain, headache, emotional lability, weight loss, nervousness, dry mouth, nausea/vomiting, asthenia, fever, diarrhea, infection, dyspepsia, agitation, dizziness, palpitations, BP elevated, tachycardia, tremor, dyskinesia, constipation, libido changes, impotence, visual disturbances, motor/phonic tic exacerbation, photosensitivity, somnolence, dyspnea, sweating, dysmenorrhea

AE (epinephrine): Serious: pulmonary edema, arrhythmias, HTN, angina, cerebral hemorrhage (IV use), tissue necrosis (SC or IM use); Common: palpitations, tachycardia, nausea/vomiting, pallor, sweating, Dizziness, weakness, tremor, headache, apprehension, nervousness, anxiety

AE (fluoxetine): Serious: worsening depression, suicidality, serotonin syndrome, neuroleptic malignant syndrome, extrapyramidal symptoms, withdrawal syndrome, mania, seizures, hyponatremia, SIADH, hypoglycemia, serum sickness, vasculitis, anaphylactoid reactions, severe rash, erythema multiforme, pulmonary fibrosis, abnormal bleeding/altered platelet fxn, priapism, acute angle-closure glaucoma, growth suppression, neonatal persistent pulmonary HTN (>20 wk gestation), neonatal serotonin syndrome (3rd trimester use), neonatal withdrawal (3rd trimester use), hypotension; Common: nausea, headache, insomnia, nervousness, anxiety, asthenia, diarrhea, anorexia, dizziness, dry mouth, tremor, dyspepsia, sweating, ejaculatory dysfunction, constipation, flu syndrome, libido decr., rash, abnormal vision, urinary disorder

AE (lisdexamfetamine): Serious: dependency/abuse, withdrawal if abrupt D/C (long-term use), psychosis, mania, aggressive behavior, Tourette syndrome, severe HTN, MI, stroke, sudden death, cardiomyopathy (long-term use), seizures, growth suppression (long-term use), anaphylactic reaction, hypersensitivity reaction, Stevens-Johnson syndrome, angioedema; Common: abdominal pain, appetite decr., dizziness, dry mouth, irritability, insomnia, nausea/vomiting, diarrhea, weight loss, anxiety, rash, affect lability, agitation, hyperhidrosis, BP incr., pyrexia, somnolence, motor/phonic tic exacerbation, visual disturbances, tremor, dyspnea

AE (lithium): Serious: coma, seizures, ventricular arrhythmias, severe bradycardia, syncope, Brugada syndrome unmasked, goiter, hypothyroidism, hyperparathyroidism, pseudotumor cerebri, Raynaud phenomenon, diabetes insipidus; Common: tremor, polyuria, polydipsia, weight gain, diarrhea, vomiting, drowsiness, cognitive impairment, impaired coordination, muscle weakness, anorexia, nausea, blurred vision, dry mouth, fatigue, hair loss, reversible leukocytosis, acne, edema

AE (methylphenidate): Serious: dependency/abuse, psychosis, mania, aggressive behavior, Tourette syndrome, arrhythmias, MI, stroke, sudden death, seizures, growth suppression (long-term use), hypersensitivity reaction, exfoliative dermatitis, erythema multiforme, thrombocytopenic purpura, leukopenia, neuroleptic malignant syndrome, cerebral arteritis, hepatic coma; Common: nervousness, insomnia, anorexia, abdominal pain, weight loss (long-term use), tachycardia, nausea, motor tics, headache, palpitations, dizziness, fever, urticarial, transient depression, drowsiness, dyskinesia, angina, BP changes, visual disturbances, ALT/AST elevated

AE (pentobarbital): Serious: respiratory depression, Stevens-Johnson syndrome, angioedema, lupus erythematosus; Common: somnolence, agitation, confusion, hyperkinesia, ataxia, CNS depression, hallucinations, dizziness, apnea, bradycardia, hypotension, syncope, nausea, vomiting, constipation, headache

CI (pentobarbital): depressed respiratory fxn, porphyria; caution if suicidal, hepatic impairment, drug abuse hx

AE (phenobarbital): Serious: respiratory depression, erythema multiforme, Stevens-Johnson syndrome, angioedema, megaloblastic anemia, TTP, blood dyscrasias, suicidality; Common: drowsiness, lethargy, hyperactivity, nausea, vomiting, somnolence, porphyria exacerbation, rash, urticarial, pain, swelling, thrombophlebitis, necrosis, physical dependence, hepatitis

AE (quetiapine): Serious: severe hypotension, syncope, extrapyramidal symptoms, tardive dyskinesia, dystonia, neuroleptic malignant syndrome, hyperthermia, hypothermia, seizures, hypothyroidism, severe hyperglycemia, DM, priapism, agranulocytosis, leukopenia, neutropenia, lens changes, cataracts, stroke, QT prolongation, worsening depression, suicidality, severe dysphagia, anaphylactic reactions, Stevens-Johnson syndrome, neonatal extrapyramidal sx (3rd trimester use), neonatal withdrawal (3rd trimester use); Common: headache, somnolence, hypertriglyceridemia, hypercholesterolemia, dizziness, constipation, orthostatic hypotension, tachycardia, dry mouth, ALT/AST elevated, dyspepsia, asthenia, fatigue, nausea/vomiting, insomnia, rash, irritability, tremor, abdominal pain, rhinitis, anemia, weight gain, appetite incr., fever, back pain, menstrual irregularities, hyperprolactinemia, impaired body temperature regulation

AE (risperidone): Serious: severe hypotension, syncope, severe extrapyramidal symptoms, tardive dyskinesia, neuroleptic malignant syndrome, severe hyperglycemia, DM, seizures, priapism, stroke, TIA, QT prolongation, hypersensitivity reaction, severe dysphagia, angioedema, anaphylactic reactions, erythema multiforme, leukopenia, neutropenia, agranulocytosis, suicidality, hypothermia, hyperthermia, neonatal extrapyramidal sx (3rd trimester use), neonatal withdrawal (3rd trimester use); Common: somnolence, appetite incr., fatigue, insomnia, rhinitis, URI, nausea/vomiting, cough, urinary incontinence, salivation, constipation, fever, extrapyramidal effects, dystonia, abdominal pain, anxiety, dizziness, headache, dry mouth, tremor, rash, akathisia, dyspepsia, tachycardia, weight gain, visual disturbances, hyperprolactinemia, confusion, gynecomastia, photosensitivity, epistaxis, dyslipidemia

AE (ziprasidone): Serious: neuroleptic malignant syndrome, severe extrapyramidal symptoms, tardive dyskinesia, dystonia, QT prolongation, torsades de pointes, seizures, syncope, stroke, priapism, severe HTN, severe hyperglycemia, DM, serotonin syndrome, hyperthermia, allergic reactions, severe dysphagia, leukopenia, neutropenia, agranulocytosis, neonatal extrapyramidal sx (3rd trimester use), neonatal withdrawal (3rd trimester use); Common: somnolence, headache (IM use), nausea, constipation, dyspepsia, akathisia, dizziness, respiratory disorders, extrapyramidal effects, asthenia, diarrhea, weight gain, rash, urticarial, dry mouth, visual disturbances, sialorrhea, tachycardia, orthostatic hypotension, menstrual irregularities, hyperprolactinemia, photosensitivity

CI (amitriptyline): acute recovery from MI, avoid abrupt withdrawal; caution cardiovascular disease, urinary retention, prostatic hypertrophy, angle-closure glaucoma, IOP, incr., seizure disorder, thyroid disease, DM, asthma, hepatic impairment, schizophrenia, bipolar disorder, electroconvulsive tx, alcohol abuse, suicide risk, GI/GU obstruction, high environmental temperature

CI (aripiprazole): caution if cardiovascular disease, MI hx, ischemic heart disease, heart failure, hypovolemia, dehydration, orthostatic hypotension, aspiration pneumonia risk, elderly pts, cerebrovascular disease, dementia, seizure hx, poor CYP2D6 metabolizer, DM, DM risk, high environmental temperature, PKU (phenylalanine-containing forms), pts <25 yo (depression use), drug-induced leukopenia or neutropenia hx, leukopenia

CI (atomoxetine): MAO inhibitor use w/in 14 ds, angle-closure glaucoma, cardiac structural abnormalities, cardiomyopathy, severe arrhythmias, severe CAD, pheochromocytoma or hx; caution if cardiovascular disease or hx, tachycardia, HTN, hypotension, cerebrovascular disease, hepatic impairment, depression, bipolar disorder, suicide risk, poor CYP2D6 metabolizer

CI (chlorpromazine): CNS depression, bone marrow depression, severe hypotension; caution if hepatic impairment, hypersens. to sulfites, leukopenia, drug-induced leukopenia or neutropenia hx, high environmental temperature

CI (dexmethylphenidate): hypersens. to methylphenidate, Tourette syndrome or family hx, motor tics, agitation, cardiac structural abnormalities, cardiomyopathy, severe arrhythmias, severe CAD, glaucoma; caution if cardiovascular disease or hx, HTN, psychosis, bipolar disorder, seizure hx, seizure risk, substance abuse hx, hyperthyroidism, long-term use

CI (dextroamphetamine): breastfeeding, symptomatic cardiovascular disease, advanced arteriosclerosis, cardiac structural abnormalities, cardiomyopathy, severe arrhythmias, mod-severe HTN, agitation, hyperthyroidism, glaucoma, drug abuse hx, avoid abrupt withdrawal; caution in elderly pts, if cardiovascular disease or hx, mild HTN, psychosis, bipolar disorder, Tourette syndrome or tics, seizure hx, seizure risk

CI (dextroamphetamine/amphetamine): breastfeeding, cardiovascular disease, symptomatic, advanced arteriosclerosis, cardiac structural abnormalities, cardiomyopathy, severe arrhythmias, mod-severe HTN, agitation, hyperthyroidism, glaucoma, drug abuse hx, avoid abrupt withdrawal; caution if cardiovascular disease or hx, mild HTN, psychosis, bipolar disorder, Tourette syndrome or tics, seizure hx/risk

CI (epinephrine): angle-closure glaucoma, shock, organic brain syndrome, labor and delivery, coronary insufficiency; caution if cardiac disease, HTN, DM, hyperthyroidism, cerebrovascular disease, psychiatric disorder, hypersens. to sulfites

CI (fluoxetine): avoid abrupt withdrawal; caution in pts <25 yo, if pregnancy >20 wk gestation, hepatic impairment, DM, volume depletion, hyponatremia, seizure disorder, hypomania/mania, IOP incr., angle-closure glaucoma, alcohol use (lisdexamfetamine)

CI (lisdexamfetamine): symptomatic cardiovascular disease, cardiac structural abnormalities, cardiomyopathy, severe arrhythmias, mod-severe HTN, agitation, hyperthyroidism, glaucoma, drug abuse hx, breastfeeding, avoid abrupt withdrawal; caution if cardiovascular disease or hx, mild HTN, psychosis, bipolar disorder, Tourette syndrome or tics, seizure hx, seizure risk

CI (lithium): Brugada syndrome; caution in renal impairment, volume depletion, severe debilitation, thyroid disorder, concurrent CNS depressant use, alcohol use

CI (methylphenidate): MAO inhibitor use w/in 14 ds, pts <6 yo, Tourette syndrome or family hx, motor tics, agitation, cardiac structural abnormalities, cardiomyopathy, severe arrhythmias, severe CAD, glaucoma; caution if cardiovascular disease or hx, HTN, psychosis, bipolar disorder, seizure hx, seizure risk, substance abuse hx, hyperthyroidism, PKU (phenylalanine-containing forms)

CI (phenobarbital): porphyria hx, severe hepatic impairment, respiratory dysfunction, avoid abrupt withdrawal; caution if depression or hx, uremia

CI (quetiapine): avoid abrupt withdrawal, arrhythmia hx, hypokalemia, hypomagnesemia, congenital QT prolongation; caution if QT prolongation family hx, impairment, seizure hx, seizure threshold lowered, cardiovascular disease, neuroleptic malignant syndrome hx, suicide risk, hypotension, hypovolemia, dehydration, aspiration pneumonia risk, dysphagia, DM, DM risk, hyperlipidemia, tardive dyskinesia, breast CA, drug-induced leukopenia or neutropenia hx, leukopenia

CI (risperidone): caution if renal/hepatic impairment, neuroleptic malignant syndrome hx, seizure hx, cardiac disease, cerebrovascular disease, hypotension, hypovolemia, dehydration, aspiration pneumonia risk, PKU (phenylalanine-containing forms), DM, DM risk, drug-induced leukopenia or neutropenia hx, leukopenia, suicide risk; may impair body temperature regulation

CI (ziprasidone): prolonged QT interval, recent MI, uncompensated heart failure, hypokalemia, hypomagnesemia, arrhythmia hx; caution if hepatic impairment, renal impairment (IM use), neuroleptic malignant syndrome hx, seizure disorder, cardiac disease, cerebrovascular disease, hypotension, hypovolemia, dehydration, aspiration pneumonia risk, DM or risk, drug-induced leukopenia or neutropenia hx, leukopenia

Amitriptyline	PRC C, Lact -
Elavil *10,25,50,75,100, 125,150*	**Depression**: 9-12 yrs: 1-3 mg/kg/d PO div tid; Start: 1 mg/kg/d PO div tid x3 d, incr. 0.5 mg/kg/d q2-3 d; Max: 5 mg/kg/d up to 200 mg/d; >12 yrs: 50-100 mg/d PO div qd-tid; Start: 10 mg PO tid and 20 mg qhs; incr. 10-25 mg/d q2-3 d; Max: 200 mg/d; Info: taper dose gradually to D/C
Aripiprazole	PRC C, Lact ?
Abilify *2,5,10, 15,20,30; 1/mL*	**Schizophrenia** (13y+): 10 mg PO qd; Start: 2 mg PO qd x2 ds, then 5 mg PO qd x2 ds; give subsequent dose incr. in 5 mg increments; Max: 30 mg/d; Info: doses >10 mg/d rarely more effective; periodically reassess need for tx; D/C if ANC <1000; consider D/C if unexplained decr. in WBC **Bipolar disorder,** manic/mixed (10y+): 10 mg PO qd; Start: 2 mg PO qd x2 ds, then 5 mg PO qd x2 d; give subsequent dose incr. in 5 mg increments; Max: 30 mg/d; Info: for acute and maint. monotherapy or valproate or lithium adjunct; D/C if ANC <1000; consider D/C if unexplained decr. in WBC Autistic disorder irritability sx (6y+): 5-10 mg PO qd; Start: 2 mg PO qd, incr. up to 5 mg/d qwk; Max: 15 mg/d; Info: periodically reassess need for tx; D/C if ANC <1000; consider D/C if unexplained decr. in WBC
Atomoxetine	PRC C, Lact ?
Strattera *10,18,25,40, 60,80,100*	**ADHD**: 80 mg PO qam; Start: 40 mg PO qam x3 d, then incr. to 80 mg PO qam, may incr. to 100 mg/d after 2-4wk if needed; Max: 100 mg/d; Info: requires slower titration if pt is poor CYP2D6 metabolizer or on strong CYP2D6 inhibitor; doses >40 mg/d may be div bid; periodically reassess need for tx during maintenance
Chlorpromazine	PRC C, Lact ?
Thorazine *10,25,50, 100,200; IM; IV*	**Severe behavioral disorders,** 6mo-5y: 2.5-6 mg/kg/d PO div q4-6h; Max: 50 mg/d PO, 40 mg/d IM; Alt: 2.5-4 mg/kg/d IM div q6-8h; 5-

	12y: 2.5-6 mg/kg/d PO div q4-6h; Max: 200 mg/d PO, 75 mg/d IM; Alt: 2.5-4 mg/kg/d IM div q6-8h; >12y: 200-400 mg/d PO div tid-qid; Start: 10-25 mg PO tid; may incr. by 20-50 mg/d after 1-2 d, then q3-4 d; Max: 1000 mg/d; Info: D/C if ANC <1000; consider D/C if unexplained decr. in WBC **Nausea/vomiting,** 6mo-5y: 0.55 mg/kg IM q6-8h prn; Max: 40 mg/d IM; Alt: 0.55 mg/kg PO q4-6h prn; 5-12y: 0.55 mg/kg IM q6-8h prn; Max: 75 mg/d IM: Alt: 0.55 mg/kg PO q4-6h prn; >12y: 10-25 mg PO q4-6h prn; Alt: 25 mg IM x1, then 25-50 mg IM q3-4h prn; Info: switch to PO ASAP if IM started; D/C or decr. dose if hypotension occurs; D/C if ANC <1000; consider D/C if unexplained decr. in WBC
Dexmethylphenidate	PRC C, Lact -
Focalin *2.5,5,10* **Focalin XR** *5,10,15,20, 25,30,35,40 ER*	**ADHD**, >6y: 2.5-10 mg PO bid; Start: 2.5 mg PO bid, incr. 5-10 mg/d q7 d; Max 20 mg/d; ADHD, >6y: 10-30 mg PO qd; Start: 5 mg PO qam, then may incr. by 5 mg/d q7 ds; Max 30 mg/d Info: to convert from methylphenidate start at 50% of current methylphenidate daily dose; space doses at least 4h apart
Dextroamphetamine	PRC C, Lact +
Dexedrine *2.5,5,7.5, 10,15,20,30; 5,10,15 ER*	**ADHD**, immediate-release form, 3-5 yo: 2.5-40 mg/d PO div qd-tid; Start: 2.5 mg PO qam, incr. 2.5 mg/d qwk; Max: 40 mg/d; >6 yo: 5-40 mg/d PO div qd-tid; Start: 5 mg PO qam or bid; incr. 5 mg/d qwk; Max: 60 mg/d; Info: give divided doses at 4-6h intervals; doses >40 mg/d rarely more effective ADHD, extended-release form, >6 yo: 5-40 mg ER PO qam; Start: 5 mg ER PO qam, incr. 5 mg/d qwk; Max: 60 mg/d ER; Info: doses >40 mg/d rarely more effective; do not cut/crush/chew

Dextroamphetamine/Amphetamine	PRC C, Lact +
Adderall *5,7.5,10, 12.5,15,20,30;*	**ADHD** immed-release, 3-5y: 2.5-40 mg/d PO div qd-tid; Start: 2.5 mg PO qam, incr. 2.5 mg/d qwk; >6y: 5-40 mg/d PO div qd-tid; Start: 5 mg PO qam or bid, incr. 5 mg/d qwk; Info: give divided doses at 4-6h intervals; doses >40 mg/d rarely more effective
Adderall XR *5,10, 15,20,25,30 ER*	ADHD extend-release 6-12y: 10 mg PO qam; Start: 5-10 mg PO qam, incr. 5-10 mg/d qwk; Max: 30 mg/d; 13-17y: 10-20 mg PO qam; Start: 10 mg PO qam, incr. 10 mg/d qwk; Max: 40 mg/d; Info: may convert from IR to ER at same total daily dose qam; doses >20 mg/d rarely more effective
Epinephrine	PRC C, Lact -
Adrenalin/Epinephrine *Inj 0.01mg/ml (1:100,000), 0.1mg/ml (1:10,000), 1mg/ ml (1:1.000)* **EpiPen,** *0.3 mg auto-injector* **EpiPen Jr,** *0.15 mg auto-injector*	**PALS**: asystole/PEA, VF/pulseless VT: 0.01 mg/ kg (1:10,000) IV/IO q3-5min prn, alt 0.1 mg/ kg (1:1000) ETT q3-5 min prn, max 1 mg/dose IV/IO, 10 mg/dose ETT; anaphylaxis: 0.01 mg/ kg (1:1000) IM q5-20min x3 doses prn, max 0.5 mg/dose IM, 1.5 mg/kg/min IV. If no response IM, give 0.01 mg/kg (1:10,000) IV x1, then 0.1 µg/kg/min IV prn. May use EpiPen auto-injector x 1 dose if >30 kg; EpiPen Jr x 1 dose if 15-30 kg.
Fluoxetine	PRC C, Lact ?
Prozac *10,20,40; 20/5 mL*	**Major depressive disorder**, 8-18y: 10-20 mg PO qd; Start: 10 mg PO qd x7 d; Info: slower titration in lower wt pts; taper dose gradually to D/C Obsessive-compulsive disorder, 7-17y: 20-60 mg PO qd; Start: 10 mg PO qd, incr. 10 mg/d q14 d; Info: slower titration, max 20-30 mg/ d in lower wt pts; taper dose gradually to D/C
Lisdexamfetamine	PRC C, Lact ?
Vyvanse *20,30,40, 50,60,70*	**ADHD**, 6-17y: 30 mg PO qam; Max: 70 mg/d; Info: may incr. dose 10-20 mg/d qwk; use lowest effective dose; periodically reassess need for tx
Lithium	PRC D, Lact +
Lithium *150,300,600; 300,450 ER; 300/5 mL*	**Bipolar disorder**: consult child psychiatrist

Methylphenidate	PRC C, Lact -
Methylphenidate *5,10,20; 20 ER; 5,10/5 mL* *Concerta 18,27,36,54 ER* *Metadate CD 10,20,30,40,50,60 ER* *Metadate ER 10,20 ER* *Methylin 5,10,20; 2.5,5,10 CH; 5,10/5 mL* *Methylin ER 10,20 ER* *Ritalin 5,10,20* *Ritalin LA 10,20,30,40 ER* *Ritalin SR 20 ER*	**ADHD**, >6y: 0.3-2 mg/kg/d PO div bid-tid; Start: 0.3 mg/kg PO bid or 2.5-5 mg PO bid, incr. 0.1 mg/kg/dose or 5-10 mg/d q7 ds; Max: 2 mg/kg/d up to 60 mg/d; Alt: 20 mg ER qd-bid; Info: ER not recommended for initial tx; IR duration 3-5h, ER 4-8h; give 30-45min before meals, last dose before 6 pm; do not cut/crush/chew ER See manufacturer info for dosing of brands
Methylphenidate hydrochloride	PRC C, Lact -
Quillivant XR *liq sol 60, 120, 180 mL*	>6 y 20 mg/od in the morning. The dose may be titrated weekly in increments of 10-20 mg. Daily doses >60 mg neither studied nor recommended; Before administering vigorously shake the bottle for at least 10 sec
Pentobarbital	PRC D, Lact ?
Nembutal *IM, IV*	**Procedural sedation**: 2-6 mg/kg IM x1; Max: 100 mg; Alt: 1-3 mg/kg IV x1; Info: onset: 10-15min IM, 1min IV; duration: 1-4h IM, 15min IV
Phenobarbital	PRC D, Lact ?
Luminal, Generics *Inj 65mg/ml, 130mg/ml*	**Status epilepticus**: 10-20 mg/kg IV x1, then 5-10 mg/kg IV q15-30 min; seizure disorder: <2mo: 3-5 mg/kg PO/IV daily div qd-bid; 2mo-2yo: 5-8 mg/kg PO/IV daily div qd-bid; >2yo: 3-5 mg/kg PO/IV daily div qd-bid
Quetiapine	PRC C, Lact ?
Seroquel *25,50,100, 150,200,300,400*	**Schizophrenia**, 13-17y: 400-800 mg/d PO div bid-tid; Start: 25 mg bid x1 d, then 50 mg bid x1 d, then incr. by 100 mg/d up to 200 mg PO bid by d 5, then may incr. by 50-100 mg/d prn; Max: 800 mg/d; Info: periodically reassess need for tx; D/C if ANC <1000; consider D/C if unexplained <WBC **Bipolar disorder,** 10-17y: 400-600 mg/d PO div bid-tid; Start: 25 mg bid x1 d, then 50 mg bid x1 d, then incr. by 100 mg/d up to 200 mg PO bid by d 5, then may incr. by 50-100 mg/d prn; Max: 600 mg/d; Info: for

	acute monotherapy or acute lithium or valproate adjunct; D/C if ANC <1000; consider D/C if unexplained decr. WBC
Risperidone	PRC C, Lact +
Risperdal *0.25,0.5, 1,2,3,4; 0.25,0.5, 1,2,3,4 ODT; 1/mL*	**Schizophrenia,** 13-17y: 1-6 mg/d PO div qd-bid; Start: 0.5 mg PO qd, then incr. 0.5 mg/d q3-7 d to target 3 mg/d; Max: 6 mg/d; Info: doses >3 mg/d rarely more effective, may incr. ADR risk; periodically reassess need for tx; D/C if ANC <1000; consider D/C if unexplained decr. in WBC; do not cut/chew ODT form **Bipolar disorder,** 10-17y: 0.5-6 mg/d PO div qd-bid; Start: 0.5 mg PO qd, then incr. 0.5-1 mg/d at intervals >24h to target 2.5 mg/d; Max: 6 mg/d; Info: doses >2.5 mg/d rarely more effective, may incr. ADR risk; periodically reassess need for tx; D/C if ANC <1000; consider D/C if unexplained decr. in WBC; do not cut/chew ODT form **Autism** irritability sx, 5-16y, 15-20 kg: 0.5-1 mg/d PO div qd-bid; Start: 0.25 mg PO qd x4 d, then incr. 0.25 mg/d q2wk prn; Max: 1 mg/d; 5-16y, >20 kg: 0.5-2.5 mg/d PO div qd-bid; Start: 0.5 mg/d PO div qd-bid x4 d, then incr. 0.5 mg/d q2wk prn; Max: 2.5 mg/d if <45 kg; 3 mg/d if >45 kg; Info: D/C if ANC <1000; consider D/C if unexplained decr. in WBC; do not cut/chew ODT form
Ziprasidone	PRC C, Lact ?
Geodon *20,40,60,80*	**Schizophrenia, bipolar disorder:** consult with child psychiatrist

16.13 Dermatology

MA/EF (acyclovir): inhibits DNA polymerase; incorporates into viral DNA
MA/EF (clindamycin): binds to 50S ribosomal subunit, interfering w/ protein synthesis
MA/EF (doxycycline) bacteriostatic; inhibits protein synthesis; exact MA in periodontitis unknown; inhibits collagenase activity; 20 mg formulation not effective as antibacterial
MA/EF (hydrocortisone) exact mechanism of anti-inflammatory action unknown; inhibits multiple inflammatory cytokines; produces multiple glucocorticoid and mineralocorticoid
MA/EF (ivermectin): contains a broad-spectrum antiparasitic agent, ivermectin; increases permeability of the cell membrane causes paralysis and death in certain parasites effects

AE (acyclovir): Oral: Serious: hallucinations, psychosis, encephalopathy, seizures, coma, leukopenia, thrombocytopenia, angioedema, anaphylaxis, erythema multiforme, Stevens-Johnson syndrome, toxic epidermal necrolysis, hepatitis, renal failure, hemolytic uremic syndrome, TTP; Common: nausea, vomiting, diarrhea, headache, malaise, dizziness, arthralgia, rash, lethargy, confusion, agitation, elevated BUN/Cr, photosensitivity
AE (acyclovir): Cream/Ointment: Serious: none reported; Common: burning, pruritus
AE (clindamycin): Serious: Clostridium difficile associated diarrhea, thrombocytopenia, anaphylaxis, Stevens-Johnson syndrome, granulocytopenia, esophagitis; Common: diarrhea, nausea, vomiting, abdominal pain, rash, pruritus, jaundice, urticarial, hypotension, thrombophlebitis (IV use)
AE (doxycycline): Serious: tooth discoloration (pts <8 yo), photosensitivity, superinfection, Clostridium difficile associated diarrhea, anaphylaxis, angioedema, lupus erythematosus, serum sickness-like reaction, vasculitis, pericarditis, autoimmune hepatitis, hepatotoxicity, nephrotoxicity, esophagitis (capsule forms), esophageal ulcers (capsule forms), pancreatitis, erythema multiforme, Stevens-Johnson syndrome, toxic epidermal necrolysis, exfoliative dermatitis, thrombocytopenia, neutropenia, hemolytic anemia, pseudotumor cerebri, bulging fontanels (infants), Jarisch-Herxheimer reaction (brucellosis or spirochetal infection use), fetal harm (in utero exposure); Common: headache, nausea, dyspepsia, joint pain, diarrhea, URI sx, rash, dysmenorrhea, photosensitivity,
AE (hydrocortisone): Serious: adrenal insufficiency, Cushing syndrome, anaphylaxis, infection, immunosuppression, steroid psychosis, GI ulceration/perforation, HTN, CHF, DM, steroid myopathy, tendon rupture, seizures, ICP incr., exophthalmos, osteopenia/osteoporosis (long-term use), glaucoma (long-term use), cataract formation (long-term use), growth suppression (long-term use), pseudotumor cerebri, pancreatitis; Common: sodium and fluid retention, nausea, vomiting, dyspepsia, appetite change, edema, headache, vertigo, dizziness, mood swings, anxiety, insomnia, hyperglycemia, hypokalemia, hypocalcemia, BP elevated, IOP incr., muscle weakness, menstrual irregularities, sweating incr., facial erythema, ecchymosis, acne, Cushing syndrome (long-term use), skin atrophy (long-term use), impaired wound healing (long-term use)
AE (ivermectin): conjunctivitis, ocular hyperemia, irritation, dandruff, dry skin, burning
CI Oral (acyclovir): caution if renal impairment, concurrent nephrotoxic agents, dehydration, electrolyte abnormalities, significant hypoxia, neurologic disease, hepatic impairment
CI Cream (acyclovir): none
CI (clindamycin): ulcerative colitis; caution if recent abx-assoc. colitis hx, hepatic or renal impairment
CI (doxycycline): pregnancy, pts <8 yo; caution if hepatic impairment, SLE, candidiasis hx, candidiasis risk, recent abx-assoc. colitis hx
CI (hydrocortisone): systemic fungal infection, neonates or premature infants (benzyl alcohol-containing INJ forms); caution if TB infection, ocular HSV, Strongyloides infection, measles or varicella exposure, immunosuppressed, active infection, HTN, CHF, DM, osteoporosis, hypothyroidism, PUD, ulcerative colitis, diverticulitis, recent intestinal anastomosis, seizure disorder, myasthenia gravis, psychiatric disorder, hepatic impairment,

renal impairment, anaphylaxis hx, avoid abrupt withdrawal **CI** (ivermectin): pt <6mo; hypersensitivity	
Acyclovir	PRC B, Lact -
Zovirax *400, 800 mg tab; 200 mg cap; 200 mg/5mL susp; 5% cream* **Acyclovir IV**	**Herpes labialis** (>12y): apply cream 5x/d x4 d, starting at sx onset Neonatal HSV (<3mo): 60 mg/kg/d IV div q8h x14-21d (21d in disseminated or CNS disease) **HSV encephalitis** (3mo-12y): 60 mg/kg/d IV div q8h x21d; (>12y): 30 mg/kg/d IV div q8h x21d **Genital/mucocutaneous HSV, immunocompetent** 3mo-2y: 15 mg/kg/d IV div q8h x5-7 d, max 60 mg/kg/d, 2-12y, 1st episode: 1200 mg/d PO div q8h x7-10 d, max 80 mg/kg/d PO; 60 mg/kg/d IV; alt: 15 mg/kg/d IV div q8h x5-7d; 2-12y, recurrence: 1200 mg/d PO div q8h x 5d, max 80 mg/kg/d; alt: 1600 mg/d PO div q12h; 2-12y, **suppression**: 80 mg/kg/d PO div q8h, max 1000 mg/d; alt: 400 mg PO bid; 200 mg PO 3-5x/d; reassess tx need at1y; >12y, 1st episode: 1000-1200 mg/d PO div 3-5x/d x7-10d, max 1200 mg/d PO; 60 mg/kg/d IV; alt: 40-80 mg/kg/d PO div q6-8h x5-10d; 15 mg/kg/d IV div q8h x5-7d; may extend tx if not healed in 10 d; >12y, recurrence: 1000-1200 mg/d PO div q8h x3-5d; >12 y, suppression: 800-1200 mg/d PO div q12h; reassess tx need at1y
Clindamycin	PRC B, Lact +
Cleocin *75,150,300; 75/5 mL; IM; IV*	**Mild-moderate bacterial infections,** infants/ children: 10-25 mg/kg/d PO div q6-8h; Max: 1.8 g/d PO; 4.8 g/d IV/IM; Alt: 15-25 mg/kg/d IV/IM div q6-8h; 350 mg/m2/d IV/IM div q6-8h; 30-40 mg/kg/d PO div q6-8h for susceptible Staph aureus skin/soft **tissue infections; adolescents**: 150-300 mg PO q6h; Max: 1.8 g/d PO; 4.8 g/d IV/IM; Alt: 15-25 mg/kg/d IV/IM div q6-8h; 350 mg/m2/d IV/IM div q6-8h; 30-40 mg/kg/d PO div q6-8h for susceptible Staph aureus skin/soft tissue infections

Doxycycline	PRC D, Lact +
Doxycycline *20,50,75,100,150; 75,100,150 DR; 25/5 mL; IV*	**Bacterial infections**, >8y: 2.2 mg/kg PO/IV qd; Start: 2.2 mg/kg PO/IV q12h x1 d; Max: 100 mg/dose; Info: duration varies by indication **Acne vulgaris**, >8y: 2.2 mg/kg PO qd; Start: 2.2 mg/kg PO q12h x1 d; Max: 100 mg/dose; Info: for adjunct tx
Hydrocortisone	PRC C, Lact -
Cortef *5,10,20*	**Chronic adrenal insufficiency**: 0.5-0.7 mg/kg/d PO div tid-qid; Max: 25-30 mg/d **Corticosteroid-responsive conditions**: 2.5-10 mg/kg/d PO div tid-qid; Max: 20-240 mg/d **Congenital adrenal hyperplasia**: 20-25 mg/m2/d PO div bid-tid; Info: give w/food or milk
Ivermectin	PRC C, Lact ?
Sklice lot *0.5% in 4oz tube*	**Head lice**: Lotion for topical treatment. Apply to dry hair in an amount sufficient (up to one tube) to thoroughly coat the scalp and hair for 10 min and then rinse off with water

16.14 Ophthalmology

MA/EF (atropine) antagonizes acetylcholine receptors (anticholinergic)
MA/EF (clonidine) stimulates α-2 adrenergic receptors (centrally-acting antihypertensive)
MA/EF (nedocromil) inhibits release of inflammatory cell mediators (mast cell stabilizer)
MA/EF (Olopatadine): selectively antagonizes histamine H1 receptors; inhibits histamine release from mast cells
MA/EF (timolol): non-selectively antagonizes beta-1 and beta-2 adrenergic receptors
AE (atropine): Serious: anaphylaxis, severe bradycardia, heat stroke; Common: headache, dry mouth, nausea, insomnia, dizziness, restlessness, blurred vision, mydriasis, constipation, delirium, tachycardia, palpitations, ataxia, tremor, dry hot skin
AE (clonidine): Serious: severe rebound HTN, severe hypotension, bradycardia, AV block, syncope, tachycardia, depression, allergic reaction, angioedema; Common: dry mouth, drowsiness, dizziness, constipation, sedation, hypotension, bradycardia, fever, weakness, nausea/vomiting, fatigue, nervousness, agitation, sexual dysfunction, headache, withdrawal symptoms
AE (nedocromil): Serious: none reported; Common: ocular burning/stinging, headache, ocular irritation, unpleasant taste, nasal congestion, photophobia, rhinitis
AE (Olopatadine): Serious: none reported; Common: headache, burning, dry eye, foreign body sensation, hyperemia, keratitis, eyelid edema, asthenia, pharyngitis, rhinitis, sinusitis, taste changes, hypersensitivity reaction, flu syndrome

AE (timolol): Serious: CHF, heart block, severe bradycardia, Raynaud phenomenon, bronchospasm, hypersensitivity reaction, anaphylaxis, lupus erythematosus, myasthenia gravis exacerbation; Common: bradycardia, fatigue, dizziness, headache, dyspnea, pruritus, ocular irritation, Raynaud phenomenon, nightmares, impotence
CI (atropine): acute angle-closure glaucoma, obstructive uropathy, paralytic ileus, toxic megacolon, asthma, myasthenia gravis; caution if high environmental temperature
CI (clonidine): avoid abrupt withdrawal; caution if cardiovascular disease, severe CAD, recent MI, cardiac conduction disturbances, hemodynamically unstable, renal impairment, depression hx, cerebrovascular disease
CI (nedocromil), (Olopatadine): none
CI (timolol): sinus bradycardia, 2nd or 3rd degree AV block, uncompensated heart failure, cardiogenic shock, sick sinus syndrome w/o pacemaker, asthma, asthma hx, severe COPD, avoid abrupt withdrawal; caution if peripheral vascular disease, bronchospastic disease, major surgery, DM, thyroid disorder, WPW syndrome, pheochromocytoma, renal impairment, hepatic impairment, pregnancy 2nd or 3rd trimester, myasthenia gravis, severe anaphylactic reaction hx

Atropine	PRC C, Lact -
Atropine Sulfate *Inj 0.04, 0.1, 0.3, 0.4, 0.5, 0.6, 0.8, 1mg/ml*	**PALS, bradycardia**: 0.02 mg/kg IV/IO x1, min 0.1 mg/dose, max 0.5 mg/dose (child), 1 mg/dose (adolescent); may repeat dose x1 **Organophosphate nerve agent poisoning**: <2 yo: 0.05 mg/kg IM or 0.02 mg/kg IV q5-10min prn; Start: 0.05 mg/kg IM x1 for mild/moderate sx, 0.1 mg/kg IM for severe sx; Info: give atropine first if also using pralidoxime (2-PAM); cont. atropinization until muscarinic sx gone; 2-10 yo: 1 mg IM/IV q5-10min prn; Start: 1 mg IM x1 for mild/moderate sx, 2 mg IM x1 for severe sx; Info: give atropine first if also using pralidoxime (2-PAM); cont. atropinization until muscarinic sx gone; >10 yo: 2 mg IM/IV q5-10min prn; Start: 2 mg IM x1 for mild/moderate sx, 4 mg IM x1 for severe sx; Info: give atropine first if also using pralidoxime (2-PAM); cont. atropinization until muscarinic sx gone **Organophosphate or carbamate insecticide poisoning:** <2 yo: 0.05 mg/kg IM or 0.02 mg/kg IV q10-30min prn; Info: doses <0.1 mg assoc. w/ paradoxical bradycardia; give atropine first if also using pralidoxime (2-PAM); cont. atropinization until

	muscarinic sx gone; 2-10 yo: 1-2 mg IM/IV q10-30min prn; Start: 1 mg IM/IV x1; Info: give atropine first if also using pralidoxime (2-PAM); cont. atropinization until muscarinic sx gone; >10 yo: 1-2 mg IM/IV q10-30min prn; Start: 2 mg IM/IV x1; Info: give atropine first if also using pralidoxime (2-PAM); cont. atropinization until muscarinic sx gone
Clonidine	PRC C, Lact ?
Catapres *0.1, 0.2,0.3*	**HTN**: 5-25 µg/kg/d PO div q6h; Start: 5-10 µg/kg/d div q6h, may incr. dose gradually q5-7 d; Max: 0.9 mg/d **ADHD**, 27-40.5 kg: 0.003-0.005 mg/kg/d PO div tid-qid; Start: 0.05 mg PO qhs, then may incr. by 0.05 mg/d q3-7 ds; Max: 0.05 mg/dose, 0.2 mg/d; 40.5-45 kg: 0.003-0.005 mg/kg/d PO div tid-qid; Start: 0.05 mg PO qhs, then may incr. by 0.05 mg/d q3-7 d; Max: 0.1 mg/dose, 0.3 mg/d; >45 kg: 0.003-0.005 mg/kg/d PO div tid-qid; Start: 0.1 mg PO qhs, then may incr. by 0.1 mg/d q3-7 d; Max: 0.1 mg/dose, 0.4 mg/d **Tourette syndrome**: 0.15-0.3 mg/d PO div bid; Start: 0.05 mg PO qhs, may incr. by 0.05 mg/d q7 d; Max: 0.3 mg/d; Info: give 1/3 of daily dose in am, 2/3 in pm; Info for all use: taper dose gradually over 2-4 d to D/C
Nedocromil	PRC B, Lact ?
Alocril *2% sol*	**Allergic conjunctivitis,** >3y: 1-2 gtt in eye(s) bid
Olopatadine	PRC C, Lact ?
Patanol *0.1% sol*	**Allergic conjunctivitis:** 1 gtt in eye(s) bid; Info: admin. doses 6-8h apart
Timolol	PRC C, Lact -
Timolol *5,10,20*	Adult dosing: **HTN**: 10-20 mg PO bid; start: 10 mg PO bid, may incr. dose q7 d; Max: 60 mg/d; Info: taper dose gradually over 1-2wk to D/C

	Migraine headache prophylaxis: 10-60 mg/d PO div bid-tid; start: 10 mg PO bid; Max: 15 mg/dose; Info: D/C if no response in 6-8wk; taper dose gradually over 1-2wk to D/C

16.15 ENT

MA/EF (azelastine) antagonizes central and peripheral histamine H1 receptors (non-selective antihistamine)
MA/EF (cetirizine) selectively antagonizes peripheral histamine H1 receptors
MA/EF (cromolyn inhaled)inhibits mast cell degranulation (mast cell stabilizer)
MA/EF (Cyproheptadine) non-selectively antagonizes central and peripheral histamine H1 receptors
MA/EF (diphenhydramine) non-selectively antagonizes central and peripheral histamine H1 receptors, suppresses the medullary cough center (antitussive); possesses anticholinergic properties, resulting in antidyskinetic, antiemetic and sedative effects
MA/EF (Fluticasone) exact mechanism of anti-inflammatory action unknown; inhibits multiple inflammatory cytokines; produces multiple glucocorticoid and mineralocorticoid effects
AE (azelastine): Serious: anaphylactoid reactions; Common: bitter taste, headache, somnolence, dysesthesia, nasal burning, URI, dry mouth, paroxysmal sneezing, nausea, fatigue, dizziness, epistaxis, weight gain, cough, conjunctivitis
AE (cetirizine): Serious: bronchospasm, anaphylactic/anaphylactoid reactions, hepatotoxicity, cholestasis, seizures, hemolytic anemia, thrombocytopenia, syncope, severe hypotension; Common: drowsiness, fatigue, abdominal pain, headache, dry mucous membranes, diarrhea, pharyngitis, dizziness, nausea, vomiting
AE (cromolyn inhaled): Serious: bronchospasm, anaphylaxis; Common: throat irritation, dry throat, bitter taste, cough, wheezing, nausea, dizziness, headache
AE (Cyproheptadine): Serious: agranulocytosis, thrombocytopenia, heat stroke; Common: dry mouth, drowsiness, nausea, vomiting, abdominal pain, dizziness, headache, fatigue, urinary retention, rash, urticaria, weight gain, diarrhea, photosensitivity
AE (diphenhydramine): Serious: anaphylactic/anaphylactoid reactions, hemolytic anemia, thrombocytopenia, agranulocytosis, leukopenia, pancytopenia, arrhythmias, seizures, toxic psychosis, acute labyrinthitis, heat stroke; Common: drowsiness, dizziness, incoordination, headache, epigastric discomfort, thickened bronchial secretions, dry mucous membranes, paradoxical CNS stimulation, constipation, dysuria, urinary retention, hypotension, blurred vision, diplopia, palpitations, tachycardia, photosensitivity, diaphoresis, erectile dysfunction
AE (fluticasone) propionate nasal: Serious: nasal septal perforation, nasal ulcer, nasal/oral candidiasis, growth suppression, IOP incr., glaucoma, cataracts, hypercortisolism, adrenal suppression, anaphylaxis, angioedema, bronchospasm, wheezing, dyspnea, Common: headache. Pharyngitis, epistaxis, nasal burning, nasal irritation, nausea, vomiting, asthma symptoms, cough, dizziness, rhinorrhea, bronchitis, diarrhea, pyrexia, abdominal pain,
AE (fluticasone) inhaled: Serious: bronchospasm, angioedema, anaphylactoid reactions, adrenal suppression, hypercortisolism, growth suppression, eosinophilia, Churg-Strauss

syndrome, hyperglycemia, glaucoma, cataracts, osteoporosis, behavioral disturbances; Common: URI, headache, throat irritation, sinusitis, oral candidiasis, pharyngitis, hoarseness, dysphonia, cough, rhinitis, nausea/vomiting, myalgia/arthralgia, rash, pruritus
CI (azelastine): caution if CNS depressant or alcohol use
CI (cetirizine): hypersens. to hydroxyzine, pts <2 yo; caution if CNS depressant use, hepatic impairment, renal impairment, pts <6 yo
CI (cromolyn inhaled): acute asthma, status asthmaticus; caution if arrhythmias
CI (Cyproheptadine): newborns or premature infants, breastfeeding, angle-closure glaucoma, bladder neck obstruction, PUD; caution in pts <2 yo, hepatic impairment, high environmental temperature
CI (diphenhydramine): pts <2 yo; caution in pts <6 yo, if CNS depressant use, IOP incr., angle-closure glaucoma, hyperthyroidism, cardiovascular disease, HTN, asthma, COPD, lower resp. tract sx, GI obstruction, PUD, prostatic hypertrophy, bladder neck obstruction, poor CYP2D6 metabolizer, high environmental temperature
CI (fluticasone) propionate nasal: unhealed nasal septal ulcer, unhealed nasal surgery or trauma wound; caution if untreated local or systemic infection, TB infection, ocular HSV infection, measles or varicella exposure, recurrent epistaxis, IOP incr., glaucoma, cataracts, recent long-term systemic corticosteroid tx

Azelastine	PRC C, Lact ?
Astelin, Astepro Nasal *137 µg/spray*	**Allergic rhinitis,** 5-11 yo: 1 spray per nostril bid; >12 yo: 1-2 sprays per nostril bid **Vasomotor rhinitis,** >12 yo: 2 sprays per nostril bid
Cetirizine	PRC B, Lact ?
Zyrtec *5,10; 5,10 CH; 1/mL*	**Allergic rhinitis, chronic idiopathic urticarial,** 2-5yo: 2.5-5 mg PO qd; Max: 5 mg/d; >6yo: 5-10 mg PO qd; Max: 10 mg/d
Cromolyn inhaled	PRC B, Lact ?
Cromolyn inhaled *20/2 mL neb*	**Persistent asthma,** >2y: 20 mg NEB qid, decr. gradually to bid after stabilized **Exercise-induced asthma**: 20 mg NEB x1, 10-60 min before exercise
Cyproheptadine	PRC B, Lact ?
Periactin *4; 2 mg/5 mL syrup*	**Allergic rhinitis or urticaria,** 2-6y: start 0.25 mg/kg/d PO div q8-12h, then 2 mg PO q8-12h; Max: 12 mg/d; 7-14y: start 0.25 mg/kg/d PO div q8-12h, then 4 mg PO q8-12h; Max: 16 mg/d **Anorexia nervosa,** >13y: start 2 mg PO qid, incr. to 8 mg PO qid maintenance over 3wk period

Diphenhydramine	PRC B, Lact -
Benadryl *25,50; 12.5/5mL; Inj 10mg/ml, 50mg/ml*	**Anaphylaxis**: 1-2mg/kg IV/IM, max 50mg single dose, rep prn q2-3h, max 400mg/d **Allergy sx,** 2-5y: 6.25 mg PO/IM/IV q4-6h prn; Max: 37.5 mg/d; 6-11y: 12.5-25 mg PO/IM/IV q4-6h prn; Max: 150 mg/d; >12y: 25-50 mg PO/IM/IV q4-6h prn; Max: 100 mg/dose; 400 mg/d
Fluticasone	PRC C, Lact ?
Flonase (nasal) *50 µg/spray* **Flovent HFA** *44,110,220 µg/spray MDI* **Flovent Diskus** *50,100,250 µg/blister DPI*	**Allergic rhinitis,** >4y: 1-2 sprays per nostril qd; Start: 1 spray per nostril qd; Max: 2 sprays per nostril/d **Asthma** maintenance, prior tx, 4-11y: 88 µg inhaled bid; Max: 176 µg/d; prior bronchodilator alone, >12y: 88-440 µg inhaled bid; Start: 88 µg inhaled bid; Max: 880 µg/d; prior inhaled steroid, >12 yo, 88-440 µg inhaled bid; Start: 88-220 µg inhaled bid; Max: 880 µg/d; prior oral steroid, >12 yo, 440-880 µg inhaled bid; Start: 440 µg inhaled bid; Max: 1760 µg/d; Info for all: rinse mouth after use; taper oral steroids gradually after >1wk; titrate to lowest effective dose
Loratadine	PRC B, Lact -
Claritin, Alavert *10; 10 ODT; 1/mL*	Allergic rhinitis and chronic idiopathic urticaria, 2-6y: 5 mg PO qd; Info: ODT form not recommended; >6y: 10 mg PO qd; Info: some pts w/urticaria may benefit from higher doses, weigh risk/benefit

16.16 Urology

MA/EF synthetic arginine vasopressin (antidiuretic hormone) analogue; exerts antidiuretic effects and increases plasma Factor VIII and von Willebrand factor levels
AE: Serious: hyponatremia, water intoxication, seizures, anaphylaxis, thrombosis; Common: flushing, headache, rhinitis, nausea, abdominal pain, dizziness, cough, epistaxis, chills, conjunctivitis
CI: CrCl <50, hyponatremia or hx, von Willebrand disease type IIB; caution if CAD, HTN, CHF, fluid and electrolyte imbalance, habitual or psychogenic polydipsia, cystic fibrosis, thrombosis risk, young children

Desmopressin	PRC B, Lact -
DDAVP *0.1,0.2; SC; IV*	**Central diabetes insipidus**, <4y: 0.1-0.8 mg/d PO div bid; Start: 0.05 mg PO qd; 4-12y: 0.1-1.2 mg/d PO div bid-tid; Start: 0.05 mg PO bid; Max: 1.2 mg/d; >12y: 0.1-1.2 mg/d PO div bid-tid; Start: 0.05 mg PO bid; Max: 1.2 mg/d PO, 4 µg/d SC/IV; Alt: 1-2 µg SC/IV bid; parenteral dose is approx. 1/10 of intranasal dose; Info: give 1st PO dose 12h after last intranasal dose when switching to PO; restrict fluid intake **Nocturnal enuresis**, >6y: 0.2-0.6 mg PO qhs; Start: 0.2 mg PO qhs; Max: 0.6 mg/d; Info: restrict fluid intake >1h before admin. until next morning or >8h after admin.; hold tx if acute illness w/ fluid and electrolyte imbalance risk **Hemophilia A or von Willebrand disease, type 1**, >3mo: 0.3 µg/kg IV x1; Info: for pts w/ FVIII levels >5%; may repeat in 8-24h; if preop, give 30min before surgery
DDAVP nasal *0.1 mg/mL sol; 10 µg/spray*	**Central diabetes insipidus**, 3mo-12y: 5-30 µg/d IN div qd-bid; Start: 2.5 µg IN qd-bid, incr. in 2.5 µg increments; >12y: 10-40 µg/d IN div qd-tid; Start: 5 µg IN qd-bid, incr. in 2.5 µg increments; Info: use rhinal tube delivery for doses not in 10 µg increments; restrict fluid intake **Hemophilia A or von Willebrand disease, type 1**: 2-4 µg/kg IN x1; Info: for pts w/ FVIII levels >5%; may repeat dose in 8-24h; if preop, give 2h before surgery

16.17 Oncology

MA/EF (chlorambucil) alkylates and crosslinks DNA
MA/EF (cyclophosphamide) alkylates and crosslinks DNA
MA/EF (dexamethasone) exact mechanism of anti-inflammatory action unknown; inhibits multiple inflammatory cytokines; produces multiple glucocorticoid and mineralocorticoid effects
MA/EF (phenytoin) modulates neuronal voltage-dependent sodium and calcium channels
MA/EF (rituximab) binds to B-lymphocyte CD20 surface antigens (monoclonal antibody)
AE (chlorambucil): Serious: bone marrow failure, myelosuppression, leukemia, neutropenia, thrombocytopenia, pancytopenia, secondary malignancy, infertility, sterility, erythema multiforme, Stevens-Johnson syndrome, toxic epidermal necrolysis, hepatotoxicity, interstitial pneumonitis, pulmonary fibrosis, seizures, peripheral neuropathy, angioneurotic edema; Common: lymphopenia, neutropenia, thrombocytopenia, anemia, fever, rash, nausea, vomiting, diarrhea, abdominal pain, amenorrhea, stomatitis
AE (cyclophosphamide): Serious: secondary malignancy, sterility, hemorrhagic cystitis, urinary bladder fibrosis, CHF, hemorrhagic myocarditis, immunosuppression, infection, anaphylactic reactions, Stevens-Johnson syndrome, toxic epidermal necrolysis, anemia, leukopenia, thrombocytopenia, interstitial pneumonitis, interstitial pulmonary fibrosis, SIADH; Common: alopecia, sterility, amenorrhea, nausea, vomiting, anorexia, diarrhea, stomatitis, hemorrhagic cystitis, anemia, leukopenia, thrombocytopenia, rash, headache
AE (dexamethasone): Serious: adrenal insufficiency, steroid psychosis, immunosuppression (long-term use), peptic ulcer, CHF, anaphylaxis, osteoporosis (long-term use), pseudotumor cerebri, pancreatitis; Common: nausea, vomiting, dyspepsia, appetite change, edema, headache, dizziness, mood swings, insomnia, anxiety, hypokalemia, HTN, hyperglycemia, Cushing syndrome (long-term use), menstrual irregularities, ecchymosis, acne, skin atrophy (long-term use), impaired wound healing (long-term use)
AE (phenytoin): Serious: ventricular fibrillation (IV use), hypotension, severe (IV use), cardiovascular collapse (IV use), AV conduction abnormalities (IV use), hepatotoxicity, thrombocytopenia, leukopenia, agranulocytosis, pancytopenia, megaloblastic anemia, exfoliative dermatitis, Stevens-Johnson syndrome, toxic epidermal necrolysis, rash w/ eosinophilia and systemic sx, tissue necrosis (IV use), purple glove syndrome (IV use), anaphylaxis, lymphoma, lupus erythematosus, osteomalacia, toxic delirium, suicidality, periarteritis nodosa; Common: nausea, vomiting, rash, nystagmus, ataxia, slurred speech, dizziness, confusion, paresthesia, blurred vision, somnolence, constipation, headache, insomnia, gingival hyperplasia, taste changes, tremor, lymphadenopathy, coarse facies, hyperglycemia, osteomalacia, phlebitis (IV use), Peyronie disease
AE (rituximab): Serious: severe or fatal infusion reaction, tumor lysis syndrome, anaphylactic/anaphylactoid reactions, severe hypersensitivity reaction, Stevens-Johnson syndrome, toxic epidermal necrolysis, pemphigus, lichenoid dermatitis, vesiculobullous rash, serious infection, PML, post-tx HBV reactivation, fulminant hepatitis, MI, arrhythmias, cardiac failure, nephrotoxicity, GI obstruction/perforation, leukopenia, neutropenia, anemia, thrombocytopenia, hypogammaglobulinemia, bronchiolitis obliterans, acute

AE (rituximab): cont. pneumonitis, prolonged hypogammaglobulinemia; Common: infusion reaction, fever/chills, lymphopenia, infection, asthenia, nausea, headache, night sweats, pruritus/rash/urticarial, abdominal pain, leukopenia, neutropenia, thrombocytopenia, transient hypophosphatemia, cough, pain, URI, diarrhea, vomiting, dizziness, myalgia/arthralgia, hypotension, HTN, hyperglycemia, anemia, peripheral edema, LDH elevated, hyperuricemia, muscle spasms, insomnia
CI (chlorambucil): pregnancy not recommended; caution if hepatic impairment, myelosuppression, concurrent myelosuppressive agents, recent XRT, seizure disorder, head injury
CI (cyclophosphamide): bone marrow depression, pregnancy 1st trimester, breastfeeding; caution if hepatic or renal impairment, leukopenia, thrombocytopenia, recent XRT, recent cytotoxic drug use, adrenalectomy, wound healing
CI (dexamethasone): systemic fungal infection; caution if CHF, seizure disorder, DM, HTN, TB infection, osteoporosis, hepatic impairment
CI (phenytoin): SA block (IM or IV use), 2nd or 3rd degree AV block (IM or IV use), sinus bradycardia (IM or IV use), Adams-Stokes syndrome (IM or IV use); caution if hypotension (IM or IV use), cardiovascular disease (IM or IV use), hepatic/renal impairment, DM, pregnancy, porphyria, alcohol use, thyroid disease, HLA-B*1502-positive, depression or hx, avoid abrupt withdrawal
CI (rituximab): hypersens. to murine proteins; caution if arrhythmias, angina, pulmonary disease, high tumor burden, HBV carrier, latent or chronic infection

Chlorambucil	PRC D, Lact +
Leukeran *2*	**Nephrotic syndrome**: 0.1-0.2 mg/kg PO qd; Info: regimens vary; use w/low dose prednisone or other corticosteroid
Cyclophosphamide	PRC D, Lact +
Cytoxan *25,50; IV*	**Rheumatoid arthritis**: 1.5-3 mg/kg PO daily
Dexamethasone	PRC C, Lact -
Decadron *0.25,0.5,0.75, 1,1.5,4,6; 0.5/5 mL; 1/mL*	**Adrenal insufficiency**: 0.03-0.3 mg/kg/d PO div q6-12h **Croup**: 0.6 mg/kg PO x1; Max: 10 mg/dose; Alt: 0.15 mg/kg PO x1; higher dose regimen may also be divided into 4 doses given q6h

Phenytoin	PRC D, Lact -
Dilantin *Inj 50mg/ml; 100, 200, 300 ER tab, 125mg/5ml susp*	**Status epilepticus:** 15-20 mg/kg IV x1, may give additional 10 mg/kg IV x1 after 20min if no response; max 1500 mg/d; begin maint dose 12h after load; Seizure disorder: <6mo: 5-8 mg/kg/d PO/IV div bid-tid; 6mo-4yo: 8-10 mg/kg/d PO/IV div bid-tid; 4-7yo: 7.5-9 mg/kg/d PO/IV div bid-tid; 7-10yo: 7-8 mg/kg/d PO/IV div bid-tid; 10-16yo: 6-7 mg/kg/d PO/IV div bid-tid (all ages, start 5 mg/kg/d; adjust dose base on levels). ER caps have 8% less drug than chewables and susp.
Rituximab	PRC C, Lact ?
Rituxan *IV*	**Rheumatoid arthritis**: consult with pediatric rheumatologist

17 Appendix

17.1 Abbreviations

-	negative
+	positive
µg	microgram
µmol	micromoles
^{0}C	degree celsius
(OH)2D	dihydroxyvitamin D
OHD	hydroxyvitamin D
AAP	American Academy of Pediatrics
ABCs	airway, breathing and circulation
ABG	arterial blood gas
ACOG	American College of Obstetrics and Gynecology
ACTH	adrenocorticotropic hormone
ADHD	attention deficit hyperactivity disorder
ADHR	autosomal dominant hypophosphatemic rickets
AE	adverse effect
AFP	alpha-fetoprotein
AIDS	acquired immune deficiency syndrome
AKA	also known as
Alk Phos	alkaline phosphatase
ALL	acute lymphocytic leukemia
ALT	alanine aminotransferase
AML	acute myeloid leukemia
AMPK	adenosine monophosphate-activated protein kinase
AN	anorexia nervosa
ANA	antinuclear antibodies
Ant. Trunk	anterior trunk
AOM	acute otitis media
aPTT	activated partial thromboplastin time
ARHR	autosomal recessive hypophosphatemic rickets
ARV	anti-retroviral
AS	aortic stenosis
ASA	aminosalicylic acid
ASD	atrial septal defect
ASO	antistreptolysin O
AST	aspartate aminotransferase
ATN	acute tubular necrosis
AV	atrioventricular
AVM	arteriovenous malformations
β-hCG	beta human chorionic gonadotropin
BAE	bilateral atrial enlargement
BCG	bacille Calmette Guérin
BED	binge eating disorder
BG	blood gases
BID	twice daily
BIW	twice a week
BMA	bone marrow aspiration
BMI	body mass index
BN	bulimia nervosa
BP	blood pressure
BPI	behavioral peer interventions
BPT	behavioral parent training

BSA	body surface area
BT	blood transfusion
BUN	blood urea nitrogen
BVH	biventricular cardiac hypertrophy
C. trachomatis	Chlamydia trachomatis
Ca	calcium
CAH	congenital adrenal hypoplasia
CBC	complete blood count
CBT	cognitive behavioral therapy
Ccr	creatine clearance
CD	concentration desired
CD	Crohn's disease
CDC	centers for disease control and prevention
CF	cystic fibrosis/cardiac failure
CHF	congestive heart failure
CI	contraindications
Cl	chloride
CLD	chronic lung disease
cm	centimeter
CMP	comprehensive metabolic panel
CMPA	cow milk protein allergy
CNS	central nervous system
CoA	coenzyme A
Cont.	continued
CP	concentration present
CPAP	continuous positive airway pressure
CPR	cardiopulmonary resuscitation

Cr	creatinine
CRP	C-reactive protein
CSF	cerebrospinal fluid
CT	computed tomography
CVA	cerebrovascular accident
CXR	chest radiograph (x-ray)
d	day
D10W	dextrose 10% in water
D5W	dextrose 5% in water
DD	dysthymic disorder
DD	developmental disabilities
DDAVP	1-deamino-8-D-arginine vasopressin
DFA	direct fluorescent antibody
DHEA	dehydroepiandrosterone
DIC	disseminated intravascular coagulation
DKA	diabetic ketoacidosis
dL	deciliter
DM	diabetes mellitus
DMARDs	disease-modifying antirheumatic drugs
DNA	deoxyribonucleic acid
DOC	deoxycorticosterone
DOT	directly observed therapy
DSM-IV-TR	Diagnostic and Statistical Manual of Mental Disorders-fourth edition (text revision)
E. coli	Escherichia coli
EBNA	Epstein-Barr nuclear antigen
EBV	Epstein-Barr virus
ECF	extracellular fluid

ECG	electrocardiogram
ECMO	extra-corporeal membrane oxygenation
ECT	electroconvulsive therapy
EDNOS	eating disorders not otherwise specified
EDs	eating disorders
EEG	electroencephalography
EF	effects
eg	for example (L: exempli grati)
EGA	estimated gestational age
ELISA	enzyme-linked immunosorbent assay
EM	erythema migrans
EMB	ethambutol
esp.	especially
ESR	erythrocyte sedimentation rate
ET	endotracheal tube
ETCOc	end-tidal carbon monoxide concentration corrected for ambient CTO
ETT	endotracheal tube
F	female
FBE	full blood examination
FDA	food and drug administration
FEF	forced expiratory flow
FEV1	forced expiratory volume in 1 second
Fig	figure
FLACC	face, legs, activity, cry, consolability
FSGS	focal segmental glomerular sclerosis
FSH	follicle-stimulating hormone
FTL	full-thickness loss
FTT	failure to thrive
FVC	forced vital capacity
g	gram
G6PD	glucose 6-phosphate dehydrogenase
GAD	generalized anxiety disorder
GAG	glycosaminoglycans
GBS	group B Streptococcus
GCS	Glasgow coma scale
GER	gastroesophageal reflux
GERD	gastroesophageal reflux disease
GFR	glomerular filtration rate
GGT	gamma-glutamyl transpeptidase
GI	gastrointestinal
GIR	glucagon infusion rate
GLUT-2	glucose transporter 2
GTT	glucose tolerance test
H. influ-enzae	Haemophilus influenzae
h	hours
HADH	hydroxyacyl CoA dehydrogenase
Hb	hemoglobin
hCG	human chorionic gonadotropin
HCO3	bicarbonate
HCT	hematocrit

HEENT	head, eyes, ears, nose, and throat
HHRH	hereditary hypophosphatemic rickets with hypercalciuria
HI	hyperinsulinism
HIV	human immunodeficiency virus
HNF4A	hepatic nuclear factor 4 alpha
HR	heart rate
HSV	herpes simplex virus
HTC	hematocrit
HTN	hypertension
HVA	homovanillic acid
hx	history
I/O	input and output
IBD	inflammatory bowel disease
ICF	intracellular fluid
ICH	intracranial hemorrhage
ICP	increased intracranial pressure
ICS	immotile cilia syndrome
IDM	infant of a diabetic mother
Ig	immunoglobulin
IgA	immunoglobulin A
IgE	immunoglobulin E
IGF II	insulin-like growth factor II
IgG	immunoglobulin G
IgM	immunoglobulin M
IGRA	interferon-release assay
M	intramuscular
NH	isoniazid
O	intraosseous

IPEX syndrome	immunodysregulation polyendocrinopathy enteropathy X-linked syndrome
ISSD	infantile sialic acid storage disorder
ITP	idiopathic thrombocytopenic purpura
IU	international unit
IV	intravenous
IVH	intraventricular hemorrhage
J/kg	joule per kilogram
JIA	juvenile idiopathic arthritis (formerly JRA)
K	potassium
KAc	potassium acetate
KATP	adenosine triphosphate [ATP] potassium channel
kcal	kilocalorie
KCl	potassium chloride
kg	kilogram
KPhos	potassium phosphate
L. monocytogenes	Listeria monocytogenes
L	liter
Lact	lactation risk category
LAE	left atrial enlargement
LAMP2	lysosome-associated membrane protein 2
LDH	lactate dehydrogenase
LE	lower extremity
LH	luteinizing hormone
LICS	left intercostal space

LLSB	lower left sternal border
LMSB	left main stem bronchus
LOC	loss of or level of consciousness
LP	lumbar puncture
LR	lactated ringer solution
LSB	left sternal border
LTBI	latent tuberculosis infection
LTRA	leukotriene receptor antagonists
LTRI	lower respiratory tract infection
LUSB	left upper sternal border
LVH	left ventricular hypertrophy
M. catarrhalis	Moraxella catarrhalis
M	male
m	meter
MA	mechanism of action
MAOIs	monoamine oxidase inhibitors
MCHC	mean corpuscular hemoglobin concentration
MCNS	minimal change nephrotic syndrome
MCV	mean corpuscular volume
MDD	major depressive disorder
mEq	milliequivalent
mg	milligrams
MI	myocardial infarction
min	minutes
mL	milliliter
mm	millimeter
mmol	millimoles
MODY	maturity-onset diabetes of the young
MPS	mucopolysaccharidosis
MP-SMX	trimethoprim-sulfamethoxazole
MR	mentally retarded
MRI	magnetic resonance imaging
N. meningitis	Neisseria meningitis
N	normal
Na	sodium
NaCl	sodium chloride
NG tube	nasogastric tube
ng	nanogram
NIPS	neonatal infant pain scale
nmol	nanomoles
NOS	not otherwise specified
NPO	nothing by mouth
NS	nephrotic syndrome
NS	normal saline
NSAIDS	nonsteroidal anti-inflammatory drugs
NSR	normal sinus rhythm
OCD	obsessive compulsive disorder
ODD	oppositional defiant disorder
OGTT	oral glucose tolerance test
OME	otitis media with effusion
ORS	oral rehydration solution
ORT	oral rehydration therapy
PaCO2	partial pressure of carbon dioxide in the blood
PALS	pediatric advanced life support

PaO_2	partial pressure of oxygen in the blood
PCO_2	partial pressure or tension of carbon dioxide in the blood
PCP	pneumocystis pneumonia
PCR	polymerase chain reaction
PCV	packed cell volume
PDA	patent ductus arteriosus
PDD	pervasive developmental disorder
PEA	pulseless electrical activity
PEFR	peak expiratory flow rate
PFTs	pulmonary function tests
pH	potential of hydrogen
Pi	inorganic phosphorus
PICU	pediatric intensive care unit
PKU	Phenylketonuria
PNH	paroxysmal nocturnal hemoglobinuria
PO	by mouth, per os
Post. Trunk	posterior trunk
PPD	purified protein derivative
PRBC	packed red blood cells
PRC	pregnancy risk category
PRKAG2	protein kinase, amp-activated, noncatalytic, gamma2
PS	pulmonic stenosis
Pseudo-hypoaldo	pseudohypoaldosteronism
PSVT	paroxysmal supraventricular tachycardia
PT	prothrombin time
PTH	parathyroid hormone
PTL	partial-thickness loss
PTSD	posttraumatic stress disorder
PUFA	polyunsaturated fatty acids
PVC	premature ventricular contractions
PVL	periventricular leukomalacia
PVMs	pulmonary vascular markings
PVR	pulmonary vascular resistance
PZA	pyrazinamide
RAD	right axis deviation
RAE	right atrial enlargement
RAST	radioallergosorbent test
RBBB	right bundle branch block
RBC	red blood cells
RBUS	renal and bladder ultrasonograph
RD	relatively decreased
RDA	recommended dietary allowances
RDS	respiratory distress syndrome
RDW	red cell distribution width
RF	rheumatoid factor
RICS	right intercostal space
RIF	rifampin
ROP	retinopathy of prematurity
ROSC	return of spontaneous circulation
RSV	respiratory syncytial virus
RV	right ventricular
RVH	right ventricular hypertrophy

S. pneumoniae	Streptococcus pneumoniae
SA	surface area
SABA	short-acting β-agonists
SAD	separation anxiety disorder
SC	subcutaneous
SD	subdermal
sec	seconds
SEM	systolic ejection murmur
SGA	small for gestational age
SIDS	sudden infant death syndrome
SLC16A1	the pyruvate transporter
SLE	systemic lupus erythematosus
SMX	sulfamethoxazole
SpO2	saturation of peripheral oxygen
SSRIs	selective serotonin reuptake inhibitors
STAT	immediately (Latin: statim)
SVT	supraventricular tachycardia
sx	symptoms
T3	triiodothyronine
T3RU	triiodothyronine resin uptake
T4	thyroxine
TB	tuberculosis
TBG	thyroxine-binding globulin
Temp	temperature
TFT	thyroid function test
TIBC	total iron-binding capacity
TMP	trimethoprim
TNHI	Transient neonatal hyperinsulinemic hypoglycemia
TPMT	thiopurine methyltransferase
TRH	thyrotropin-releasing hormone
TSB	total serum bilirubin
TSH	thyroid stimulating hormone
TST	tuberculin skin test
TTG	tissue transglutaminase
U	units
UA	urinalysis
UC	ulcerative colitis
UCP2	mitochondrial uncoupling protein 2
UE	upper extremity
ULSB	upper left sternal border
UPr	urine protein
URSB	upper right sternal border
USPHS	U.S. Public Health Service
UTI	urinary tract infection
VCA	viral capsid antigen
VDDR	vitamin D-dependent rickets
VF	ventricular fibrillation
VMA	vanillylmandelic acid
VSD	ventricular septal defect
VT	ventricular tachycardia
VUR	vesicoureteral reflux
vWF	von Willebrand disease
w/o	without
WBC	white blood cell
WPW	Wolff-Parkinson-White syndrome
x/wk	time/week

XLH	x-linked hypophosphatemic rickets
yr/ yrs	year/ years
ZDV	zidovudine

17.2 Useful Links

American Academy of Pediatrics
http://www.aap.org/

American Pediatric Society-Society for Pediatric Research
http://www.aps-spr.org/home.asp

Academic Pediatric Association
http://www.ambpeds.org/

Pediatric Associates, LLC; Vineland-, New Jersey
http://www.pediatricassociatesvineland.com

Pediatric Associates of Barrington
http://www.pediatric-associates.net/

Pediatric Associates
http://www.pediatricassociates.us/

Pediatric Associates of Dallas
http://paddallas.com/

Northern Virginia Pediatric Associates
http://www.northernvirginiapediatrics.com

PEDIATRICS Journal
http://pediatrics.aappublications.org/

American Association for Pediatric Ophthalmology and Strabismus
http://www.aapos.org/

Pediatric Academic Societies (PAS)
http://www.pas-meeting.org/

Pediatric Endocrine Society
http://www.lwpes.org/

The Society for Pediatric Dermatology
http://www.pedsderm.net/

The Society for Pediatric Radiology
http://www.pedrad.org/

Pediatric Infectious Diseases Society
http://www.pids.org/

North American Society for Pediatric Gastroenterology, Hepatology and Nutrition
http://www.naspghan.org/

Child Neurology Society
http://www.childneurologysociety.org/

International Pediatric Association
http://www.ipa-world.org/

European Society for Paediatric Research
http://www.espr.info/

European Paediatric Association (EPA UNEPSA)
http://www.epa-unepsa.org/

Numerics

A

B

Trade name = bold *Drug name = italic*

S

T